'There was a time when the notion that diet [affects] brain health was controversial. Today, it is from the news. The incredible *Grain Brain* by Dr. David Perlmutter is a significant reason for this change.' – **Robb Wolf**, *New York Times* bestselling author of *The Paleo Solution* and *Wired to Eat*

'*Grain Brain, Revised Edition*, is brilliant, accessible, and life changing. By following the scientific advice, you can have healthier brain and healthier body starting today.' – **Daniel G. Amen, MD**, author of *Memory Rescue* and *Change Your Brain, Change Your Body*

'Dr. Perlmutter has compiled an important and highly useful update to his bestselling book that has helped so many understand the pernicious influence that grains can have on your health.' – **Dr. Joseph Mercola**, *New York Times* bestselling author and author of *Fat for Fuel*

'Dr. Perlmutter outlines an innovative approach to our most fragile organ, the brain. He is an absolute leader in the use of alternative and conventional approaches in the treatment of neurologic disorders. I have referred him patients with wonderful results. He is on the cutting edge and can help change the way we practice medicine.' – **Mehmet Oz, MD**

'Dr. Perlmutter takes us on a detailed tour of the destructive effects that 'healthy whole grains' have on our brains. Modern wheat, in particular, is responsible for destroying more brains in this country than all the strokes, car accidents, and head trauma combined. Dr. Perlmutter makes a persuasive case for this wheat-free approach to preserve brain health and functioning, or to begin the process of reversal.' – **William Davis, MD**, author of *Wheat Belly*

'Dementia and many other brain diseases are not inevitable, nor are they genetic. They are directly and powerfully linked to a diet high in sugar and grains. *Grain Brain* not only proves this, it also gives you everything you need to know to protect your brain – or a loved one's – now.' – **Christiane Northrup, MD**, author of *Women's Bodies, Women's Wisdom*

'This book is a treasure. It is filled with self-empowering wisdom and easily understood leading-edge science. It can help you to avoid the devastating effects of an unhealthy diet and the dietary factors which are involved.

By learning from the information presented in Dr. Perlmutter's book, you can avoid multiple health and neurological problems.' – **Bernie Siegel, MD**, author of *Faith, Hope, and Healing* and *The Art of Healing*

'A provocative, eye-opening scientific account of how diet profoundly influences nerve health and brain function. *Grain Brain* explains how the American diet rich in gluten and inflammatory foods is linked to neurological conditions. Dr. Perlmutter outlines a blueprint for optimal health and a more resilient brain through proper nutrition and lifestyle. *Grain Brain* is a must-read!' – **Gerard E. Mullin, MD**, Associate Professor of Medicine, The Johns Hopkins School of Medicine, and author of *The Inside Tract: Your Good Gut Guide to Great Digestive Health*

'Dr. Perlmutter is the leading integrative medicine neurologist in North America today. His ability to fully integrate conventional medicine diagnosis and treatment with the latest innovations in nutritional and environmental medicine is phenomenal. As a teacher and clinician, he has fundamentally changed how physicians and patients think about neurological degeneration and, happily, regeneration.' – **Joseph Pizzorno, MD**, coauthor of *Encyclopedia of Natural Medicine*

'Dr. Perlmutter provides sound advice, supported by the latest and most well respected medical research.' – **Russell. B. Roth, MD**, Past President, American Medical Association

'A galvanizing call to arms against a gluten-heavy diet . . . Perlmutter's credentials as a board-certified neurologist and American College of Nutrition Fellow make him a uniquely qualified voice in the debate about which foods are best for the brain and body.' – ***Kirkus Reviews***

'Mind-blowing and disruptive to some long-standing beliefs about what our bodies require for optimal health . . . GRAIN BRAIN lays out an easy-to-understand roadmap packed with the latest science.' – **Max Lugavere, *Psychology Today***

'A tour de force that is destined to save many lives. As I read this important and well-written book I found myself nodding my head vigorously in agreement at practically every page. [*Grain Brain*] gives us what we need to know to be well again. Please read it.' – ***Health Central***

GRAIN BRAIN

The Surprising Truth About Wheat, Carbs,

and Sugar — Your Brain's Silent Killers

Revised Edition

DR DAVID PERLMUTTER

WITH KRISTIN LOBERG

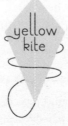

First published in Great Britain in 2014 by Yellow Kite
An imprint of Hodder & Stoughton
An Hachette UK company

First published in the USA in 2013, 2018 by Little, Brown Spark,
an imprint of Little, Brown and Company,
a division of Hachette Book Group, Inc.

Reissued in 2019 by Yellow Kite

3

A CIP catalogue record for this title is available from the British Library

Trade Paperback ISBN 978 1 473 69558 0

Printed and bound by CPI Group (UK) Ltd, Croydon, CR0 4YY

Hodder & Stoughton policy is to use papers that are natural,
renewable and recyclable products and made from wood grown in
sustainable forests. The logging and manufacturing processes are expected
to conform to the environmental regulations of the country of origin.

Yellow Kite
Hodder & Stoughton Ltd
Carmelite House
50 Victoria Embankment
London EC4Y 0DZ

www.yellowkitebooks.co.uk
www.hodder.co.uk

The original dedication in the 2013 edition of
Grain Brain read as follows:

To my father, who at age ninety-six begins each day
by getting dressed to see his patients —
despite having retired more than a quarter century ago.

Five years later, I dedicate this anniversary edition
to his memory.

Your brain . . .

weighs three pounds and has one hundred thousand miles of blood vessels.

contains more connections than there are stars in the Milky Way.

is the fattest organ in your body.

could be suffering this very minute without you having a clue.

Contents

PART I

THE WHOLE GRAIN TRUTH

Contents

PART II

GRAIN BRAIN REHAB

PART III

SAY GOODBYE TO GRAIN BRAIN

GRAIN BRAIN

Introduction

Against the Grain

Maintaining order rather than correcting disorder is the ultimate principle of wisdom. To cure disease after it has appeared is like digging a well when one feels thirsty, or forging weapons after the war has already begun.

— *Huangdi Neijing,* 2ND CENTURY BC

WHEN THIS BOOK first came out in 2013, it challenged the dietary dogma of the day. The premise focused on reducing carbohydrates, eliminating gluten, and increasing the consumption of high-quality dietary fat. Such a protocol flew in the face of the prevailing wisdom of what made for a healthful diet. I pushed the limits not just with respect to severely cutting sugars and carbs and adding more dietary fat, but in promoting ketosis and employing the power of intermittent fasting. This led to mainstream discussions about these topics as they relate to salubrious dietary choices and general habits. I like to think I started a revolution. And it must continue, especially now that I've lost my dear dad to Alzheimer's disease.

In truth, however, I wasn't the one who ignited this revolution. I didn't have a global marketing plan back then. What propelled the movement were readers who implemented these changes in their eating habits and experienced positive results. Those results then motivated them to make other favorable shifts in their habits beyond diet. All those little changes added up to immense transformation; the micro grew into the macro. They upped the overall quality of their life and shared their story with others.

Nothing is more powerful than the spread of ideas through good old-fashioned word-of-mouth. My hope with this revised edition is to reach both those who read the original work and those who are just meeting me and my ideas for the first time. Welcome. I've written this for both audiences, and I hope it speaks to you in ways that empower you to take control—and ownership—of your health today like never before.

I took some heat for my contrarian advice (my advice doesn't help the wheat and sugar industries), but the results manifested by following the recommendations in *Grain Brain* made clear the fundamental soundness of its principles. Countless readers who struggled lifelong with a variety of chronic health conditions—from anxiety, attention deficit hyperactivity disorder (ADHD), and brain fog to inflammatory diseases, mood disorders and depression, neurodegenerative decline, diabetes, and obesity—were finally able to shift their health destiny, for the better. You can learn about some of these stories of transformation online at DrPerlmutter.com or on my YouTube channel, DavidPerlmutterMD. I'll also be showcasing more testimonials throughout this book as sidebar boxes (look for "A True GB Story").

Grain Brain has become a global phenomenon, with more than 1 million copies in print and translated into 30 languages. It continues to astonish me, and I am forever humbled by the opportunity to participate in so many positive health outcomes, reaching people I never could have previously in my private practice. The book's success has also opened the door for me to travel globally and meet with health-care practitioners, top research scientists, and lay populations alike. One of my most gratifying experiences occurred in 2017 when I shared my views on brain health at the World Bank, a presentation that was broadcasted to 150 sites around the planet. I've participated in countless other public and private events, lectures at medical schools, and high-profile media including print and television, to continue to amplify and support the guidelines originally contained in the *Grain Brain* protocol.

But I must go further with this new edition.

The basic operating system underlying the practice of medicine in America today is myopically focused on treating our ills with highly profitable remedies directed at symptom management.[1] Causality is ignored. Preventing disease is derogated and relegated to the province of alternative modalities. Watching our elected leaders debate the merits of funding the ever-changing iterations of a health-care plan designed to treat illnesses presents a poignant irony, as it has little to do with health and everything to do with sickness. But it has become clear that both sides of the aisle enthusiastically agree that Americans must have access to their pills—and lots of them.

From my perspective, getting the word out that people can make simple changes to prevent a disease like Alzheimer's for which there is no meaningful treatment not only makes sense, but is imperative. The word *doctor* means "teacher." And now that so many physicians seem steeped in providing drug remedies, it is the right time to take a step back, review current science, and get the word out that the patients for whom we care can make choices, today, to remain healthy.

A lot has happened in nutritional and brain science since 2013, and publications from our most highly respected academic institutions have now fully validated the principles that I originally put forth in *Grain Brain* and that I'll address in this updated edition. Even the U.S. government has modified its dietary guidelines to reflect this research, backpedaling away from endorsing low-fat, low-cholesterol diets and moving closer to my way of eating. Times are a-changin'!

In 2013, certain myths still circulated in health circles like bad rumors. We were still living in a world that considered all dietary fat to be somehow associated with risk for disease (obesity included), gluten sensitivity was a conversation held only in the context of celiac disease, and no scientist dared to push simple lifestyle modifications to stimulate the growth and proliferation of new brain cells. Five years later, we have more evidence to show what contributes to brain decline and diseases like Alzheimer's.

In the original edition of *Grain Brain*, I posited that the main reason for avoiding gluten-containing foods was because of their role in exacerbating inflammation in the human body. In this revised edition, we will not only revisit the original research that set the foundation, but we will review newer research that clearly defines the mechanism related to inflammation from gluten. In fact, in 2015, a study published in the journal *Nutrients* revealed that gliadin, a protein found in gluten, is associated with increased gut permeability in all humans.[2] This research was based on the groundbreaking discoveries of Dr. Alessio Fasano at Harvard, who unraveled the mechanism whereby gluten induces these changes in the gut lining. Increased gut permeability intensifies the production of the chemical mediators of inflammation. And make no mistake about it, systemic inflammation—meaning widespread inflammation in the body, including the intestines—is damaging for the brain. This connection between the gut and the brain is a pillar upon which *Grain Brain* is built.

An important theme that I am going to revisit is how we look at the balance between neurogenesis—the growth and development of brain cells and neuronal tissue—and inflammation:

Neurogenesis - Inflammation

My goal is to show you how certain habits reduce inflammation while at the same time enhancing neurogenesis, so that rather than destroying brain cells you are sparking the growth of new ones.

One of the most contentious ideas posited in *Grain Brain* was that people can have significant negative reactions, even neurological symptoms, as a result of being sensitive to gluten. Nonetheless, to this day we continue to see aggressive, and seemingly authoritative, online commentary indicating that if you don't have celiac disease or a bona fide wheat allergy, there is no benefit to going gluten-free. These pervasive publications indicate that no one is sensitive to gluten except for the very small percentage of individuals who have the autoimmune condition we call celiac disease or who are otherwise allergic to wheat. I can only imagine who supports this kind of non-scientific nonsense, which does such a disservice to so many. There is now universal recognition that so-called non-celiac gluten sensitivity is a real entity. Indeed, as published in 2017 in the highly respected *Journal of the American Medical Association*, Harvard researchers made it quite clear that non-celiac gluten sensitivity is a common problem and can be associated with not only gastrointestinal issues but even extraintestinal issues as well, some of which involve the brain, as seen in the following table.[3]

Gastrointestinal and Extraintestinal Manifestations of Non-celiac Gluten Sensitivity

Intestinal Symptoms	Extraintestinal Symptoms
Abdominal pain	Anemia
Bloating	Anxiety
Constipation	Arthralgia (joint pain)
Diarrhea	Arthritis
Flatulence	Ataxia (unsteady gait)
Lactose intolerance	Depression
	Rash (e.g., eczema)
	Fatigue
	Headache
	Irritability
	Myalgias (muscle pain)
	Peripheral neuropathy

While the general consensus around the ills of too much sugar and carbs has grown, we still have a giant problem on our hands that has not changed: The rates of dementia, including Alzheimer's disease, continue to rise sharply on a global, massive scale. As Drs. Michal Schnaider-Beeri and Joshua Sonnen wrote in their 2016 paper for the journal *Neurology:* "Despite great scientific efforts to find treatments for Alzheimer disease (AD), only 5 medications are marketed, with limited beneficial effects on symptoms, on a limited proportion of patients, without modification of the disease course."[4]

My mission to end this illness will not finish while I'm still roaming the planet. Brain health has been my passion, professionally, for the past forty-plus years and personally since my father was diagnosed and subsequently died from Alzheimer's disease—the most common form of dementia that has no treatment, let alone cure, despite the billions of dollars thrown at it in research circles. It now affects one out of every ten people in America aged sixty-five or older. And what doesn't get any significant attention is the fact that women are affected by this disease twice as often as men. We've made some great progress in other areas like heart disease, stroke, HIV/ AIDS, and certain cancers. But consider this: Between 2000 and 2014, there was a dramatic reduction in people dying of these ailments, yet during that same time period, deaths related to Alzheimer's disease increased a staggering 89 percent.[5]

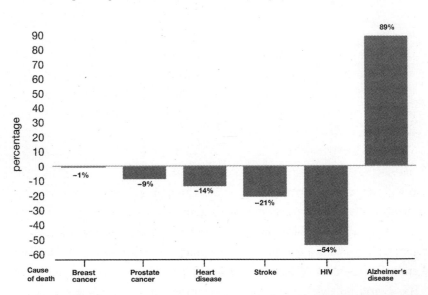

Percentage Changes in Selected Causes of Death (All Ages) Between 2000 and 2014

It pains me to even mention the financial toll of this crisis. To think that we are spending up to $215 billion a year on dementia care in this country—far more than we're spending on any other disease—is infuriating when we consider that the vast majority of these dementia cases could have been prevented with simple lifestyle modifications early in the life cycle. I should also add that we cannot put a value on the emotional expense to loved ones and caregivers. This year, the global cost of dementia care has topped $1 trillion, and incredibly, this figure is predicted to double by the year 2030.[6] That means that right now, global expenditures for dementia health-care exceed the market value of companies like Apple and Google. And if dementia care was looked at in the context of an economy, globally it would be the eighteenth largest economy. Again, this is a largely preventable disease striking a new patient every three seconds.

The numbers are rising in places where incidence of dementia has been historically low compared with Western nations. Based on current projections, Eastern Europe will have about a 26 percent increase in dementia cases by 2050, and in Africa the prevalence will skyrocket by 291 percent. In Central America, the increase is predicted to be 348 percent. This goes to show we're not looking at a genetic problem. While there are genes that do raise one's risk for Alzheimer's disease, purely genetic cases are dwarfed by those from environmental and behavioral influences. Worldwide, the majority of dementia patients live in upper-middle-income or high-income countries, and by 2050, a staggering 73 percent of the 131 million dementia patients will be represented by individuals from the highest brackets of the income scale, as seen in the figure on the next page.[7]

The idea that lifestyle choices profoundly influence a person's risk for developing Alzheimer's disease is not new and was certainly not first proposed in *Grain Brain*. Our most respected journals, such as the *Journal of the American Medical Association*, have for many years been publishing research showing that the choices we make influence our brains' destiny. Case in point: In 2009 researchers analyzed a group of nearly two thousand elderly individuals without dementia who were followed from 1992 through 2006.[8] They asked a simple question: What did these folks eat and how much activity did they get? Their findings were compelling. They demonstrated that those individuals who were the most active and had a diet that was mostly "Mediterranean type" experienced a significant reduction in the risk for becoming patients with Alzheimer's disease. Since that study, numerous others have made the same conclusions, prompting the Mayo Clinic to post

World Bank Income Group	Number of people with dementia (millions)		
	2015	2030	2050
Low Income	1.2	2.0	4.4
Lower Middle Income	9.8	16.4	31.5
Upper Middle Income	16.3	28.4	54.0
High Income	19.5	28.0	42.2
World	46.8	74.7	131.5

an article on its site in 2018 by one of its leading neurologists and faculty members stating that a Mediterranean diet can help protect the brain and reduce the risk of developing dementia.[9] As we did in the original book, we will explore in depth how this is possible, but now with more up-to-date understanding and validation of our original contentions. We also know from this study and others that multiple interventions come into play for Alzheimer's risk, such as physical activity, restorative sleep, and nutritional supplements.

There's so much to explore, so let's get to it, starting with a look back to simpler times many millennia ago. I painted this picture previously, but it's so powerful that it begs to be repeated.

BRAIN HEALTH BEGINS WITH YOU

IF YOU COULD ASK YOUR GRANDPARENTS or great-grandparents what people died from when they were growing up, you'd likely hear the words "old age." Or you might learn the story of someone who got a nasty germ and passed away prematurely from tuberculosis, cholera, or dysentery. What you won't hear are things like diabetes, cancer, heart disease, and dementia. You also would not hear about numerous people suffering from conditions like anxiety and depression, ADHD, chronic pain, and any of the multitude of auto-immune disorders, from fibromyalgia to multiple sclerosis. These are the ailments of modern life, *despite* access to modern medicine.

Since the mid-twentieth century, we've had to attribute someone's immediate cause of death to a single disease or condition rather than use the term "old age" on a death certificate. Today, those single illnesses tend to be the kind that go on and on in a chronic, degenerating state and involve multiple complications and symptoms that accumulate over time. Which is why eighty- and ninety-year-olds don't usually die from a specific ailment. Like an old house in ongoing disrepair, the materials weather and rust, the plumbing and electrical systems falter, and the walls begin to crack from tiny fissures you cannot see. Throughout the home's natural decline, you do the needed maintenance wherever necessary. But it will never be like new unless you tear down the structure and start over again. Each attempt at patching and fixing buys you more time, but eventually the areas in desperate need of a total remodel or complete replacement are everywhere. And, as with all things in life, the human body simply wears out. An enfeebling illness sets in and slowly progresses until the body finally goes kaput.

This is especially true when it comes to brain disorders, including the most dreaded of them all: Alzheimer's disease. It's a modern medical bogey-man that's never far from the headlines. If there is one health worry that seems to eclipse all others as people get older, it's falling prey to Alzheimer's or some other form of dementia that leaves you unable to think, reason, recall, and remember. Research shows how deep this angst runs. Numerous polls taken around the world indicate that people fear dementia more than cancer and other leading causes of death. Fear of death itself takes a back seat to the prospect of dementia. And this fear doesn't just affect older people. Younger generations begin worrying about their brain health the moment someone in their family or circle of friends shows decline. In the words of my friend and colleague Dr. Dale Bredesen, "Everyone knows a cancer survivor; no one knows an Alzheimer's survivor."

There are plenty of perpetual myths about the basket of brain-degenerating maladies, which include Alzheimer's: *It's in the genes, it's inevitable with age, and it's a given if you live into your eighties and beyond.*

Not so fast.

I'm here to tell you that the fate of your brain is not in your genes. It's not unavoidable. And if you're someone who suffers from another type of brain disorder, such as chronic headaches, depression, epilepsy, or extreme moodiness, the culprit may not be encoded in your DNA.

It's largely in the food you eat.

Yes, you read that right: Brain dysfunction starts in your daily bread, and I'm going to prove it. I'll state it again because I realize it sounds absurd: Modern grains are silently destroying your brain. By "modern," I'm not just referring to the refined white flours, pastas, and rice that have already been demonized by the anti-obesity folks; I'm referring to all the grains that so many of us have embraced as being healthful—whole wheat, whole grain, multigrain, seven-grain, live grain, stone-ground, and so on. Basically, I am calling what is arguably our most beloved dietary staple a terrorist group that bullies our most precious organ, the brain. I will demonstrate how fruit and other carbohydrates—especially those laden with sugars, real and artificial—could be health hazards with far-reaching consequences that not only will wreak physical havoc on your brain, but also will accelerate your body's aging process from the inside out and screw with its metabolic engines. This isn't science fiction; it's documented fact.

It is my objective in updating *Grain Brain* to provide information that is sound and based on evolutionary, modern scientific, and physiological perspectives. As before, this book goes outside the box of the layman's accepted dogma—and away from vested corporate interests. I don't have a lot of friends in industries whose bottom lines I threaten. It proposes a new way of understanding the root cause of brain disease and offers a promising message of hope: Brain disease can be largely prevented through the choices you make in life. So if you haven't figured it out by now, I'll be crystal clear: This is not just another diet book or generic how-to guide to all things preventive health. This is a game-changer. At the end of the day, we should all want the same things for ourselves: freedom from chronic conditions that are attributed to how we choose to live. To quote Dr. Bredesen again: "The profound power of lifestyle components to prevent and reverse illness is a gift we have only begun to open." Years ago, if you had asked me if cognitive decline and even symptoms of Alzheimer's disease were reversible, I would have said categorically no. Today, I say a resounding yes—if you do the work and change your ways.

Every day we hear about something new in our various wars against chronic disease, particularly with regard to illnesses that are predominantly avoidable through your habits. You'd have to be living under a rock not to know that we are getting fatter and fatter every year despite all the information sold to us about how to stay slim and trim. You'd also be hard-pressed to find someone who doesn't know about our soaring rates of type 2 diabetes. Or the fact that heart disease remains our number one killer, trailed closely by cancer.

Eat your vegetables. Brush your teeth. Sweat once in a while. Get plenty of rest. Don't smoke. Laugh more. Be a member of a community. There are certain tenets to health that are pretty commonsensical and that we all know we should practice routinely. But somehow, when it comes to preserving our brain's health and mental faculties, we tend to think it's not really up to us—that somehow it's our destiny to develop brain disorders during our prime and grow senile in our elder years, or that we'll escape such a fate through the luck of good genes or medical breakthroughs. Certainly, we would probably do well to stay mentally engaged after retirement, complete crossword puzzles, stay socially active, keep reading, and go to museums. And it's not as though there's a blatantly obvious, direct correlation between brain dysfunctions and specific lifestyle choices as there is between, say, smoking two packs of cigarettes a day and getting lung cancer, or gorging on French fries and becoming obese. As I said, we have a habit of categorizing brain ailments separately from the other afflictions we attribute to bad habits.

I'm going to change this perception by showing you the relationship between how you live and your risk of developing an array of brain-related problems, some that can strike when you're a toddler and others that get diagnosed at the other end of your life span. I believe that the shift in our diet that has occurred over the past century—from high-fat, low-carb to today's low-fat, high-carb diet, consisting primarily of refined grains and other damaging carbohydrates—is the origin of many of our modern scourges linked to the brain, including chronic headaches, insomnia, anxiety, depression, epilepsy, movement disorders, schizophrenia, ADHD, and those "senior moments" that quite likely herald serious cognitive decline and full-blown, irreversible, untreatable, and incurable brain disease. I'll reveal to you the detrimental effect that grains could be having on your brain *right now* without your even knowing or feeling it.

The idea that our brains are sensitive to what we eat has been circulating in our most prestigious medical literature. This information begs to be known by the public, which is increasingly duped by an industry that sells foods commonly thought of as "nutritious." It also has led doctors and scientists like me to question what we considered to be "healthy." Are carbohydrates and processed polyunsaturated vegetable oils such as canola, corn, cottonseed, peanut, safflower, soybean, and sunflower to blame for our spiraling rates of cardiovascular disease, obesity, and dementia? Is a high–saturated fat and high-cholesterol diet actually good for the heart and brain? Can we really change our DNA with food despite the genes we've inherited? It's fairly well known now that a small percentage of the population's digestive systems are sensitive to gluten, the protein found in wheat, barley, and rye; but is it possible for virtually *everyone's* brain to have a negative reaction to this ingredient?

Questions like these really began to bother me before I first wrote *Grain Brain* as damning research started to emerge while my patients got sicker. As a practicing neurologist at the time who cared day in and day out for individuals searching for answers to debilitating brain conditions, as well as families struggling to cope with the loss of a loved one's mental faculties, I felt compelled to get to the bottom of this. Perhaps it's because I'm not just a board-certified neurologist but also a fellow of the American College of Nutrition—one of the only doctors in the country with both of these credentials. I now serve on the American College of Nutrition's Board of Directors. I'm also a founding member and fellow of the American Board of Integrative and Holistic Medicine. This enables me to have a unique perspective on the relationship between what we eat and how our brains function. This is not well understood by most people, including doctors who were educated years before this new science was established. It's time we paid attention. It's time someone like me came out from behind the microscope and the door to the clinical exam room and, frankly, blew the whistle. After all, the statistics are astounding.

For starters, diabetes and brain disease are this country's costliest and most pernicious diseases, yet they are largely preventable and are uniquely tied together: Having diabetes doubles your risk for Alzheimer's disease. In fact, if there's one thing this book clearly demonstrates, it's that many of our illnesses that involve the brain share common denominators. Diabetes and dementia may not seem related at all, but I'm going to show you how close every one of our potential brain dysfunctions is to conditions that we rarely attribute to the brain. I'm also going to draw surprising connections between vastly different brain disorders, such as Parkinson's and a propensity to engage in violent behavior, that point to root causes of an array of afflictions that involve the brain. Newer research is even showing that the road to serious cognitive decline from consuming too many sugary foods doesn't even have to involve diabetes. In other words, the higher the blood sugar, the faster the cognitive decline—regardless of being diabetic or not!

While it's well established that processed foods and refined carbohydrates have contributed to our challenges with obesity and so-called food allergies, no one has explained the relationship between grains and other ingredients and brain health and, in the broader outlook, DNA. It's pretty straightforward: Our genes determine not just how we process food but, more important, how we *respond* to the foods we eat. There is little doubt that one of the largest and most wide-reaching events in the ultimate decline of brain health in modern society has been the introduction of wheat into the human diet. While it's true that our Neolithic ancestors consumed minuscule amounts of this grain, what we now call wheat bears little resemblance to the wild einkorn variety that our forebears consumed on rare occasions. With modern hybridization and gene-modifying technology, the 197 pounds of wheat and other grains that the average American consumes each year share almost no genetic, structural, or chemical likeness to what hunter-gatherers might have stumbled upon.[10] And therein lies the problem: We are increasingly challenging our physiology with ingredients for which we are not genetically prepared.

For the record, this is not a book about celiac disease (a rare autoimmune disorder that involves gluten but affects only a small number of people). If you're already thinking that this book isn't for you because (1) you haven't been diagnosed with any condition or disorder or (2) you're not sensitive to gluten as far as you know, I implore you to read on. This is about *all* of us. Gluten is what I call a "silent germ." It can inflict lasting damage without your knowing it.

Beyond calories, fat, protein, and micronutrients, we now understand that food is a powerful epigenetic modulator—meaning it can change our DNA's behavior for better or worse. Indeed, beyond simply serving as a source of calories, protein, and fat, food actually regulates the expression of many of our genes. And we have only just begun to understand the damaging consequences of wheat consumption from this perspective.

Most of us believe that we can live our lives however we choose, and then when medical problems arise, we can turn to our doctors for a quick fix in the form of a pill. This convenient scenario fosters an illness-centered approach on the part of physicians as they play their role as the purveyors of drugs. But this approach is tragically flawed on two counts. First, it is focused on illness, not wellness. Second, the treatments themselves are often fraught with dangerous consequences. As an example, a 2012 report in the American Medical Association's *Archives of Internal Medicine,* now called *JAMA Internal Medicine,* revealed that postmenopausal women who were put on statin drugs to lower their cholesterol had a nearly 48 percent increased risk of developing diabetes compared to those who weren't given the drug.[11] This one example becomes more critical when you consider that becoming diabetic doubles your risk for Alzheimer's disease. In a more recent study, published in 2015, Finnish researchers calculated a 46 percent increased risk of type 2 diabetes among more than 8,500 men aged forty-five to seventy-three taking statins.[12] The increased risk was attributable to decreases in insulin sensitivity and insulin secretion. Think about that for a moment: These statin drugs, which are heavily marketed to help reduce the risk of a cardiovascular event, can increase the risk for diabetes, which is powerfully linked to heart attack risk and heart disease in general. I should note that the exact mechanism by which statins affect insulin sensitivity and insulin secretion is not entirely clear; statins likely accelerate progression to diabetes via molecular pathways that impact insulin sensitivity and secretion—regardless of diet.

These days, we are seeing an ever-increasing public awareness of the effects of lifestyle choices on health as well as disease risk. We often hear of the "heart smart" diet or recommendations to increase dietary fiber as a strategy to reduce colon cancer risk. We listen to "anti-cancer" messages in the media daily. But why is precious little information made available about how we can keep our brains healthy and stave off brain diseases? Is it because the brain is tied to the ethereal concept of the mind, and this erroneously distances it from our ability to control it? Or is it that pharmaceutical companies are invested in discouraging the idea that lifestyle choices have an influence on brain health? Fair warning: I'm not going to have kind things to say about our pharmaceutical industry. I know far too many stories of people abused by it rather than helped by it. You'll be reading some of these stories in the pages ahead.

This book is about those lifestyle changes you can make today to keep your brain healthy, vibrant, and sharp, while substantially reducing your risk for debilitating brain disease in the future. I have dedicated more than four decades to the study of brain diseases. My workday centers on creating integrative programs designed to enhance brain function in those afflicted with devastating disease. On a daily basis I hear from families and other loved ones whose lives have been turned upside down by illness. It's heart-wrenching for me as well. My father finally passed in 2015 after a long bout with Alzheimer's disease, so to say my crusade is personal is an understatement. He had been a brilliant neurosurgeon trained at the prestigious Lahey Clinic. That was the same year I closed my medical practice and took to spreading my message through teaching, the media, and the global lecture circuit.

The information that I will reveal to you is not just breathtaking; it's undeniably conclusive. You'll be shifting how you eat—and live—immediately.

And you'll be looking at yourself in a whole new light. Right about now, you might be asking, *Is the damage already done?* Have you doomed your brain from all those years of having your cake and eating it too? Don't panic. More than anything, I intend to empower you by equipping you with a remote control to your future brain. It's all about what you do from this day forward.

Drawing on decades of clinical and laboratory studies (including my own), as well as extraordinary results I've seen over the past forty years in my practices, I'll tell you what we know and how we can take advantage of this knowledge. I'll also offer a comprehensive action plan to transform your cognitive health and add more vibrant years to your life. And the benefits don't stop at brain health. I can promise that this program can help any of the following (note: some of these are additions to my original list, for new science speaks!):

- ADHD
- allergies and food sensitivities
- anxiety and chronic stress
- autoimmunity
- chronic constipation or diarrhea
- chronic fatigue
- chronic headaches and migraines
- depression
- diabetes
- epilepsy
- focus and concentration problems
- frequent colds or infections
- hypertension and dyslipidemia (high blood fats)
- inflammatory conditions and diseases, including arthritis
- insomnia

- intestinal problems, including celiac disease, gluten sensitivity, irritable bowel syndrome, ulcerative colitis, and Crohn's disease

- memory problems and mild cognitive impairment, frequently a precursor to Alzheimer's disease

- mood disorders

- overweight and obesity

- Tourette's syndrome

- and much more

Even if you don't suffer from any of the above conditions, this book can help you preserve your well-being and mental acuity. It is for both the old and the young, including women who plan to become or are pregnant. Studies are now showing that babies born to women who are sensitive to gluten live with an increased risk of developing schizophrenia and other psychiatric disorders later in life.[13] That's a huge, chilling finding that all expectant moms need to know.

I've seen dramatic turnarounds in health, such as the twenty-three-year-old man whose crippling tremors vanished after a few easy changes to his diet, and the countless case studies of epileptic patients whose seizures ended the day they replaced grains with more healthy fats and protein. Or the thirty-something woman who experienced an extraordinary transformation in her health after suffering from a litany of medical challenges. Before coming to see me, she not only experienced crushing migraines, depression, and heartbreaking infertility, but also had a rare condition called dystonia that contorted her muscles into strange positions and nearly incapacitated her. Thanks to a few simple dietary tweaks, she allowed her body and brain to recover back to perfect health... and a perfect pregnancy. These stories speak for themselves and are emblematic of millions of other stories of people who live with unnecessary life-depleting conditions. I see a lot of patients who have "tried everything" and who have had every neurological exam or scan available to them in the hope of finding a cure for their condition. With a few simple prescriptions that don't involve drugs, surgery, or even talk therapy, the vast majority of them heal and find a path back to health. You'll find all these prescriptions in the upcoming pages.

A brief note about the book's organization: I've divided the material into three parts, starting with a comprehensive questionnaire designed to show you how your daily habits might be affecting the function and long-term health of your brain. Part I, "The Whole Grain Truth," takes you on a tour of your brain's friends and enemies, the latter of which render you vulnerable to dysfunction and disease. Turning the classic and now obsolete American food pyramid upside down, I'll explain what happens when the brain encounters common ingredients like wheat, fructose (the natural sugar found in fruit), and certain fats, proving that an extremely low-carbohydrate but high-fat diet is ideal (we're talking no more than 20 to 25 grams of *net* carbs a day—the amount in one serving of whole fibrous fruit). I will also be prescribing a strict ketogenic diet for those who want to accelerate and maximize their results. This may sound preposterous, but I'll be recommending that you start swapping out your daily bread with butter and eggs. You'll soon be consuming more saturated fat and cholesterol and rethinking the aisles in your grocery store. Anyone who's already been diagnosed with high cholesterol and prescribed a statin will be in for a rude awakening: I'm going to explain what's really going on in your body and tell you how to remedy this condition easily, deliciously, and without drugs.

In compelling detail, backed by science, I'll put a new spin on the topic of inflammation—showing you that in order to control this potentially deadly biochemical reaction that lies at the heart of brain disease (not to mention all our degenerative illnesses from head to toe), your diet will need to change. I'll show you how your food choices can bring inflammation under control by actually changing the expression of your genes. And it's not as helpful to consume antioxidants as you think. Instead, we need to eat ingredients that turn on the body's own innate antioxidant and detoxification pathways. Part I includes an exploration of the latest research on how we can change our genetic destiny and actually control the "master switches" in our DNA. The research is so captivating that it will inspire the most exercise-averse fast-food junkie; studies that have come out in the last couple of years alone are compelling enough to turn couch potatoes into 5K participants. Part I ends with a more in-depth look at some of our most pernicious psychological and behavioral disorders, such as ADHD and depression, as well as headaches. I'll explain how many cases can be remedied without drugs.

In part II, "Grain Brain Rehab," I present the science behind the habits that support a healthy brain, which includes three primary areas: nutrition and supplements, exercise, and sleep. The lessons gained in this part will help you execute my month-long program outlined in part III, "Say Goodbye to Grain Brain." Included are menu plans, recipes, and weekly goals. I've updated many of the recipes to feature new dishes. For additional support and ongoing updates, you can go to my website at DrPerlmutter.com. There, you'll be able to access the latest studies, read my blog, watch *The Empowering Neurologist* vlogs and interviews with world-renowned scientists and thinkers in this field, and access materials that will help you tailor the information to your personal preferences. Some of the resources (e.g., lists of gluten-containing products and carb content of common foods) will also be accessible online, so they will be easy to download and pin up in your kitchen or on your refrigerator as a reminder. My website has become a destination for anyone wanting to gain further insights into the themes of this book, as well as share stories and learn from others' experiences. You can sign up for my newsletter and link to social media sites like Facebook, Twitter, and Instagram, as well as my YouTube channel.

Exactly what is "grain brain"? I think you already have a clue. It can best be understood by reflecting back on a now-vintage public service announcement. If you were paying attention to advertising in the mid-1980s, you might recall the commercials for a large-scale anti-narcotics campaign that featured an egg in a frying pan with the memorable tagline *This is your brain on drugs*. The penetrating image suggested that the effect of drugs on the brain was like that of a hot pan on an egg. *Sizzle, sizzle.*

This pretty much sums up my assertion about our brains on refined wheat, carbs, and sugar. Let me prove it to you. Then it's up to you to decide if you'll take this all seriously and welcome a brighter, more disease-free future. We've all got a lot to lose if we don't heed this message, and a lot to gain if we do.

Self-Assessment

What Are Your Risk Factors?

WE TEND TO think of brain disease as something that can strike us at any time, for no good reason other than genetic predisposition or bad luck. Unlike heart disease, which progresses over time due to a combination of certain genetic and lifestyle factors, brain ailments seem like conditions that befall us by chance. Some of us escape them, while others become "afflicted." But this thinking is wrong. Brain dysfunction is really no different from heart dysfunction. It develops over time through our behaviors and habits. On a positive note, this means we can consciously prevent disorders of our nervous system and even cognitive decline much in the way we can stave off heart disease: by eating right and getting our exercise. The science now tells us, in fact, that many of our brain-related illnesses, from depression to dementia, are closely related to our nutritional and behavioral choices. Yet only one in one hundred of us will get through life without any mental impairment, let alone a headache or two.

Before I delve into the science behind the bold statement that brain disorders often reflect poor nutrition, as well as a lot of other aggressive assertions, let's start with a simple questionnaire that reveals what habits could be silently harming you right now. The goal of the questionnaire is to gauge your risk factors for current neurological problems, which can manifest in migraines, seizures, mood and movement disorders, sexual dysfunction, and ADHD, as well as serious mental decline in the future. Respond to these statements as honestly as possible. Don't think about the connections to brain disease implied by my statements; just respond truthfully. In upcoming chapters you'll begin to understand why I used these particular statements and where you stand in your risk factors. Note that if you feel like you're in between true and false, and would answer "sometimes," then you should choose true.

1. I eat bread (any kind).   TRUE/FALSE

2. I drink fruit juice (any kind).   TRUE/FALSE

3. I have more than one serving of fruit a day.   TRUE/FALSE

4. I choose agave or an artificial sweetener over sugar.   TRUE/FALSE

5. I get out of breath on my daily walk.   TRUE/FALSE

6. My cholesterol is below 150.   TRUE/FALSE

7. I have insulin resistance or diabetes.   TRUE/FALSE

8. I am overweight.   TRUE/FALSE

9. I eat pasta, crackers, and pastries.   TRUE/FALSE

10. I drink milk.   TRUE/FALSE

11. I don't exercise regularly.   TRUE/FALSE

12. Neurological conditions run in my family.   TRUE/FALSE

13. I don't take a vitamin D supplement.   TRUE/FALSE

14. I eat a low-fat diet.   TRUE/FALSE

15. I take a statin.   TRUE/FALSE

16. I avoid high-cholesterol foods.   TRUE/FALSE

17. I drink soda (diet or regular).   TRUE/FALSE

18. I don't drink wine.   TRUE/FALSE

19. I drink beer.   TRUE/FALSE

20. I eat cereal (any kind).   TRUE/FALSE

A perfect score on this test would be a whopping zero "true" answers. If you answered true to one question, your brain—and your entire nervous system—is at greater risk for disease and disorder than if you scored a zero.

And the more trues you tallied up, the higher your risk. If you scored more than a ten, you're putting yourself into the hazard zone for serious neurological ailments that can be prevented but cannot necessarily be cured once you are diagnosed.

TESTING, TESTING, 1-2-3

"What are my risks?" It's a question I am asked countless times every day. The good news is that we now have the means to medically profile individuals to determine their risk for developing certain diseases—from Alzheimer's to obesity (which is now a well-documented risk factor for brain disease)—and to follow them along their journey to mark their progress. The laboratory studies listed below are available today, are economical, and are generally covered by most insurance plans. I've fully revised this section to reflect my updated testing recommendations. I no longer prescribe gluten sensitivity tests—you should assume that you're sensitive to it and avoid it entirely. This is an important difference between the first edition of the book and this new edition. You'll learn more about these tests in later chapters, as well as ideas for improving your results (your "numbers"). The reason I list them here, however, is that many of you want to know right away what tests your doctor can perform that will help you get a true sense of your risk factors for brain disease. Don't hesitate to bring this list with you to your next doctor's visit and request the following lab work.

* **Fasting blood glucose:** A commonly used diagnostic tool to check for prediabetes and diabetes, this test measures the amount of sugar (glucose) in your blood after you have not eaten for at least eight hours. A level between 70 and 100 mg/dL is considered normal; above this, your body is showing signs of insulin resistance and diabetes, and an increased risk for brain disease. Ideally, you want to have a fasting blood glucose of less than 95 mg/dL.

* **Hemoglobin A1C:** Unlike a test of blood sugar, this test reveals an "average" blood sugar over a ninety-day period and provides a far better indication of overall blood sugar control. Because it can indicate the damage

done to brain proteins due to blood sugar (something called "glycated hemoglobin"), it's one of the greatest predictors of brain atrophy (brain shrinkage). A good A1C value is between 4.8 and 5.4 percent. Note that it can take time to see this number improve, which is why it's typically measured only every three to four months. Later on, we'll see how chronic high blood sugar is now a major risk factor for cognitive decline *with or without a diagnosis of diabetes*. We'll also see that lowering this number (if yours happens to be high) is absolutely not the job of a pharmaceutical drug, despite what mainstream media will have you believe. You can control your A1C through one simple action: losing the excess weight. And you can do that (and so much more) on this program.

- **Fasting insulin:** Long before blood sugar begins to climb as a person becomes diabetic, the fasting insulin level will rise, indicating that the pancreas is working overtime to deal with the excess of dietary carbohydrate. It is a very effective early warning system for getting ahead of the diabetes curve, and so has tremendous relevance for preventing brain disease. You want this number to be below 8 uIU/ml (ideally, below 3).

- **Homocysteine:** Higher levels of this amino acid, produced by the body, are associated with many conditions, including atherosclerosis (narrowing and hardening of the arteries), heart disease, stroke, and dementia; it can often be easily lowered with specific B vitamins. Having a homocysteine level of just 14 µmol/L—a value exceeded by many of my patients when first examined—was described in the *New England Journal of Medicine* as being associated with a doubling of the risk for Alzheimer's disease (an "elevated" homocysteine level is anything above 10 µmol/L in the blood). Although the relationship between high plasma levels of homocysteine (Hcy) and higher risk for Alzheimer's disease has been controversial in the past, new meta-analyses from well-designed studies published in 2015 and 2016 now demonstrate a causal link between plasma total homocysteine and the risk for Alzheimer's disease that calls for further investigation.[14] They also show a pattern among Alzheimer's patients whereby they have high Hcy and low levels of two B vitamins in particular: folic acid and B_{12}. The 2015 study stated that "high Hcy and low folic acid levels may be risk factors of AD." A

2017 study done in China found the same results among older Chinese adults: Low blood levels of folate and vitamin B_{12} and elevated Hcy were associated with mild cognitive impairment and AD, and the association was stronger for AD.[15] (Folate is the form of vitamin B_9 found naturally in foods; folic acid, on the other hand, is the form of B_9 used in supplements.) Homocysteine levels are almost always easy to improve (see chapter 7). Your level should be 8 μmol/L or less. Note that high levels of homocysteine have also been shown to triple the rate of telomere shortening. Telomeres are those caps on the ends of your chromosomes that protect your genes; their length is a biological indication of how fast you are aging.

• **C-reactive protein (CRP):** This is a marker of inflammation. You want to see less than 3.0 mg/L. CRP may take several months to improve, but you may well see positive changes even after one month on the program.

• **Vitamin D (optional):** This is a critical brain *hormone* (it's not a vitamin). In 2014, new recommendations from the U.S. Preventive Services Task Force were published advising against vitamin D testing, stating that it's not helpful to know your levels because experts cannot agree on what the number means. While it's fine to forgo testing, I still recommend taking a vitamin D supplement to ensure you're getting adequate amounts. It's impossible to overdose on vitamin D using my guidelines (see chapter 7), and it's a key component to many functions in the body that play into brain health. You can't go without it!

Even if you don't choose to have these tests done today, having a general understanding of them and what they mean will help you embrace the principles of *Grain Brain*. I will be referring to these tests and their implications throughout the book.

PART I

THE WHOLE
GRAIN TRUTH

If the thought of your brain suffering over a bowl of savory pasta or plate of sweet French toast seems far-fetched, brace yourself. You probably already knew that processed sugars and carbs weren't all that great for you, especially in excess, but so-called healthy carbohydrates like whole grains and natural sugars? Welcome to the whole grain truth. In this part, we're going to explore—with all the latest science—what happens when the brain is bombarded by carbohydrates, many of which are packed with inflammatory ingredients like gluten that can irritate your nervous system. The damage can begin with daily nuisances like headaches and unexplained anxiety and progress to more sinister disorders such as depression and dementia.

We'll also look at the role common metabolic challenges like insulin resistance and diabetes play in neurological dysfunction, and see how we likely owe our obesity and Alzheimer's epidemics to our undying love for carbs and stark disdain for fat and cholesterol.

By the end of this part, you'll have a new appreciation for dietary fat and an educated apprehension when it comes to most carbohydrates. You'll also learn that there are things you can do to spur the growth of new brain cells, gain control of your genetic destiny, and protect your mental faculties.

CHAPTER 1

The Cornerstone of Brain Disease

What You Don't Know About Inflammation

The chief function of the body is to carry the brain around.

— THOMAS A. EDISON

IMAGINE BEING TRANSPORTED BACK to the Paleolithic era of early humans who lived in caves and roamed the savannas tens of thousands of years ago. Pretend, for a moment, that language is not a barrier and you can communicate easily. You have the opportunity to tell them what the future is like. From a cross-legged perch on a dirt floor in front of a warm fire, you start by describing the wonders of our high-tech world, with its planes, trains, and automobiles, city skyscrapers, computers, televisions, smartphones, and the information highway that is the Internet. Humans have already traveled to the moon and back, and now have their sights set on Mars and general spacefaring. At some point, the conversation moves to other lifestyle topics and what it's like to really live in the twenty-first century. You dive into describing modern medicine with its stupendous array of drugs to treat problems and combat diseases and germs. Serious threats to survival are few and far between. Not many people need to worry about predacious tigers, famine, and pestilence. You explain what it's like to shop at grocery stores and supermarkets, a totally foreign concept to these individuals. Food is plentiful, and you mention things like cheeseburgers, French fries, soda, pizza, bagels, bread, cinnamon rolls, pancakes, waffles, scones, pasta, cake, chips, crackers, cereal, ice cream, and candy. You can eat fruit all year long and access virtually any kind of food at the touch of a button or just a short drive away. Refrigeration, flash-freezing, and mass transit have revolutionized life. Water and juice come in bottles for transportability. Although you try to avoid brand names, it's hard to resist because they have become such a part of life—Starbucks, Wonder Bread, Pepperidge Farm, Pillsbury, Lucky Charms, Skittles, Domino's, Subway, McDonald's, Lay's, Gatorade, Ben & Jerry's, Cheerios, Yoplait, Cheez-It, Coca-Cola, Hershey's, Tropicana, and Budweiser.

They are in awe, barely able to picture this future. Most of the features you chronicle are unfathomable; they can't even visualize a fast-food restaurant or bread basket. The term "junk food" is impossible to put into words these people understand. Before you can even begin to mention some of the milestones that humans had to achieve over millennia, such as farming and herding, and later food manufacturing and processing, they ask about the challenges modern people deal with. The obesity epidemic, which has gotten so much attention in your media lately, comes first to mind. This isn't an easy matter for their lean and toned bodies to grasp, and neither is your account of the chronic illnesses that plague society—heart disease, diabetes, depression, autoimmune disorders, cancer, and dementia. These are totally unfamiliar to them, and they ask a lot of questions. What is an "autoimmune disorder"? What causes "diabetes"? What is "dementia"? At this point you're speaking a different language. In fact, as you give them a rundown of what kills most people in the future, doing your best to define each condition, you are met with looks of confusion and disbelief. You painted a beautiful, exotic picture of the future in these people's minds, but then you tore it down with causes of death that seem to be more frightening than dying from an infection or being eaten by a predator higher up on the food chain. The thought of living with a chronic condition that slowly and painfully leads to death sounds awful. And when you try to convince them that ongoing, degenerative disease is possibly the trade-off for potentially living much longer than they do, your prehistoric ancestors don't buy it. And, soon enough, neither do you. Something seems wrong with this picture.

As a species, we are genetically and physiologically identical to these humans who lived before the dawn of agriculture. And we are the product of an optimal design—shaped by nature over thousands of generations. We may not call ourselves hunters and gatherers anymore, but our bodies certainly behave as such from a biological perspective. Now, let's say that during your time travel back to the present day, you begin to ponder your experience with these ancestors. It's easy to marvel at how far we've come from a purely technological standpoint, but it's also a no-brainer to consider the struggles that millions of your contemporary comrades suffer needlessly. You may even feel overwhelmed by the fact that preventable, noncommunicable diseases account for more deaths worldwide today than all other diseases combined. This is tough to swallow. Indeed, we may be living longer than our ancient relatives, but we could be living much better—enjoying our lives sickness-free, increasing our healthy life span—especially during the second half of life, when the risk of illness rises. While it's true that we are living longer than previous generations, most of our gains are due to improvements in infant mortality and child health. In other words, we've gotten better at surviving the accidents and illnesses of childhood. We haven't, unfortunately, gotten better at preventing and combating illnesses that strike us when we're older. And while we can certainly make a case for having much more effective treatments now for many ailments, that still doesn't erase the fact that millions of people have conditions that could have been avoided. When we applaud the average life expectancy in America today, we shouldn't forget about quality of life.

When I was in medical school decades ago, my education revolved around diagnosing disease and knowing how to treat or, in some cases, cure each disease with a drug or other therapy. I learned how to understand symptoms and arrive at a solution that matched those symptoms. A lot has changed since then, because we are not only less likely to encounter easily treatable and curable illnesses, but also better able to understand many of our modern, chronic diseases through the lens of a common denominator:

inflammation. So, rather than spotting infectious diseases and addressing symptoms with known underlying culprits, such as germs, viruses, or bacteria, doctors are faced with myriad conditions that don't have clear-cut answers. I can't write a prescription to eradicate someone's cancer, vanquish inexplicable pain, instantly reverse diabetes, or restore a brain that's been washed away by Alzheimer's disease. I can certainly try to mask or lessen symptoms and manage the body's reactions, but there's a big difference between treating an illness at its root and just keeping symptoms at bay. Now that one of my own kids is a physician, I see how times have changed in medical education and training. Today's young doctors have not only learned how to diagnose and treat; they are equipped with ways of *thinking* that help them address today's epidemics, many of which are rooted in inflammatory pathways run amok.

Before I get to the connection between inflammation and the brain, let's consider what I think is arguably one of the most monumental discoveries of our era: *The origin of brain disease is in many cases predominantly dietary.* Although several factors play into the genesis and progression of brain disorders, to a large extent numerous neurological afflictions often reflect the mistake of consuming too many carbs and too few healthy fats. The best way to comprehend this truth is to consider the most dreaded neurological ailment of all—Alzheimer's—and view it within the context of a type of diabetes triggered by diet alone. We all know that poor diet can lead to obesity and diabetes, but a busted brain?

ALZHEIMER'S DISEASE: A NEW TYPE OF DIABETES?

Flash back to your moment with those hunters and gatherers. Their brains are not too different from yours. Both have evolved to seek out foods high in fat and sugar. After all, it's a survival mechanism. The problem is that your hunting efforts end quickly because you live in the age of plenty, and you're more likely to find processed fats and sugars. Your caveman counterparts are likely to spend a long time searching, only to come across fat from animals and natural sugar from plants and berries if the season is right (and those plants and berries are far less sugary than what you picture when you think of fruit). So while your brain might operate similarly, your sources of nutrition are anything but. In fact, take a look at the following graphic, which depicts the main differences between our diet and that of our forebears.

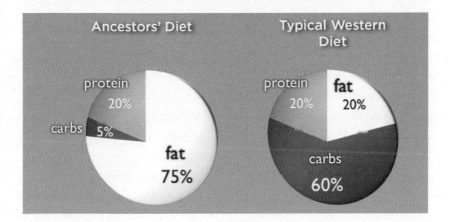

And what, exactly, does this difference in dietary habits have to do with how well we age and whether or not we suffer from a neurological disorder or disease?

Everything.

The studies describing Alzheimer's as a third type of diabetes began to emerge in 2005,[1] but the link between poor diet—notably a high-carb one—and Alzheimer's has only more recently been brought into sharper focus with newer research showing how this can happen.[2] These studies are both convincingly horrifying and empowering at the same time. To think we can prevent Alzheimer's just by changing the food we eat is, well, eye-opening. This has many implications for preventing not just Alzheimer's disease but all other brain disorders, as you'll discover in the upcoming chapters. But first, a brief lesson on what diabetes and the brain have in common. The moniker "type 3 diabetes" sounds a little confusing at first, but all the types of diabetes share one feature in common: a bad relationship with insulin, one of the body's most important substances for cellular metabolism.

Evolutionarily, our bodies have designed a brilliant way to turn the fuel from food into energy for our cells to use. For almost the entire existence of our species, glucose — the body's major source of energy for most cells — has been scarce. This pushed us to develop ways to store glucose and convert other things into it. The body can manufacture glucose from fat or protein if necessary through a process called gluconeogenesis. But this requires more energy than the conversion of starches and sugar into glucose, which is a more straightforward reaction.

The process by which our cells accept and utilize glucose is an elaborate one. The cells don't just suck up glucose passing by them in the bloodstream. This vital sugar molecule has to be allowed into the cell by insulin, which is a hormone produced by the pancreas. Its job is to ferry glucose from the bloodstream into muscle, fat, and liver cells. Once there, it can be used as fuel. Normal, healthy cells have a high sensitivity to insulin. But when cells are constantly exposed to high levels of insulin as a result of a persistent intake of glucose (much of which is caused by an overconsumption of hyper-processed foods filled with refined sugars that spike insulin levels beyond a healthy limit), our cells adapt by reducing the number of receptors on their surfaces to respond to insulin. In other words, our cells desensitize themselves to insulin as if they are revolting against its deluge. This causes insulin resistance, which allows the cells to ignore the insulin and fail to retrieve glucose from the blood. The pancreas then responds by pumping out *more insulin*. So higher levels of insulin become needed for sugar to go into the cells. This creates a cyclical problem that eventually culminates in type 2 diabetes. By definition people with diabetes have high blood sugar because their body cannot transport sugar into cells, where it can be safely stored for energy. And this sugar in the blood presents many problems — too many to mention. Like a poisonous venom, the toxic sugar inflicts a lot of damage, leading to blindness, infections, nerve damage, heart disease, and, yes, Alzheimer's and even death. Throughout this chain of events, inflammation runs rampant in the body.

I should also point out that insulin can be viewed as an accomplice to the events that unfold when blood sugar cannot be managed well. Unfortunately, insulin doesn't just escort glucose into our cells. It's also an anabolic hormone, meaning it stimulates growth, promotes fat formation and retention, and encourages inflammation. When insulin levels are high, other hormones can be affected adversely, either increased or decreased due to insulin's domineering presence. This, in turn, plunges the body further into unhealthy patterns of chaos that cripple its ability to recover its normal metabolism.[3]

Genetics are certainly involved in whether or not a person becomes diabetic, and genetics can also determine at what point the body's diabetes switch gets turned on, once its cells can no longer tolerate the high blood sugar. For the record, type 1 diabetes is a separate disease thought to be an autoimmune disorder—accounting for only 5 percent of all cases. People with type 1 diabetes make little or no insulin because their immune system attacks and destroys the cells in the pancreas that produce insulin, so daily injections of this important hormone are needed to keep blood sugars balanced. Unlike type 2, which is usually diagnosed in adults after their bodies have been abused by too much glucose over time, type 1 diabetes is typically diagnosed in children and adolescents. And unlike type 2, which is reversible through diet and lifestyle changes, there is no cure for type 1 yet, though it can be managed relatively well through drugs and diet. That said, it's important to keep in mind that even though genes strongly influence the risk of developing type 1 diabetes, the environment can play a role, too. It has long been known that type 1 results from both genetic and environmental influences, but the rising incidence over the last several decades has led some researchers to conclude that environmental factors could be more instrumental in the development of type 1 than previously thought.

SAD BUT TRUE

More than 193,000 people younger than age twenty have diabetes (either type 1 or type 2).[4] Type 2 diabetes used to be known as "adult-onset diabetes," but with so many young people being diagnosed, the term had to be dropped. And new science shows that the progression of the disease happens more rapidly in children than in adults. It's also more challenging to treat in the younger generation. Diabetes is the seventh leading cause of death in the United States. Alzheimer's disease is the sixth.[5]

What we're beginning to understand is that at the root of "type 3 diabetes" is the phenomenon in which neurons in the brain become unable to respond to insulin, which is essential for basic tasks, including memory and learning. We also think that insulin resistance, as it relates to Alzheimer's disease, may spark the formation of those infamous plaques that are present in diseased brains. These plaques are the buildup of an odd protein that essentially hijacks the brain and takes the place of normal brain cells. Some researchers believe that insulin deficiency is central to the cognitive decline of Alzheimer's disease—brain cells can't get their insulin because they are resistant to it! And the fact that we can associate insulin resistance with brain disease is why talk of "type 3 diabetes" is starting to circulate among researchers. It's all the more telling to note that obese people are at a much greater risk of impaired brain function, and that those with diabetes are at least twice as likely to develop Alzheimer's disease. And those with prediabetes or metabolic syndrome—a cluster of biochemical abnormalities associated with the development of type 2 diabetes as well as cardiovascular disease—have an increased risk of pre-dementia or mild cognitive impairment (MCI), which often progresses to full-blown Alzheimer's disease.

This statement is not meant to imply that diabetes directly and always causes Alzheimer's disease, only that they share the same origin. They both often spring from overconsuming foods that force the body to develop biological pathways leading to dysfunction and, further down the road, illness. While it's true that one person with diabetes and another person with dementia may look and act differently, they have a lot more in common than we previously thought. And what I find really interesting (and which I mentioned earlier) is that newer studies are showing that people with high blood sugar—whether or not they have diabetes—have a higher rate of cognitive decline than those with normal blood sugar. This was true in one particularly disturbing longitudinal study from 2018 following more than five thousand people over ten years.[6] Their rate of cognitive decline—regardless of whether or not they were diabetic—hinged on blood sugar levels. The higher the blood sugar, the faster the decline—even in the non-diabetics.

In the last twenty years, we've witnessed a parallel rise in the number of type 2 diabetes cases and the number of people who are considered obese.

Now, however, we're starting to see a pattern among those with dementia, too, as the rate of Alzheimer's disease increases in sync with type 2 diabetes. I don't think this is an arbitrary observation. It's a reality we all have to face as we shoulder the weight of soaring health-care costs and an aging population. New estimates indicate that Alzheimer's will more than triple in prevalence and likely affect 16 million Americans by 2050, a crippling number for our health-care system and one that will dwarf our obesity epidemic.[7] There were an estimated 50 million people worldwide living with dementia in 2017, and this number will almost double every twenty years, reaching 75 million in 2030 and 131.5 million in 2050. Today, someone in the United States develops Alzheimer's dementia every 66 seconds. By mid-century, someone in the United States will develop the disease every 33 seconds (remember, someone in the world develops dementia every 3 seconds).[8] The prevalence of type 2 diabetes, which accounts for 90 to 95 percent of all diabetes cases in the United States, has tripled in the past forty years, and millions of people go undetected and untreated for a long time. By anyone's definition, this is absolutely an epidemic. No wonder the U.S. government is anxiously looking to researchers to improve the prognosis and avert a catastrophe. According to the Centers for Disease Control and Prevention (CDC), more than 30 million people have diabetes, which amounts to nearly 10 percent of the U.S. population; other reports have calculated that the percentage among adults is more like 12 to 14 percent, depending on the criteria used.[9] An estimated 7.2 million adults, eighteen years or older, are undiagnosed (23.8 percent of people with diabetes).

THE SILENT BRAIN ON FIRE

One of the most frequent questions I hear from families of Alzheimer's patients is *How did this happen? What did my mother (or father, brother, sister, husband, wife) do wrong?* I am careful how I respond at such a heartbreaking time in a family's life. Watching my own father wither away slowly, day after day, continues to be a constant reminder of the multitude of emotions that a family experiences. There is frustration fused with helplessness, and anguish mingled with regret. But if I had to tell people (myself included) the absolute truth given what we know today, I'd say that their loved one may have done one or more of the following:

- lived with chronic high blood sugar levels even in the absence of diabetes

- eaten too many carbohydrates throughout life, especially those with refined sugars, flours, and grains

- opted for a low-fat diet that minimized cholesterol

- lived with chronic hypertension (high blood pressure) especially at midlife

- saddled the body with chronically elevated levels of widespread, "silent" inflammation

When I tell people that gluten sensitivity represents one of the greatest and most under-recognized health threats to humanity, the response I hear is pretty much the same: "You can't be serious. Not everyone is sensitive to gluten. Of course, if you have celiac disease, but that's a small number of people." And when I remind people that all the latest science points to the bane of gluten in triggering not just dementia but epilepsy, headaches, depression, schizophrenia, ADHD, and even decreased libido, a common thread prevails in the response: "I don't understand what you mean." They say this because all they know about gluten focuses on intestinal health— not neurological wellness.

We're going to get up close and personal with gluten in the next chapter. Gluten isn't just an issue for those with bona fide celiac disease. As many as 40 percent of us can't properly process gluten, and the remaining 60 percent could be in harm's way. The question we need to be asking ourselves is this: *What if we're all sensitive to gluten from the perspective of the brain?* Unfortunately, gluten is found not only in wheat breads and cereals but also in the most unexpected products—from ice cream to hand cream. Increasing numbers of studies are confirming the link between gluten sensitivity and neurological dysfunction. This is true even for people who have no problems digesting gluten and who test negative for gluten sensitivity. I see this every day in my work. Many of the individuals who reach out to me for guidance do so once they have "tried everything" and have been to scores of other doctors in search of help. Whether it's headaches and migraines, Tourette's syndrome, seizures, insomnia, anxiety, ADHD, depression, or just some odd set of neurological symptoms with no definite label, one of the first things I do is prescribe the total elimination of gluten from their diets. And the results continue to astound me.

A True GB Story

In early 2016 I weighed in at 244 pounds. I had started cutting out sugar, but I really needed help with a healthy diet. My son-in-law told me about *Grain Brain,* and I ordered it immediately! I started changing my diet right away. The weight just flew off me and I felt so much better. In time I began to notice the change in my memory, too! I suffer from severe osteoarthritis of the spine and just about every other bone. I really needed to lose that weight and learn how to eat the right things. I will never change my new eating habits! - Linda P.

Researchers have known for some time now that the cornerstone of all degenerative conditions, including brain disorders, is inflammation. But what they hadn't documented until now are the instigators of that inflammation—the first missteps that prompt this deadly reaction. And what they are finding is that gluten, and a high-carbohydrate diet for that matter, are among the most prominent stimulators of inflammatory pathways that reach the brain. What's most disturbing about this discovery, however, is that we often don't know when our brains are being negatively affected. Digestive disorders and food allergies are much easier to spot because symptoms such as gas, bloating, pain, constipation, and diarrhea emerge relatively quickly. But the brain is a more elusive organ. It could be enduring assaults at a molecular level without your feeling it. Unless you're nursing a headache or managing a neurological problem that's clearly evident, it can be hard to know what's going on in the brain until it's too late. When it comes to brain disease, once the diagnosis is in for something like dementia, turning the train around is hard.

The good news is that I'm going to show you how to control your genetic destiny even if you were born with a natural tendency to develop a neurological challenge. This will require that you free yourself from a few of the myths that so many people continue to cling to. The two biggest ones: (1) a low-fat, high-carb diet is healthy and (2) dietary cholesterol is unhealthy.

The story doesn't end with the elimination of gluten. Gluten is just one piece of the puzzle. In the upcoming chapters, you'll understand why cholesterol is one of the most important players in maintaining brain health and function. Study after study shows that high cholesterol reduces your risk for brain disease and increases longevity.[10] By the same token, high levels of dietary fat (the good kind, no trans fats here) have been proven to be key to health and peak brain function.

Say what? I realize you may doubt these statements because they run so contrary to what you've been taught to believe. One of the most prized and respected studies ever done in America, the famous Framingham Heart Study, has added volumes of data to our understanding of certain risk factors for disease, including, most recently, dementia. It commenced in 1948 with the recruitment of 5,209 men and women between the ages of thirty and sixty-two from the town of Framingham, Massachusetts, none of whom had yet suffered a heart attack or stroke or even developed symptoms of cardiovascular disease.[11] Since then, the study has added multiple generations stemming from the original group, which has allowed scientists to carefully monitor these populations and gather clues to physiological conditions within the context of myriad factors—age, gender, psychosocial issues, physical traits, and genetic patterns. In the mid-2000s, researchers at Boston University set out to examine the relationship between total cholesterol and cognitive performance, and they looked at 789 men and 1,105 women who were part of the original group. All of the individuals were free of dementia and stroke at the beginning of the study and were followed for sixteen to eighteen years. Cognitive tests were performed every four to six years, evaluating things like memory, learning, concept formation, concentration, attention, abstract reasoning, and organizational abilities—all the features that are compromised in patients with Alzheimer's disease.

According to the study's report, published in 2005, "There was a significant positive linear association between total cholesterol and measures of verbal fluency, attention/concentration, abstract reasoning, and a composite score measuring multiple cognitive domains."[12] Moreover, "participants with 'desirable' total cholesterol (less than 200) performed less well than participants with borderline high total cholesterol levels (200 to 239) and participants with high total cholesterol levels (greater than 240)." The study concluded that "lower naturally occurring total cholesterol levels are associated with poor performance on cognitive measures, which placed high demand on abstract reasoning, attention/concentration, word fluency, and executive functioning." In other words, the people who had the *highest* cholesterol levels scored higher on cognitive tests than those with lower levels. Evidently, there is a protective factor when it comes to cholesterol and the brain. We'll be exploring how this is possible in chapter 3.

The research keeps coming from various labs around the world, flipping conventional wisdom on its head. In 2012, researchers with the Australian National University in Canberra published one of the first studies of its kind in the journal *Neurology* (the medical journal of the American Academy of Neurology) showing that people whose blood sugar is on the high end of the "normal range" have a much greater risk for brain atrophy, or shrinkage, a follow-up study published in 2016 and the 2018 review paper I called out a few pages ago confirmed these findings.[13] This ties directly into the story of type 3 diabetes. We've known for a long time that brain disorders and dementia are associated with brain shrinkage. But knowing now that such shrinkage can happen as a result of blood sugar spikes in the "normal" range has tremendous implications for anyone who eats blood sugar–boosting foods (that is, carbohydrates). So often people will tell me that they are fine because their blood sugar is normal. But what is normal? The lab test may indicate that an individual is "normal" by established standards, but new science is forcing us to reconsider normal parameters. Your blood sugar may be "normal," but if you could peek into your pancreas, you might be aghast at how much it's struggling to pump out enough insulin to keep you on an even keel. For this reason, getting a fasting insulin test, which is done first thing in the morning before eating a meal, is critical. An elevated level of insulin in your blood at this time is a red flag—a sign that something isn't metabolically right. You could be on the verge of diabetes, already depriving your brain of its future functionality.

The original Australian study involved 249 people aged sixty to sixty-four who had blood sugar in the so-called normal range, and who underwent brain scans at the start of the study and again an average of four years later. Those with higher blood sugar levels within the normal range were more likely to show a loss of brain volume in regions involved with memory and cognitive skills. The researchers even managed to factor out other influences, such as age, high blood pressure, smoking, and alcohol use. Still, they found that blood sugar on the high end of normal accounted for 6 to 10 percent of the brain shrinkage. The follow-up 2016 study involved slightly more participants (287) with the same results: Higher blood sugar equates with brain atrophy. These studies again suggest that blood sugar levels could have an impact on brain health even for people who do not have diabetes.[14]

Blood sugar and insulin imbalances are epidemic. One in two Americans suffers from diabesity—the term now used to describe a range of metabolic imbalances from mild insulin resistance to prediabetes to full-blown diabetes. The hardest fact of all to accept is that many of these people don't even know they have this dangerous condition that typically starts with being overweight or obese. They will carry on and come to learn of their predicament when it's far too late. My mission is to interrupt such an unfortunate destiny. We want to focus not on calling all the king's horses and all the king's men, but on coaxing Humpty Dumpty down from the wall before disaster strikes. This will require a shift in a few daily habits.

If the thought of going on a low-carb diet is terrifying (you're already biting your nails at the thought of nixing all the delicious foods you've come to love), don't give up yet. I promise to make this as easy as possible. I might take away the bread basket, but I'll replace it with other things you might have avoided under the false idea that they were somehow bad for you, such as butter, meat, cheese, and eggs, as well as an abundance of wonderfully healthful vegetables. The best news of all is that as soon as you shift your body's metabolism from relying on carbs to relying on fat and protein, you'll find a lot of desirable goals easier to achieve, such as losing weight effortlessly and permanently, gaining more energy throughout the day, sleeping better, being more creative and productive, having a sharper memory and faster brain, and enjoying a better sex life. This, of course, is in addition to safeguarding your brain.

INFLAMMATION GETS CEREBRAL

Let's get back to this idea of inflammation, which I've mentioned a few times in this chapter without a full explanation. Everyone has a rough idea what is meant by the term "inflammation" in a general sense. Whether it's the redness that quickly appears after burning your hand while cooking in the kitchen or the chronic ache of an arthritic joint, most of us understand that when there is some kind of stress in the body, our body's natural response is to create swelling and pain, hallmarks of the inflammatory process. But inflammation isn't always a negative reaction. It can also serve as an indication that the body is trying to defend itself against something it believes to be potentially harmful. Whether to speed recovery from an injury or reduce movement in a sprained ankle to allow healing, inflammation is vital to our survival.

Problems arise, however, when inflammation gets out of control. Just as one glass of wine a day can be healthy but multiple glasses every day can lead to health risks, the same holds true for inflammation. Inflammation is meant to be a spot treatment. It's not supposed to be turned on for prolonged periods of time, and never forever. But that's what's happening in millions of people. If the body is constantly under assault by exposure to irritants, the inflammation response stays on. And it spreads to every part of the body through the bloodstream; hence, we have the ability to detect this kind of widespread inflammation through blood tests that find markers of inflammation such as C-reactive protein.

When inflammation goes awry, a variety of chemicals are produced that are directly toxic to our cells. This leads to a reduction of cellular function

45

followed by cellular destruction. Unbridled inflammation is rampant in Western cultures, with leading scientific research showing that it is a fundamental cause of the morbidity and mortality associated with coronary artery disease, cancer, diabetes, Alzheimer's disease, and virtually every other chronic disease you can imagine. I love how vividly my good friend and colleague Dr. David Ludwig, a nutrition researcher, physician, and professor at Harvard Medical School, describes it: "Imagine rubbing the underside of your arm with sandpaper. Before long, the area would become red, swollen, and tender—the hallmarks of acute inflammation. Now imagine that this inflammatory process took place over many years within your body, affecting all the vital organs as a result of poor diet, stress, sleep deprivation, and other exposures. Chronic inflammation may not be immediately painful, but it silently underlies the greatest killers of our era, including heart disease, diabetes, Alzheimer's, and even cancer."

It's not much of a stretch to appreciate how unchecked inflammation would underlie a problem like arthritis, for example. After all, the common drugs used to alleviate the symptoms, such as ibuprofen and aspirin, are marketed as "anti-inflammatories." With asthma, antihistamines are used to combat the inflammatory reaction that occurs when someone is exposed to an irritant that elicits an allergic response. These days, more and more doctors are beginning to understand that coronary artery disease, a leading cause of heart attacks, may actually have more to do with inflammation than it does with high cholesterol. This explains why aspirin, in addition to its blood-thinning properties, is useful in reducing risk not only for heart attacks but also for strokes.

But the connection of inflammation to brain diseases, although well described in the scientific literature, seems somehow difficult to embrace—and it's largely unknown by the public. Perhaps one reason people can't seem to envision "brain inflammation" as being involved in everything from Parkinson's disease to multiple sclerosis, epilepsy, autism, Alzheimer's disease, and depression is that, unlike the rest of the body, the brain has no pain receptors, so we can't feel inflammation in the brain.

Focusing on reducing inflammation might seem out of place in a discussion of enhancing and preserving brain health and function. But while we are all familiar with inflammation as it relates to such disease states as arthritis and asthma, the past decade has produced an extensive body of research clearly pointing the finger of causality at inflammation when considering a variety of neurodegenerative conditions as well. In fact, studies dating back as far as the 1990s show that people who have taken nonsteroidal anti-inflammatory medications such as Advil (ibuprofen) and Aleve (naproxen) for two or more years may have more than a 40 percent reduced risk for Alzheimer's and Parkinson's disease.[15] At the same time, other studies have clearly shown dramatic elevation of cytokines, the cellular mediators of inflammation, in the brains of individuals suffering from these and other degenerative brain disorders.[16] Today, new imaging technology is finally allowing us to see cells actively involved in producing inflammatory cytokines in the brains of Alzheimer's patients. We can even measure correlations between signs of systemic inflammation and brain shrinkage further down the road.

In 2017 a consortium of scientists from high-profile institutions (Johns Hopkins University School of Medicine, Baylor College of Medicine, and the Mayo Clinic, among others) reported in the journal *Neurology* that high levels of inflammatory markers in the blood during midlife were associated with smaller brain volumes in late life.[17] These researchers documented baseline levels of inflammation in more than 1,600 men and women in their fifties. Then, after twenty-four years, the scientists measured not only how well the participants' brains were working, but with the help of MRI technology, they measured volumes of certain brain regions associated with memory and Alzheimer's disease. And what was discovered is that higher levels of inflammation in midlife were correlated with significant brain shrinkage overall, with pronounced atrophy in the Alzheimer's-related areas of the brain and the hippocampus—by as much as 5 percent total shrinkage. Further, the number of words that an individual could recall was drastically reduced if that individual had higher levels of inflammatory markers twenty-four years earlier. (The verbal recall test worked as follows: A person was read a list of ten words and then, after several minutes, was asked to remember as many words as possible. It was essentially a measure of short-term memory.) The implications of this study are important because it means that the lifestyle we adopt when we are younger has a big role in determining our brain destiny when we are older. It is also important to note that the subjects who had the worst results were the *youngest* at the beginning of the study.

So, we are now forced to regard inflammation in a whole new light. Far more than just the cause of your painful knee and sore joints, it underpins the very process of brain degeneration. We have also come to learn that it may very well be at the heart of another epidemic condition today: depression.[18] That's right: Depression, which is now the number one cause of disability worldwide, may not necessarily be due to a chemical imbalance in the brain. It's an inflammatory disease with roots in other imbalances throughout the body. (When I witness people improve from depression by going on a gluten-free diet, it might have to do with the fact that they have decreased inflammation in their bodies.) I did not devote a lot of space to the subject of depression in the first edition. The evidence to date, however, compels me to include more on it now. To think you can treat and sometimes cure depression through diet alone is empowering.

Ultimately, the key downstream effect of inflammation in the brain that is responsible for the damage is activation of chemical pathways that increase free radical production. At the center of chronic inflammation is the concept of oxidative stress—a biological type of "rusting." This gradual corrosion happens on all tissues. It's a normal part of life; it occurs everywhere in nature, including when our bodies turn calories (energy) from food and oxygen from the air into usable energy. But when it begins to run rampant, or when the body can't keep it under healthy control, it can become deadly. Although the word *oxidation* implies oxygen, it's not the kind we breathe. The felon here is simply O because it's not paired with another oxygen molecule (O_2).

Let me take you one step further in describing the oxidation process. Most of us have heard about free radicals by now. These are molecules that have lost an electron. Normally, electrons are found in pairs, but forces such as stress, pollution, chemicals, toxic dietary triggers, ultraviolet sunlight, and ordinary body activities can "free" an electron from a molecule such that it loses its social graces and starts trying to steal electrons from other molecules. This disorder is the oxidation process itself, a chain of events that creates more free radicals and stirs inflammation. Because oxidized tissues and cells don't function normally, the process can render you vulnerable to a slew of health challenges. This helps explain why people with high levels of oxidation, which is often reflected by high levels of inflammation, have an extensive list of health challenges and symptoms ranging from a low resistance to infection to joint pain, digestive disorders, anxiety, headaches, depression, and allergies.

And, as you probably can guess, reduced oxidation lowers inflammation, which in turn helps limit oxidation. Antioxidants are important for this very reason. These nutrients, such as vitamins A, C, and E, donate electrons to free radicals, and this interrupts the chain reaction and helps prevent damage. Historically, antioxidant-rich foods such as plants, berries, and nuts were part of our diet, but the food industry today processes a lot of nutrients out of our diets that are sorely needed for optimal health and energy metabolism.

Later in this book I'm going to show you how to turn on a particular pathway in your body that not only directly reduces free radicals naturally, but also protects the brain by reducing excess free radicals produced by inflammation. Interventions designed to reduce inflammation using natural substances like turmeric have been described in medical literature dating back more than two thousand years, but it is only in the past decade that we have begun to understand this intricate and eloquent biochemistry.

Another upshot of this biological pathway is the activation of specific genes that code for the production of enzymes and other chemicals that serve to break down and eliminate various toxins to which we are exposed. One might wonder why human DNA would contain codes for the production of detoxification chemicals, because we tend to assume that our first real exposure to toxins began with the industrial era. But humans (and, in fact, all living things) have been exposed to a variety of toxins for as long as there has been life on the planet. Aside from toxins that naturally exist in our external environment, like lead, arsenic, and aluminum, as well as powerful toxins created as a form of protection by variously consumed plants and animals, our bodies produce toxins internally during the normal processes of metabolism. So these detoxification genes—now needed more than ever—have thankfully served us for a very long time. And we are just beginning to understand how natural substances you can buy at your local grocery store, such as turmeric and the omega-3 docosahexaenoic acid (DHA), can act as powerful detoxification agents by enhancing genetic expression.

It is not just what we eat that can change the expression of our genes and, therefore, help us manage inflammation. You're also going to learn about the latest studies demonstrating the ways in which exercise and sleep come into play, as these are important regulators (read: remote controllers) of our DNA. What's more, you'll learn how to grow new brain cells; I'm going to show you how and why neurogenesis—the birth of new brain cells—is under your control.

THE CRUEL IRONY: STATINS

Diet and exercise can boost our body's natural methods to manage inflammation, but is there also a case for drugs? Ironically, cholesterol-lowering statins, which are among the most commonly prescribed drugs (e.g., Lipitor, Crestor, Zocor, Mevacor, Pravachol), are now being touted as a way to reduce overall levels of inflammation. But statins *may lessen brain function and increase risk for heart disease* in some people. The reason is simple: The brain needs cholesterol to thrive, a point I've already made but will repeat to make sure you don't forget it. Cholesterol is a critical brain nutrient essential for the function of neurons, and it plays a fundamental role as a building block of the cell membrane. It acts as an antioxidant and a precursor to important brain-supporting elements like vitamin D, as well as the steroid-related hormones (e.g., sex hormones such as testosterone and estrogen). Most important, cholesterol is looked upon as an essential fuel for the neurons. Neurons themselves are unable to generate significant cholesterol; instead, they rely on delivery of cholesterol from the bloodstream via a specific carrier protein. Interestingly, this carrier protein, LDL, has been given the derogatory title of "bad cholesterol." In reality, LDL is not a cholesterol molecule at all, good or bad. It's a low-density lipoprotein (hence its acronym), and there is absolutely nothing bad about it. The fundamental role of LDL in the brain, again, is to capture life-giving cholesterol and transport it to the neuron, where it performs critically important functions.

And now we have the evidence in the scientific literature to prove that when cholesterol levels are low, the brain simply doesn't work well; individuals with low cholesterol are at much greater risk for dementia and other neurological problems. We need to change our attitudes about cholesterol and even LDL; they are our friends, not foes.

But what about cholesterol and coronary artery disease? I'm going to tackle that very conundrum in chapter 3. For now, I want to implant in your brain the idea that cholesterol is good. You'll soon see that we've been barking up the wrong tree—blaming cholesterol, and LDL especially, when coronary artery disease has more to do with *oxidized* LDL. And how does LDL become so damaged that it's no longer able to deliver cholesterol to the brain? One of the most common ways is through physical modification by glucose. Sugar molecules attach themselves to LDL and change the molecule's shape, rendering it less useful while increasing free radical production.

If what I just described to you raced past your head, don't panic. I'm going to take you by the hand through all these biological events in the upcoming chapters. I've broadly touched upon a lot of issues in this chapter as a prelude to the balance of the book, which will take you deeper into the story of *Grain Brain*. The chief questions I want you to think about are: Have we accelerated our brain's decline by following a low-fat, high-carb diet with fructose on the side? Can we really control the fate of our brains through lifestyle alone despite the DNA we've inherited? Is there too much invested interest in Big Pharma to consider the fact we can naturally prevent, treat, and sometimes cure—without drugs—a spectrum of brain-based ailments such as ADHD, depression, anxiety, insomnia, autism, Tourette's syndrome, headaches, and Alzheimer's disease? The answer to all three of these questions is a resounding yes. I'll go even further and suggest that we can prevent heart disease and diabetes, too. The current model of "treatment" for these maladies pays too much attention to the symptomatic smoke and ignores the smoldering fire. Such an approach is ineffective and unsustainable. If we're ever going to push the boundaries of human longevity, live long past 100 years old with our brains as sharp as ever, and really have something amazing to report to our prehistoric ancestors, then we're going to have to change our whole MO.

The goal of this chapter was to explain the story of inflammation and introduce you to a new way of thinking—and looking—at your brain (and body). We take it for granted that the sun rises in the east every morning and sets in the west at night. The next day, the sun does the same thing again. But what if I told you that the sun isn't moving at all? It's *we* who are spinning and moving around the sun! I trust you already knew that, but the takeaway from the analogy is that we tend to get mentally wedded to ideas that are no longer valid. After lectures, people frequently approach me to say thanks for thinking outside the box. With all due respect, that's not the point. It does the world no good for me to be seen as someone whose ideas are "outside the box." My mission is to make the box bigger so that these concepts are part of our culture and way of living. Only then will we be able to make serious, meaningful headway with our modern afflictions.

FROM BRAIN HEALTH TO TOTAL HEALTH

The inescapable fact is that we have evolved into a species that requires fat for life and health. The massive amounts of carbs we eat today are fueling a silent firestorm in our bodies and brains. And I'm not just talking about the manufactured, refined stuff that we all know is not going to win prizes for us at the doctor's office (much less on the scale). I love how Dr. William Davis puts it in his seminal work *Wheat Belly:*[19]

> Whether it's a loaf of organic high-fiber multigrain bread or a Twinkie, what exactly are you eating? We all know that the Twinkie is just a processed indulgence, but conventional advice tells us that the former is a better health choice, a source of fiber and B vitamins, and rich in "complex" carbohydrates.

Ah, but there's always another layer to the story. Let's peer inside the story. Let's peer inside the contents of this grain and try to understand why — regardless of shape, color, fiber content, organic or not — it potentially does odd things to humans.

And that's exactly where we're going next. But we're going to go one step beyond Davis's brilliant account of the modern grain and the battle of the bulge in order to see how gluten can inflict harm where we never imagined before: the brain.

CHAPTER 2

The Sticky Protein

Gluten's Role in Brain Inflammation (It's Not Just About Your Belly)

Tell me what you eat, I'll tell you who you are.

— ANTHELME BRILLAT-SAVARIN (1755–1826)

MOST EVERYONE HAS EXPERIENCED the throb of a headache and the agony of severe congestion. In many instances, we can point to a probable cause when symptoms descend on us, such as a long day in front of the computer in the case of a tension headache, or a passing cold bug when it hurts to swallow and the nose clogs up. For relief we can usually turn to over-the-counter remedies to manage our symptoms until the body returns to a normal, healthy state. But what do you do when the symptoms don't go away and the culprit is much harder to pin down? What if, like so many patients I treat, you find yourself in an unending war with nagging pain and misery for years?

For as long as she could remember, Fran struggled to chase the pulsating sensation out of her head. When I first examined her on a warm January day, Fran was as pleasant as could be for a sixty-three-year-old who endured daily migraine headaches. Of course she had tried all the usual headache medications and was taking Imitrex (sumatriptan), a powerful migraine drug, several times a week. In reviewing her medical history, I noted that in her early twenties she'd undergone "intestinal exploratory surgery" because she was suffering from "severe intestinal discomfort." As part of her evaluation, I tested her for gluten sensitivity and, not to my surprise, found that she was strongly positive in eight of the markers. I prescribed a gluten-free diet.

Four months later, I received a letter from Fran stating: "My almost daily migraine symptoms have abated since removing gluten from my diet.... The two biggest changes in my body are the lack of a very hot head in the night with resulting migraines, and the huge increase in my energy levels. Today my level of daily accomplishment is enormous compared to my life before seeing you." She went on to conclude: "Thank you, once again, for finding what seems to be the solution to my many years of migraine misery." I wish she could have gotten the years back, but at least now I could give her a pain-free future.

Another woman who came to me with a totally different set of symptoms but a similarly long history of suffering was Lauren. At just thirty years old, she told me squarely on our first meeting that she was "having some mental problems." Lauren detailed the previous twelve years, which she described as a consistent downhill ride in terms of health. She told me how her early life was quite stressful once she lost both her mother and grandmother at a young age. When she started college she was hospitalized on several occasions for "mania." During this time she would experience episodes of becoming highly talkative and overly grandiose about herself. She would then eat excessively, gain a lot of weight, and become severely depressed and suicidal. She had just started taking lithium, a medication used to treat bipolar disorder. Mental illness ran in her family; her sister had schizophrenia and her father was bipolar. Aside from Lauren's dramatic account of her mental issues, the rest of her medical history was fairly unremarkable. She had no laments of bowel issues, food allergies, or any other of the standard types of complaints associated with gluten sensitivity.

I went ahead and ordered a test for gluten sensitivity (as with Fran's case, this was during the time I still tested for gluten sensitivity; remember, testing is no longer necessary—more on this shortly). We found profoundly elevated levels of six important markers for the condition. In fact, several of these markers were more than twice the normal range. Two months after starting a gluten-free diet, Lauren wrote a letter to me that echoed what I'd been hearing from so many patients who'd gone gluten-free and experienced striking results. She stated:

> Since being off gluten, my life has taken a complete 180. The first change that comes to mind, and the most important one, is my mood. When I was eating gluten, I would struggle with feeling depressed. I would always have to fight a "dark cloud over my head." Now that I'm off gluten, I don't feel depressed. The one time I ate some by mistake, I felt depressed again the next day. Other changes I've noticed include having more energy and being able to stay focused for longer periods. My thoughts are as sharp as ever. I can make a decision and come to a logical, confident conclusion like never before. I am also free of a lot of obsessive-compulsive behavior.

Let me give you one more example of a case that's emblematic of another set of symptoms linked to the same culprit. Kurt and his mother came to see me when he was a twenty-three-year-old man suffering from abnormal movements. His mother stated that six months prior to their visit, he began "looking like he was shivering." Initially his tremors were subtle, but they increased with time. He had been to two neurologists and received two different diagnoses: one for what's called "essential tremor" and another for "dystonia." The doctors had offered him a blood pressure medication, propranolol, which is used to treat some types of tremor disorders. The other recommendation was to have the various muscles in his arms and neck injected with Botox, the botulinum toxin, to temporarily paralyze the spastic muscles. Both he and his mother had elected not to try either the pills or the injections.

What was interesting about his history were two things. First, he was diagnosed as having a learning disability in the fourth grade; his mother said that "he could not handle excessive stimulation." And second, for several years he had complaints of stomach pain with loose bowel movements to the extent that he had to see a gastroenterologist, who took a biopsy of his small intestine to test for celiac disease. It proved negative.

When I examined Kurt, his excessive movement problem was very evident. He could not control the shaking of his arms and neck and appeared to be suffering mightily. I reviewed his laboratory studies, which, for the most part, were unrevealing. He had been checked for Huntington's disease, an inherited disorder known to cause a similar movement abnormality in young people, as well as Wilson's disease, a disorder of copper metabolism also associated with a movement abnormality. All these tests were negative. Blood work for gluten sensitivity did, however, show some elevated levels of certain antibodies indicative of vulnerability. I explained to Kurt and his mother that it was important to make sure gluten sensitivity wasn't the cause of his movement disorder, and I provided them with information on how to pursue a gluten-free diet.

After several weeks I received a phone call from Kurt's mother indicating that without question his movements had calmed down. Because of his improvement he elected to stay on a gluten-free diet, and after approximately six months, the abnormal movements had all but disappeared completely. The changes that occurred in this young man are breathtaking, especially when you consider that a simple dietary change had such a life-transforming impact.

We are just beginning to see medical literature documenting a connection between movement disorders and gluten sensitivity, and physicians like me have now identified and treated a handful of individuals whose movement disorders have completely abated with a gluten-free program and for whom no other cause was identified. But, unfortunately, most mainstream doctors are not on the lookout for the dietary explanation for such movement disorders and are not aware of the latest reports. I bet most don't know that in 2015 the literature started to fill with cases in which gluten sensitivity mimics amyotrophic lateral sclerosis (ALS).[1] Imagine getting (mis)diagnosed with ALS and then finding out all you really had was gluten sensitivity. I should stress, however, that this is not common (and going gluten-free is not a cure for ALS, which is a very serious disease for which there is no treatment).

These cases are not outliers. They reflect patterns that I've witnessed in many patients. They might come to me with vastly different medical complaints, but they share a common thread: gluten sensitivity. It's my belief that gluten is a modern poison, and that the research is compelling doctors like me to notice and reexamine the bigger picture when it comes to brain disorders and disease. The good news is that knowing this common denominator now means we can treat and, in some cases, cure a wide spectrum of ailments with a single prescription: the eviction of gluten from the diet.

Walk into any health food store, and now even a regular grocery store, and you're sure to be amazed at the selection of gluten-free products. In the past couple of years, the volume of gluten-free products sold has exploded; by 2020 the global gluten-free food market is projected to be valued at more than $7.5 billion.[2] Spin-offs of everything from breakfast cereals to salad dressing are now positioned to take advantage of the ever-increasing number of individuals who are choosing foods without gluten. Why all the hype?

No doubt media attention may be playing a role. Scores of high-profile individuals, professional athletes, and celebrities have sworn by the transformative effects of going gluten-free. But a questionable side to this lifestyle has also emerged. In May 2017 headlines around the country suggested that going gluten-free in the absence of celiac disease was dangerous: LOW-GLUTEN DIET LINKED TO HEART ATTACK RISK was a headline carried by many news reports, with *The Independent* going so far as to state, "Trendy gluten-free diets loved by Gwyneth Paltrow and Russell Crowe may increase the risk of heart disease."[3] True? And what about the headlines that stated that going off gluten-containing foods would increase a person's risk of arsenic and mercury toxicity?[4] Let's take these two allegations in turn.

First, the gluten-heart debate. If you were to pull the curtain behind the frightening headlines and examine the studies referenced to arrive at such an absurd assertion, you'd find that (and I quote from one such respectable study published in *The BMJ*, formerly known as *The British Medical Journal*, and authored by various medical departments at Columbia and Harvard Universities): "Long-term dietary intake of gluten was not associated with risk of coronary heart disease. However, the avoidance of gluten may result in reduced consumption of beneficial whole grains, which may affect cardiovascular risk."[5] By and large individuals going on a gluten-free program consume less dietary fiber. They often turn to products labeled "gluten-free" that indeed may not contain that ingredient but are otherwise processed with nutritional offenders in other ways (think trans fats, sugars, and artificial additives). We know that dietary fiber is important in helping reduce inflammation and in nurturing the gut bacteria, which also play a role in reducing inflammation. The take-home message is that gluten remains a problem, as I will describe in more detail below, and that in the avoidance of gluten it is of paramount importance to, nonetheless, ensure that you are consuming copious amounts of gluten-free dietary fiber. That is the appropriate conclusion from this research, as the authors indicated.

Now, as for gluten causing arsenic and mercury poisoning, a similar thread of explanation is at play here. Consider the hyped headline: GLUTEN-FREE DIET MAY INCREASE RISK OF ARSENIC, MERCURY EXPOSURE.[6] Now think about that for a moment. It's the last word that should tell you something. After all, how could *avoiding* something increase your exposure to toxic chemicals? Indeed, the study did find higher levels of these toxins in gluten-free individuals, but it was because they ate more of other potentially contaminated foods in place of gluten-containing grains. Rice, for example, is a popular choice for people giving up gluten, and the data show a powerful risk for arsenic exposure in folks who eat a lot of rice. (To be clear, rice in all its natural forms — white, brown, wild, basmati — is technically a seed, not a grain.) In addition, we do know that fiber helps the body rid itself of toxins. And going off gluten might lead to a reduction in fiber consumption, as previously noted.

So there you have it; I felt compelled to address those matters first. Now let's get to more about what the scientific community has to say about gluten. What does it mean to be "gluten sensitive"? How does it differ from celiac disease? What's so bad about gluten? Hasn't it always been around? And just what exactly do I mean by "modern grains"? Let's take a tour.

THE GLUE OF GLUTEN

Gluten — which is Latin for "glue" — is a protein composite that acts as an adhesive material, holding flour together to make bread products, including crackers, baked goods, and pizza dough. When you bite into a fluffy muffin or roll and stretch pizza dough prior to cooking, you have gluten to thank. In fact, most of the soft, chewy bread products available today owe their gumminess to gluten. Gluten plays a key role in the leavening process, letting bread "rise" when wheat mixes with yeast. To hold a ball of what is essentially gluten in your hands, just mix water and wheat flour, create a dough by kneading the ball with your hands, and then rinse the glob under running water to eliminate the starches and fiber. What you're left with is a glutenous protein mixture.

Most Americans consume gluten through wheat and wheat-based products, but gluten is found in a variety of grains, including rye, barley, spelt, kamut, and bulgur. It's one of the most common food additives on the planet and is used not only in processed foods, but also in personal care products. As a trusty stabilizing agent, it helps cheese spreads and margarines retain their smooth texture, and it prevents sauces and gravies from curdling. Thickening hair conditioners and volumizing mascaras have gluten to thank, too. People can be as allergic to it as they can be to any protein. But let's get a better look at the scope of the problem.

Gluten is not a single molecule; it's actually made up of two main groups of proteins, the *glutenins* and the *gliadins*. A person may be sensitive to either of these proteins or to one of the twelve different smaller units that make up gliadin. Any of these could cause a sensitivity reaction leading to inflammation.

When I speak with patients about gluten sensitivity, one of the first things they say is something like, "Well, I don't have celiac disease. I've been tested!" I do my best to explain that there's a huge difference between celiac disease and gluten sensitivity. My aim is to convey the idea that celiac disease, also known as sprue, is an extreme manifestation of gluten sensitivity. Celiac disease is what happens when an allergic reaction to gluten causes damage specifically to the small intestine. It's one of the most severe reactions one can have to gluten. Although many experts estimate that 1 in every 100 people worldwide has celiac disease, this is a conservative calculation; the number is probably closer to 1 in 30, since so many individuals remain undiagnosed (an estimated 2.5 million Americans alone are undiagnosed).[7] As many as 1 in 4 people are vulnerable to the disease due to genetics alone; people of northern European ancestry are particularly susceptible. What's more, people can carry genes that code for mild versions of gluten intolerance, giving rise to a wide spectrum of gluten sensitivity. Celiac disease doesn't just harm the gut. Once the genes for this disease are triggered, sensitivity to gluten is a lifelong condition that can affect the skin and mucous membranes, as well as cause blisters in the mouth.

Extreme reactions that trigger an autoimmune condition such as celiac aside, the key to understanding gluten sensitivity is that it can involve *any* organ in the body, even if the small intestine is completely spared. So while a person may not have celiac disease by definition, the rest of the body— including the brain—is at great risk if that individual is gluten sensitive.

It helps to understand that food sensitivities in general are usually a response from the immune system. They can also occur if the body lacks the right enzymes to digest ingredients in foods. In the case of gluten, its "sticky" attribute interferes with the breakdown and absorption of nutrients. As you can imagine, poorly digested food leads to a pasty residue in your gut, which alerts the immune system to leap into action, eventually resulting in an assault on the lining of the small intestine. Those who experience symptoms complain of abdominal pain, nausea, diarrhea, constipation, and intestinal distress. Some people, however, don't experience obvious signs of gastrointestinal trouble, but they could nevertheless be experiencing a silent attack elsewhere in their body, such as in their nervous system. Remember that when a body negatively reacts to food, it attempts to control the damage by sending out inflammatory messenger molecules to label the food particles as enemies. This leads the immune system to keep sending out inflammatory chemicals, killer cells among them, in a bid to wipe out the enemies. The process often damages our tissue, leaving the walls of our intestine compromised, a condition known as "leaky gut." Once you have a leaky gut, you're highly susceptible to additional food sensitivities in the future. And the onslaught of inflammation can also put you at risk for developing various autoimmune diseases.[8]

Inflammation, which you know by now is the cornerstone of many brain disorders, can be initiated when the immune system reacts to a substance in a person's body. When antibodies of the immune system come into contact with a protein or antigen to which a person is allergic, the inflammatory cascade is provoked, releasing a whole host of damaging chemicals known as cytokines. Gluten sensitivity in particular is caused by elevated levels of antibodies against the gliadin component of gluten. When the antibody combines with this protein (creating an anti-gliadin antibody), specific genes are turned on in a special type of immune cell in the body. Once these genes are activated, inflammatory cytokine chemicals collect and can attack the brain. Cytokines are highly antagonistic to the brain, damaging tissue and leaving the brain vulnerable to dysfunction and disease — especially if the assault continues. Another problem with anti-gliadin antibodies — one that has been described for decades — is that they can directly combine with specific proteins found in the brain that look like the gliadin protein found in gluten-containing foods, but the anti-gliadin antibodies just can't tell the difference. This, again, leads to the formation of more inflammatory cytokines.[9]

Given this, it's no wonder that elevated cytokines are seen in Alzheimer's disease, Parkinson's disease, major depression, multiple sclerosis, and even autism.[10] Again, research has even shown that some people who are wrongly diagnosed with ALS (aka Lou Gehrig's disease) simply have a sensitivity to gluten, and eliminating it from the diet resolves the symptoms.[11] As Dr. Marios Hadjivassiliou, one of the most well-respected researchers in the area of gluten sensitivity and the brain at the Royal Hallamshire Hospital in Sheffield, England, reported in a 1996 article in the *Lancet*, "Our data suggest that gluten sensitivity is common in patients with neurological disease of unknown cause and may have etiological significance."[12]

For someone like me whose life's work has been dealing with challenging brain disorders "of unknown cause" on a daily basis, Dr. Hadjivassiliou's statement is especially sobering when you consider that an estimated 99 percent of people whose immune systems react negatively to gluten don't even know it. Dr. Hadjivassiliou goes on to state that "gluten sensitivity can be primarily, and at times, exclusively, a neurological disease." In other words, *people with gluten sensitivity can have issues with brain function without having any gastrointestinal problems whatsoever*. I love how Dr. Hadjivassiliou and his colleagues stated the facts in a 2002 editorial in the *Journal of Neurology*,

Neurosurgery, and Psychiatry titled "Gluten Sensitivity as a Neurological Illness":

> It has taken nearly 2,000 years to appreciate that a common dietary protein introduced to the human diet relatively late in evolutionary terms (some 10,000 years ago) can produce human disease not only of the gut but also the skin and the nervous system. The protean neurological manifestations of gluten sensitivity can occur without gut involvement and neurologists must therefore become familiar with the common neurological presentations and means of diagnosis of this disease.[13]

In addition, the editorial summed up the findings brilliantly in the conclusion, which reiterated statements made in earlier papers: "Gluten sensitivity is best defined as a state of heightened immunological responsiveness in genetically susceptible people. This definition does not imply bowel involvement. That gluten sensitivity is regarded as principally a disease of the small bowel is a historical misconception."

As you already know, I no longer recommend testing for gluten sensitivity because it's best to assume that you are sensitive to gluten and avoid it entirely—even if you have no celiac and have tested negative to gluten sensitivity in the past. In 2015, Harvard's Dr. Fasano published a landmark paper with a group of colleagues from other institutions including the Naval Medical Center, the University of Maryland, and Johns Hopkins School of Medicine.[14] In their study, led by the Navy's Dr. Justin Hollon, they showed how gliadin can wreak so much havoc and even be the culprit behind autoimmune disorders and cancer. Briefly, gliadin triggers production of another protein called zonulin, which breaks down the gut lining and increases permeability. Once the lining is compromised, substances that are supposed to stay in the gut leak into the bloodstream and incite inflammation. The discovery of zonulin's effects on the body inspired researchers to look for illnesses characterized by intestinal permeability. And lo and behold, this led to the finding that most autoimmune diseases, including celiac disease, type 1 diabetes, rheumatoid arthritis, multiple sclerosis, and inflammatory bowel disease, are distinguished by abnormally high levels of zonulin and a leaky gut. So powerful is zonulin that when scientists expose animals to the toxin, the animals develop type 1 diabetes almost immediately; the toxin induces a leaky gut, and the animals begin producing antibodies to islet cells, which are responsible for making insulin. Fasano's study concluded: "Gliadin exposure induces an increase in intestinal permeability in all individuals, regardless of whether or not they have celiac disease." Which means that all of us—whether or not we have celiac—have some level of gluten sensitivity. The gliadin protein within gluten causes a cascade of events in the gut that can result in leaky intestines with major downstream adverse health implications.

Since this book was first published, multiple studies have emerged to further show the connection between gluten, and specifically the gliadin protein, and increased permeability of the gut, which we know is a fundamental mechanism for increasing inflammation. These studies confirm over and over again that non-celiac gluten sensitivity is real and much more widespread than we could ever have imagined. So much so that in 2016, the Celiac Disease Foundation declared non-celiac gluten (wheat) sensitivity a bona fide condition following mounting physical evidence of immune system activation and intestinal damage in people who consume wheat without celiac disease or wheat allergy.[15] And the condition affects six times more people than celiac disease.[16] This declaration came on the heels of yet another study showing that people without celiac can indeed exhibit markers of intestinal cellular damage related to a severe systemic immune activation.[17] The study was led by researchers from no less authority than Columbia University Medical Center.

Measuring Gut Permeability

One of the ways we can test for a leaky gut is to look for lipopolysaccharide (LPS) in the blood. LPS is a combination of fat and sugars and is found on the outer membrane of certain bacteria in the intestines. It serves to protect these bacteria so they are not digested by bile salts from the gallbladder. These types of bacteria are abundant in the gut, representing as much as 50 to 70 percent of the intestinal flora. But LPS induces a violent inflammatory response in humans—

so violent that it's also considered an endotoxin, meaning a toxin that comes from within. Animal models used in laboratory settings for research purposes to study such diverse conditions as Alzheimer's disease, multiple sclerosis, inflammatory bowel disorders, diabetes, Parkinson's disease, rheumatoid arthritis, lupus, depression, and even autism employ LPS because of its ability to quickly push that inflammatory button in the body. Normally, LPS is blocked from gaining entrance into the bloodstream by the tight junctions that exist between the cells lining the intestine. But, as you can imagine, when the intestinal cells become leaky or permeable and those junctions are compromised, LPS is able to gain entry into the systemic circulation, where it can inflict damage and fuel inflammation. LPS levels in the blood are indicative of not only inflammation in general, but also leakiness of the bowel. In patients with Alzheimer's, ALS, major depression, and even autism, levels of LPS are often elevated.

Before we go into more detail about gluten sensitivity, let's get a clearer understanding on how we came to understand celiac disease, the most extreme version of gluten sensitivity.

CELIAC THROUGH THE CENTURIES

Although the relationship between gluten sensitivity and neurological disease has received precious little attention in the medical literature, we can trace a prominent thread of accumulating knowledge back thousands of years to a time when gluten wasn't even part of our vocabulary. The evidence, it turns out, was already mounting; we just weren't able to document it until the current century. The fact that we can finally identify a link between celiac disease, the strongest reaction to gluten, and neurological problems has implications for all of us, including those who don't have celiac. The study of celiac patients has enabled us to zoom in on the real dangers of gluten that have largely remained hidden and silent for so long.

Celiac may seem like a "new disease," but the first descriptions of the disorder date back to the first century AD, when Aretaeus of Cappadocia, one of the most distinguished ancient Greek doctors, wrote about it in a medical textbook covering various conditions, including neurological abnormalities such as epilepsy, headache, vertigo, and paralysis. Aretaeus was also the first to use the word *celiac,* which is Greek for "abdominal." In describing this malady, he said: "The stomach being the digestive organ, labours in digestion, when diarrhea seizes the patient…and if in addition, the patient's general system be debilitated by atrophy of the body, the coeliac disease of a chronic nature is formed."[18]

In the nineteenth century, the term *sprue* was introduced into the English language from the Dutch word *sprouw,* which means chronic diarrhea — one of the classic symptoms of celiac disease. The English pediatrician Dr. Samuel J. Gee was among the first to recognize the importance of diet in managing patients with celiac; he gave the first modern-day description of the condition in children in a lecture at a London hospital in 1887, noting, "If the patient can be cured at all, it must be by means of diet."

At the time, however, no one could pinpoint which ingredient was the culprit, so recommendations in dietary changes in search of a cure were far from accurate. Dr. Gee, for example, banned fruits and vegetables, which wouldn't have posed a problem, but allowed thin slices of toasted bread. He was particularly moved by the curing of a child "who was fed upon a quart of the best Dutch mussels daily," but who relapsed when the season of mussels was over (perhaps the child went back to eating toast). In the United States, the first discussion of the disorder was published in 1908 when Dr. Christian Herter wrote a book about children with celiac disease, which he called "intestinal infantilism." As others had noted previously, he wrote that these children failed to thrive and added that they tolerated fat better than carbohydrate. Then, in 1924, Dr. Sidney V. Haas, an American pediatrician, reported positive effects of a diet of bananas. (Obviously, bananas weren't the cause of the improvement, but rather, the banana diet happened to exclude gluten.)

While it's hard to imagine such a diet enduring the test of time, it remained popular until the actual cause of celiac could be determined and confirmed. This took another couple of decades, until the 1940s when the Dutch pediatrician Dr. Willem Karel Dicke made the connection to wheat flour. By then, carbohydrates in general had long been suspected, but not until a cause-and-effect observation could be made with wheat in particular did we see the direct connection. And how was this discovery actually made? During the Dutch famine of 1944, bread and flour were scarce, and Dr. Dicke noticed a dramatic decrease in the death rate among children affected by celiac — from greater than 35 percent to virtually zero. Dr. Dicke also reported that once wheat was again available, the mortality rate rose to previous levels. Finally, in 1952, a team of doctors from Birmingham, England, including Dr. Dicke, made the link between the ingestion of wheat proteins and celiac disease when they examined samples of intestinal mucosa taken from surgical patients. The introduction of the small bowel biopsy in the 1950s and '60s confirmed the gut as a target organ. (To be fair, I should note that historical experts have debated whether or not Dicke's earlier anecdotal observations in the Netherlands were completely correct, arguing that it would have been difficult if not impossible for him to record such a relapse when flour became available again. But these debaters are not dismissing the importance of identifying wheat as a culprit — they merely aim to highlight the fact that wheat isn't the *only* culprit.)

So when did we begin to see a connection between celiac and neurological issues? Again, the trail goes back much further than most people realize. More than a century ago the first anecdotal reports began to emerge, and throughout the twentieth century various doctors documented neurological conditions in patients with celiac. Early on, though, when neurological problems were found to correlate to celiac disease, by and large they were thought to represent a manifestation of nutritional deficiencies because of the gut issue. In other words, doctors didn't think that a certain ingredient was necessarily wreaking havoc on the nervous system; they just thought that the celiac condition itself, which prevented the absorption of nutrients and vitamins in the gut, led to deficiencies that triggered neurological problems like nerve damage and even cognitive impairments. And they were far from being able to grasp the role of inflammation in the story, which had yet to enter our medical library of knowledge. In 1937, the *Archives of Internal Medicine* published the Mayo Clinic's first review of neurological involvement in patients with celiac, but even then the research could not accurately describe the real cascade of events.[19] They attributed the brain involvement to "electrolyte depletion" due principally to the gut's failure to digest and absorb nutrients properly.[20]

To reach the point where we could understand and fully explain the link between sensitivity to gluten and the brain, we needed a great deal of advancements in our technology, not to mention our understanding of the role of inflammatory pathways. But the turnaround in our perspective has indeed been sensational, and relatively recent. In 2006, the Mayo Clinic again came out with a report, published in the *Archives of Neurology*, about celiac disease and cognitive impairment, but this time the conclusion was a game-changer: "A possible association exists between progressive cognitive impairment and celiac disease, given the temporal relationship and the relatively high frequency of ataxia and peripheral neuropathy, more commonly associated with celiac disease."[21] Ataxia is the inability to control voluntary muscle movement and maintain balance, most frequently resulting from disorders in the brain; peripheral neuropathy is a fancy way of saying nerve damage. It encompasses a wide range of disorders in which the damaged nerves outside of the brain and spinal cord—peripheral nerves—cause numbness, weakness, or pain.

In this particular study, the researchers looked at thirteen patients who showed signs of progressive cognitive decline within two years of the onset of celiac disease symptoms or a worsening of the disorder. (The most common reasons why these patients sought medical help for their brain impairments were amnesia, confusion, and personality changes. Doctors confirmed all cases of celiac disease by small-bowel biopsy; anyone whose cognitive decline could potentially be pinned on an alternative cause was excluded.) One thing became clear during the analysis that instantly invalidated previous thinking: The cognitive decline could not be attributed to nutritional deficiencies. What's more, doctors noted that the patients were relatively young to have dementia (the median age when signs of cognitive impairment began was sixty-four years, with a range from forty-five to seventy-nine years). As reported in the media, according to Dr. Joseph Murray, a Mayo Clinic gastroenterologist and the study investigator, "There has been a fair amount written before about celiac disease and neurological issues like peripheral neuropathy...or balance problems, but this degree of brain problem—the cognitive decline we've found here—has not been recognized before. I was not expecting there would be so many celiac disease patients with cognitive decline."

Murray went on to add that it's unlikely these patients' conditions reflected a "chance connection." Given the association between the celiac symptoms starting or worsening and the cognitive decline within just two years, the likelihood of this being a random event was very small. Perhaps the most stunning finding of all in this study was that several of the patients who were put on a gluten-free diet experienced "significant improvement" in their cognitive decline. When they completely withdrew from gluten consumption, three patients' mental faculties either improved or stabilized, leading the researchers to highlight that they may have discovered a reversible form of cognitive impairment. This is a huge finding. Why? We really don't have many forms of dementia that are readily treatable, so if we can stop and in some cases *reverse* the path to dementia, identifying celiac disease in the presence of cognitive decline should become customary. What's more, such a finding further argues against chance as an explanation for the link between celiac disease and cognitive decline. When asked about the scientific reasoning behind the link, Dr. Murray mentioned the potential impact of inflammatory cytokines—those chemical messengers of inflammation that contribute to problems in the brain.

One more item I'd like to point out from this study: When the researchers performed brain scans on these patients, they found noticeable changes in the white matter that could easily be confused with multiple sclerosis or even small strokes. This is the reason I have always prescribed a gluten-free diet in patients referred to me with a diagnosis of multiple sclerosis; on many occasions I've found patients whose brain changes were in fact not related to multiple sclerosis at all and were likely due to gluten sensitivity. And lucky for them, a gluten-free diet reversed their condition. Since the 2006 Mayo report, numerous others have documented a relationship between gluten ingestion and neurological disorders (the term "gluten ataxia" has even entered the medical lexicon).

THE BIGGER PICTURE

Recall the young man I discussed at the beginning of the chapter who was originally diagnosed with a movement disorder called dystonia. He couldn't control his muscle tone, resulting in wild and intense spasms throughout his body that prevented him from leading a normal life. Although neurological disease or side effects to drugs are often to blame in cases like this, my belief is that a lot of dystonia and other movement disorders can be attributed simply to gluten sensitivity. In my patient's situation, once we removed gluten from his diet, his tremors and convulsive twitches came to a screeching halt. Other movement disorders, such as ataxia, which I described earlier; myoclonus, another affliction characterized by spasmodic jerky contractions of muscles; and certain forms of epilepsy are often misdiagnosed—they are attributed to an unexplained neurological problem rather than to something as simple as gluten sensitivity. I've had several epileptic patients in the past who've gone from considering risky surgery and relying on daily medication regimes to manage their seizures to becoming completely seizure-free through simple dietary shifts.

Dr. Hadjivassiliou has similarly examined brain scans from headache patients and documented dramatic abnormalities caused by gluten sensitivity. Even a lay reader without a trained eye can easily see the impact. Take a look at one example:

Brain MRI images showing severe changes in the white matter (arrows) related to gluten sensitivity and headaches (left) compared to a normal study (right).

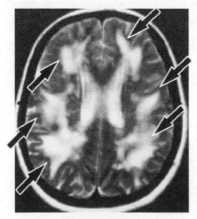 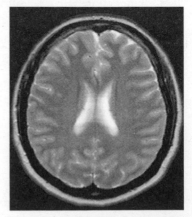

Gluten sensitive   Normal

Dr. Hadjivassiliou has repeatedly shown that a gluten-free diet can result in complete resolution of headaches in patients with gluten sensitivity. In a 2010 review for the *Lancet Neurology*, he makes a clarion call for change in how we view gluten sensitivity.[22] For him and his colleagues, nothing could be more critical than getting the word out about the connection between seemingly invisible gluten sensitivity and brain dysfunction. And I agree. Dr. Hadjivassiliou's chronicle of patients with evident signs of cognitive deficits and documented gluten sensitivity, as well as their recovery, is impossible to deny. In 2013, he co-established the Sheffield Institute of Gluten-Related Disorders in the United Kingdom; it is the world's first clinic to specialize in the neurological manifestations of gluten-related disorders.

As we've discussed, one of the most important takeaways from all the new information we've gained about celiac disease is that it's not confined to the gut. I would go so far as to say that gluten sensitivity *always* affects the brain. Neurobiologist Dr. Aristo Vojdani, a colleague who has published extensively on the topic of gluten sensitivity, has stated that the incidence of gluten sensitivity in Western populations may be as high as 30 percent.[23] And because most cases of celiac are clinically silent, the prevalence of the disease itself is now recognized to be twenty times higher than it was thought to be two decades ago. Let me share what Dr. Rodney Ford of The Children's Clinic and The Allergy Center in Christchurch, New Zealand, proposed in his 2009 article aptly titled "The Gluten Syndrome: A Neurological Disease": "The fundamental problem with gluten is its interference with the body's neural networks...gluten is linked to neurological harm in patients, both with and without evidence of celiac disease."[24] He added, "Evidence points to the nervous system as the prime site of gluten damage," and he boldly concluded that "the implication of gluten causing neurologic network damage is immense. With estimates that at least one in ten people are affected by gluten, the health impact is enormous. Understanding the gluten syndrome is important for the health of the global community."

Although you may not be sensitive to gluten in the same way an individual with celiac is, I've inundated you with data for good reason: It goes to show that we may all be sensitive to gluten from a neurological standpoint. We just don't know it yet because there are no outward signs or clues to a problem happening deep within the quiet confines of our nervous system and brain. Remember, at the heart of virtually every disorder and disease is inflammation. When we introduce anything to the body that triggers an inflammatory response, we set ourselves up for taking on much greater risk for a medley of health challenges, from chronic daily nuisances like headaches and brain fog to serious ailments such as depression and Alzheimer's. We can even make a case for linking gluten sensitivity with some of the most mysterious brain disorders that have eluded doctors for millennia, such as schizophrenia, epilepsy, depression, bipolar disorder, and, more recently, autism and ADHD. In 2015, Italian researchers added "gluten psychosis" to the medical dictionary when they reported on a troubling case of a child with psychosis that could be attributed to non-celiac gluten sensitivity.[25] To think that gluten can induce psychosis in children is simply shocking.

I'll be covering these connections later in the book. For now, I want you to get a scope of the problem, with a firm understanding that gluten can exert effects not only on the normal brain but also on the vulnerable abnormal brain. It's also important to keep in mind that each of us is unique in terms of our genotype (DNA) and phenotype (how genes express themselves in their environment). Unchecked inflammation in me could result in obesity and heart disease, whereas the same condition in you could translate to an autoimmune disorder.

Once again, it helps to turn to the literature on celiac disease, since celiac reflects an extreme case; it allows us to identify patterns in the course of the disorder that can have implications for anyone who consumes gluten, regardless of celiac. Multiple studies, for example, have shown that people with celiac have significantly increased production of free radicals, and they exhibit free radical damage to their fat, protein, and even DNA.[26] In addition, they also lose their ability to produce antioxidant substances in the body as a result of the immune system's response to gluten. In particular, they have reduced levels of glutathione, an important antioxidant in the brain, as well as vitamin E, retinol, and vitamin C in their blood—all of which are key players in keeping the body's free radicals in check. It's as if the presence of gluten disables the immune system to such a degree that it cannot fully support the body's natural defenses. Here's my question: If gluten sensitivity can compromise the immune system, what else does it open the door to?

Research has also shown that the immune system's reaction to gluten leads to activation of signaling molecules that basically turn on inflammation and induce what's called the COX-2 enzyme, which leads to increased production of inflammatory chemicals.[27] If you're familiar with drugs like Celebrex, ibuprofen, or even aspirin, you're already familiar with the COX-2 enzyme, which is responsible for inflammation and pain in the body. These drugs effectively block that enzyme's actions, thus reducing inflammation. High levels of another inflammatory molecule called TNF alpha have also been seen in celiac patients. Elevations of this cytokine are among the hallmarks of Alzheimer's disease and virtually every other neurodegenerative condition. Bottom line: *Gluten sensitivity—with or without the presence of celiac—increases the production of inflammatory cytokines, and these inflammatory cytokines are pivotal players in neurodegenerative conditions.* Moreover, no organ is more susceptible to the deleterious effects of inflammation than the brain. It's one of the most active organs in the body, yet it lacks bulletproof protective factors. Although the blood-brain barrier acts as a gatekeeper of sorts to keep certain molecules from crossing over from the bloodstream into our brain, it's not a foolproof system. Plenty of substances sneak past this portal and provoke undesirable effects. (Later in the book I'll go into richer detail about these inflammatory molecules and the ways in which we can use the power of food to combat them.)

It's time we created new standards for what it means to be "gluten sensitive." The problem with gluten is far more serious than anyone ever imagined, and its impact on society is far greater than we've ever estimated.

A GLUT OF GLUTEN IN MODERN FOOD

If gluten is so bad, how have we managed to survive so long while eating it? The quick answer is that we haven't been eating the same kind of gluten since our ancestors first figured out how to farm and mill wheat. The grains we eat today bear little resemblance to the grains that entered our diet about ten thousand years ago. Ever since the nineteenth century, when Gregor Mendel described his famous studies of crossing different plants to arrive at new varieties, we've gotten good at mixing and matching strains to create some unusual progeny in the grain department. And while our genetic makeup and physiology haven't changed much since the time of our ancestors, our food chain has had a rapid makeover during the past half century. Modern food manufacturing, including bioengineering and specifically hybridization, has allowed us to grow structurally modified grains that contain gluten that's less tolerable than the gluten that's found in grains cultivated just a few decades ago.[28] Whether this has been intended to increase yield or appeal to people's palates, or both, is anyone's guess. But one thing we do know: Modern gluten-containing grains are more problematic than ever. There continues to be debate about the extent to which modern grains, and especially modern wheat, are "different" from their ancient counterparts due to genetic manipulation and agribusiness. But again, we cannot deny the rise in gluten sensitivity and a fourfold increase in celiac disease in the past sixty years.

If you've ever felt a rush of euphoric pleasure following the consumption of a bagel, scone, doughnut, or croissant, you're not imagining it—and you're not alone. We've known since the late 1970s that gluten breaks down in the stomach to become a mix of polypeptides that can cross the blood-brain barrier. Once they gain entry, some of them can then bind to the brain's morphine receptor to produce a sensorial high. This is the same receptor to which opiate drugs bind, creating their pleasurable, albeit addicting, effect. The original scientists who discovered this activity, Dr. Christine Zioudrou and her colleagues at the National Institutes of Health, named these brain-busting polypeptides exorphins, which is short for exogenous morphine-like compounds, as distinguished from endorphins, the body's naturally produced painkillers.[29] What's most interesting about these exorphins, and further confirms their impact on the brain, is that we know they can be stopped by opiate-blocking drugs like naloxone and naltrexone—

the same drugs used to reverse the action of opiate drugs such as heroine, morphine, and oxycodone. Dr. William Davis describes this phenomenon well in his book *Wheat Belly:* "So this is your brain on wheat: Digestion yields morphine-like compounds that bind to the brain's opiate receptors. It induces a form of reward, a mild euphoria. When the effect is blocked or no exorphin-yielding foods are consumed, some people experience a distinctly unpleasant withdrawal."[30] Not all exorphins, however, have pleasant side effects.

Researchers are currently looking into how the act of digesting foods like bread and pasta produces certain exorphins that not only sneak past the intestinal lining and reach the bloodstream where they can travel throughout the body, including past the blood-brain barrier, but can also incite inflammation.[31] Exorphins could be yet another explanation for why gluten is so problematic. Exorphins that are produced during gluten digestion have also been found in the spinal fluid of people with schizophrenia and autism.[32]

Given the blissful sensations that can accompany some exorphin-yielding foods, is it any wonder that food manufacturers try to pack as much gluten into their products as possible? And is it any surprise to find so many people addicted to gluten-filled foods today—fanning the flames of not just inflammation but the obesity epidemic? I think not. Most of us have known and accepted the fact that sugar and alcohol can have feel-good properties that entice us to come back for more. But gluten-containing foods? Your whole-wheat bread and instant oatmeal? The idea that gluten can change our biochemistry, right down to our brain's pleasure and addiction center, is remarkable. And scary. It means we need to rethink how we categorize these foods if they are indeed the mind-altering agents that science proves they are.

When I watch people devour gluten-laden carbohydrates, it's like watching them light up a cigarette. Gluten is our generation's tobacco. Gluten sensitivity is far more prevalent than we realize—potentially harming all of us to some degree without our knowing it—and gluten is hiding where you least suspect it. It's in our seasonings, condiments, and cocktails, and even in cosmetics, hand cream, and ice cream. It's disguised in soups, sweeteners, and soy products. It's tucked into our nutritional supplements and brand-name pharmaceuticals. The term "gluten-free" is becoming just as vague and diluted as "organic" and "all-natural" have become.

A True GB Story

I have suffered for thirty years with various illnesses, including seizures and shaking, along with extreme anxiety. I was diagnosed with chronic fatigue syndrome and bipolar disorder. This was incredibly difficult for me, as I was a professional violinist and was forced to give this up due to these symptoms and my inability to use my hands. Initially, I found out I had terrible blood sugar and realized I had a problem with carbohydrates. I then was diagnosed with gluten sensitivity, as was most of my family. I am now on a low-carb and very high-fat (but good fat) diet and continue to make other important changes, like eating more probiotics. I have fully recovered and today find myself in better health than when I was a child. I now play concerts again and am completely free from seizures, anxiety, and lack of confidence! Beyond this, I have suffered from weight problems all my life. For a time, I was quite obese. I lost 77 pounds and have now kept it off for years! I'm forty-seven, but I look (so I'm told) and feel like I'm in my thirties! ~ Priscilla D.

For the greater part of the past 2.6 million years, our ancestors' diets consisted of wild game, seasonal plants and vegetables, and the occasional berries. As we saw in the previous chapter, today most people's diets are centered on grains and carbs—many of which contain gluten. But even casting aside the gluten factor, I should point out that one of the main reasons why consuming so many grains and carbs can be so harmful is that they raise blood sugar in ways that other foods, such as meat, fish, poultry, and vegetables, do not.

High blood sugar, you'll recall, produces high insulin, which is released by the pancreas to move sugar into the body's cells. The higher the blood sugar, the more insulin must be pumped from the pancreas to deal with the sugar. And as the insulin increases, cells become less and less sensitive to the insulin signal. Basically, cells cannot hear insulin's message. What the pancreas does, as anyone would do if a person couldn't hear your message, is speak louder—that is, it increases its insulin output, creating a life-threatening feed-forward process. Higher levels of insulin cause the cells to become even less responsive to the insulin signal, and in order to deal with lowering the blood sugar, the pancreas works overtime, increasing its insulin output further, again to maintain a normal blood sugar. Even though the blood sugar is normal, the insulin level is climbing.

Since cells are resistant to the insulin signal, we use the term "insulin resistance" to characterize this condition. As the situation progresses, the pancreas finally maximizes its output of insulin, but it's still not enough. At that point, cells lose their ability to respond to the insulin signal and, ultimately, blood sugar begins to rise, resulting in type 2 diabetes. The system has essentially broken down and now requires an outside source (diabetes drugs) to keep the body's blood sugars balanced. Remember, though, that you don't have to be diabetic to suffer from chronic high blood sugar.

When I give lectures to members of the medical community, one of my favorite slides is a photo of four common foods: a slice of whole-wheat bread, a Snickers bar, a tablespoon of pure white sugar, and a banana. I then ask the audience to guess which one produces the greatest surge in blood sugar—or which has the highest glycemic index (GI), a numerical rating that reflects a measure of how quickly blood sugar levels rise after eating a particular type of food. The glycemic index encompasses a scale of 0 to 100, with higher values given to foods that cause the most rapid rise in blood sugar. The reference point is pure glucose, which has a GI of 100.

Nine times out of ten, people pick the wrong food. No, it's not the sugar (GI = 68), it's not the candy bar (GI = 55), and it's not the banana (GI = 54). It's the whole-wheat bread at a whopping GI of 71, putting it on par with white bread (so much for thinking whole wheat is better than white). We've known for more than thirty years that wheat increases blood sugar more than table sugar, but we still somehow think that's not possible. It seems counterintuitive. But it's a fact that few foods produce as much of a surge in blood glucose as those made with wheat.

It's important to note that the rise in gluten sensitivity is not only the outcome of hyperexposure to gluten in today's engineered foods. It's also the result of too much sugar and too many pro-inflammatory foods. We can also make a case for the impact of environmental toxins, which can change how our genes express themselves and whether or not autoimmune signals start to fire. These ingredients—gluten, sugar, pro-inflammatory foods, and environmental toxins—combine to create a perfect storm in the body, and especially the brain.

If any food that foments a biological storm—despite the presence of gluten—is hazardous to our health, then we must raise another critically important question in terms of brain health: *Are carbs—even "good carbs"—killing us?* After all, carbs are often the main source of these antagonizing ingredients. Any conversation about blood sugar balance, gluten sensitivity, and inflammation has to revolve around the impact that carbohydrates can have on the body and brain. In the next chapter, we'll look at how carbs in general raise risk factors for neurological disorders, often at the expense of our brain's real lover: fat. When we consume too many carbs, we eat less fat—the very ingredient our brain demands for health.

SIGNS OF GLUTEN SENSITIVITY

As mentioned, I no longer recommend getting tested for gluten sensitivity, be it a blood test or even small-intestine biopsy. Assume that gluten is toxic to you. Period. Below is a list of symptoms and illnesses associated with gluten sensitivity, but even if you don't have any of these conditions, your body—and brain—could be suffering without your knowing or feeling it.

ADHD	autism
alcoholism	autoimmune disorders
ALS	(diabetes, Hashimoto's
anxiety	thyroiditis, rheumatoid
ataxia (loss of balance)	arthritis, etc.)

bone pain/osteopenia/
osteoporosis
brain fog
cancer
chest pain
constantly getting sick
dairy intolerance
delayed growth
depression
digestive disturbances (gas,
bloating, diarrhea,
constipation, cramping,
etc.)
heart disease

hives/rashes
infertility
irritable bowel syndrome
malabsorption of food
migraines
miscarriages
nausea/vomiting
neurological disorders
(dementia, Alzheimer's
disease, schizophrenia,
etc.)
Parkinson's disease
seizures/epilepsy
sugar cravings

THE GLUTEN POLICE

The following grains and starches contain gluten:

barley
bulgur
graham flour
kamut
rye
semolina
spelt

triticale
wheat and products made
from wheat, such as
couscous, farina, and
matzo
wheat germ

The following grains and starches are gluten-free:

amaranth
arrowroot
buckwheat
corn
millet
potato

quinoa
rice
sorghum
soy
tapioca
teff

The following foods often contain gluten (unless certified gluten-free):

baked beans (canned)
beer
blue cheeses
bouillons/broths
    (commercially prepared)
breaded foods
cereals
chocolate milk (commercially
    prepared)
cold cuts
communion wafers
egg substitute
energy bars
flavored coffees and teas
French fries (often dusted
    with flour before freezing)
fried vegetables/tempura
fruit fillings and puddings
gravy
hot dogs
ice cream
imitation crabmeat,
    bacon, etc.
instant hot drinks
ketchup
malt/malt flavoring

malt vinegar
marinades
mayonnaise
meatballs/meatloaf
nondairy creamer
oat bran (unless certified
    gluten-free)
oats (unless certified
    gluten-free)
processed cheese
    (e.g., Velveeta)
roasted nuts
root beer
salad dressings
sausage
seitan
soups
soy sauce and teriyaki
    sauce
syrups
tabbouleh
trail mix
veggie burgers
vodka
wheatgrass
wine coolers

The following are miscellaneous sources of gluten (unless certified gluten-free):

cosmetics
lipsticks/lip balm
medications
non-self-adhesive stamps
    and envelopes

shampoos/conditioners
vitamins and supplements
    (check label)

The following ingredients are often code for gluten:

amino peptide complex

Avena sativa (a form of oats)

brown rice syrup

caramel color (frequently made from barley)

cyclodextrin

dextrin

fermented grain extract

Hordeum distichon

Hordeum vulgare

hydrolysate

hydrolyzed malt extract

hydrolyzed vegetable protein

maltodextrin

modified food starch

natural flavoring

phytosphingosine extract

Secale cereal

soy protein

Triticum aestivum

Triticum vulgare

vegetable protein (HVP)

yeast extract

CHAPTER 3

Attention, Carboholics and Fat Phobics

Surprising Truths About Your Brain's Real Enemies and Lovers

No diet will remove all the fat from your body because the brain is entirely fat. Without a brain, you might look good, but all you could do is run for public office.

— GEORGE BERNARD SHAW

SOME OF MY MOST REMARKABLE CASE STUDIES involve people transforming their lives and health through the total elimination of gluten from their diets and a new appreciation for fats instead of carbs. I've watched this single dietary shift lift depression, relieve chronic fatigue, reverse type 2 diabetes, extinguish obsessive-compulsive behavior, and cure many neurological challenges, from brain fog to bipolar disorder.

But apart from gluten, there's much more to the story of carbohydrates in general and their impact on brain health. Gluten isn't the only villain. To shift your body's biochemistry to one that burns fat (including the kind that "never goes away"), tames inflammation, and prevents illness and mental dysfunction, you need to factor in another big piece of the equation: carbs versus fats. In this chapter, I'll take you on a tour of why an extremely low-carb and high-fat diet is what your body fundamentally craves and needs. I'll also explain why consuming excess carbohydrates—even those that don't contain gluten—can be just as harmful as eating a gluten-laden diet.

Ironically, ever since we "scientized" nutrition, the state of our health has declined. Decisions about what to eat and drink have gone from habits of culture and heritage to calculated choices based on shortsighted nutritional theories, with little consideration of how human beings reached modernity in the first place. And we can't forget about all the commercial interest out there. Do you think the makers of high-carbohydrate breakfast cereals (read: the entire aisle in your grocery store devoted to boxed cereals) truly have your health in mind? In my opinion, we should call it out for what it actually is: corporate support for the (faulty) scientific publications in the late 1960s that resulted in more deaths than World Wars I and II combined as it shifted us away from healthful fat to a higher-carb diet.

> One of the most profitable businesses for food manufacturers is cereal. It's one of the only industries that can turn an inexpensive ingredient (processed grains) into a pricey commodity. The R&D department for General Mills, called, ironically, the Bell Institute of Health and Nutrition, is located in Minneapolis and has a division devoted just to "cereal technology." It is home to hundreds of scientists whose sole purpose is to design new and tasty cereals that can command a high price and last for a long time on the shelves. Michael Pollan describes his visit to the facility in his book *The Omnivore's Dilemma*, in which he writes about the wild secrecy and profitability surrounding cereal. Even he could not get food scientists to talk about their projects. In 2017, nearly 290 million Americans consumed breakfast cereals, each downing about 10 pounds of it in total.[1]

Consider what you've experienced in just the past few decades. You've witnessed an untold number of ideas on what you should consume to fuel your metabolism, only to learn the opposite could be true. Take eggs, for instance. Eggs were thought to be good for you; then they were deemed to be bad for you because of their saturated fat content; and then you were exceedingly confused by messages implying that "More evidence is needed to determine the health effect of eggs." It's unfair, I know. With all this white noise, it's no wonder people feel endlessly frustrated. Even the updated federal dietary guidelines published in 2015 failed to highlight new science on many fronts, though I was glad to see that they had removed recommendations to limit intake of cholesterol-rich foods and added a reference to coffee as potentially being part of a healthy diet.[2]

This chapter should make you rejoice. I'm going to rescue you from a lifetime of trying to avoid eating fat and cholesterol and prove how these delicious ingredients preserve the highest functioning of your brain. We've developed a taste for fat for good reason: It's our brain's secret love. But in the last several decades it's been demonized as an unhealthy nutritional source, and we've regrettably become a fat-phobic, carb-addicted society— and it doesn't help that we automatically lower our intake of healthy fat when we eat lots of carbs. Advertisements, weight-loss companies, grocery stores, and popular books are touting the idea that we should be on a low-fat or as close to a no-fat, low-cholesterol diet as humanly possible. True, there are certain types of fat that are associated with health issues, and no one can deny the health threat linked squarely with commercially modified fats and oils. There is compelling scientific support that trans fats are toxic and are clearly linked to any number of chronic diseases. But the missing message is simple: Our bodies thrive when given "good fats," and cholesterol is one of these. And we don't do so well with copious amounts of carbohydrates, even if those carbs are gluten-free, whole grain, and high in fiber.

Interestingly, the human dietary requirement for carbohydrates is virtually zero; we can survive on a minimal amount of carbohydrates, which can be furnished by the liver as needed. But we can't go long without fat. Unfortunately, most of us equate the idea of eating fat to *being* fat, when in reality, obesity—and its metabolic consequences—has almost nothing to do with dietary fat consumption and everything to do with our addiction to carbs. The same is true about cholesterol: Eating high-cholesterol foods has no impact on our actual cholesterol levels, and the alleged correlation between higher cholesterol and higher cardiac risk is an absolute fallacy.

NEW EVIDENCE CONFIRMS CURSE OF HIGH BLOOD SUGAR AND HIGH BLOOD PRESSURE — DESPITE WEIGHT

When I wrote this book initially, early studies showed a relationship between high blood sugar and risk for cognitive decline, as already noted. Since then, other studies have come to the same conclusion, while further showing a link between long-term high blood pressure (hypertension) and brain decline. That means that the risk for cognitive decline is no longer tied to just obesity and metabolic disorders like diabetes. The mere consumption of carbs that raise blood sugar is enough to up one's risk. You can be of "healthy" weight, with no signs of metabolic dysfunction whatsoever, yet suffer from silent high blood sugar surges that put you in the danger zone. This message needs to ring loud and clear.

Earlier I referenced studies that found that people with high blood sugar had a faster rate of cognitive decline than those with normal blood sugar — whether or not their blood-sugar level technically made them diabetic. There are several reasons why high blood sugar can lead to dementia. For starters, the condition can weaken the blood vessels, increasing the likelihood for mini-strokes in the brain, which then trigger various forms of dementia. Second, a high intake of simple sugars can make cells, including those in the brain, insulin resistant. In turn, brain cells die.

High blood sugar can be stealthy in people who are of normal weight, but for those who are obese, it's practically a given. And that excess fat can be particularly harmful. It is far from silent, as it releases hormones and cytokines, which are inflammatory proteins that can also contribute to cognitive deterioration as inflammation levels rise and create a slow-burning fire in the body and brain. Rebecca Gottesman, professor of neurology at Johns Hopkins, has found in her research that obesity doubled a person's risk of having elevated amyloid proteins in the brain later in life. Those amyloid plaques are the hallmarks of Alzheimer's disease. In a 2014 study that started in the 1980s following thousands of Americans, some with and some without high blood pressure, Gottesman unveiled that having hypertension at midlife is a major risk factor for cognitive decline—independent of other risk factors such as obesity.[3] Gottesman published a follow-up study in 2017 that was even more conclusive: Middle-aged Americans who have vascular health risk factors, including diabetes, high blood pressure, and smoking, have a greater chance of suffering from dementia later in life.[4]

FAT GENES AND PHAT SCIENCE

Of all the lessons in this book, the one I most hope you take seriously is the following: Respect your genome. Fat—not carbohydrate—is the preferred fuel of human metabolism and has been for all of human evolution. We have consumed a high-fat diet for the past two million years, and it is only since the advent of agriculture about ten thousand years ago that carbohydrates have become abundant in our food supply. We still have a hunter-gatherer genome; it's thrifty in the sense that it's programmed to make us fat during times of abundance. The thrifty gene hypothesis was first described by geneticist James Neel in 1962 to help explain why type 2 diabetes has such a strong genetic basis and results in such negative effects favored by natural selection. According to the theory, the genes that predispose someone to diabetes— "thrifty genes"—were historically advantageous. They helped one fatten up quickly when food was available, since long stretches of food scarcity were inevitable. But once modern society changed our access to food, the thrifty genes were no longer needed but were still active—essentially preparing us for a famine that never comes. It is believed that our thrifty genes are responsible for the obesity epidemic, too, which is closely tied to diabetes.

Unfortunately, it takes forty thousand to seventy thousand years for any significant changes to take place in the genome that might allow us to adapt to such a drastic change in our diet and for our thrifty genes to even think about ignoring the instructions that say "store fat." While some of us like to believe we're plagued with genes that promote fat growth and retention, thus making weight loss and maintenance hard, the truth is we all carry the "fat gene." It's part of our human constitution and, for the majority of our existence on the planet, has kept us alive.

Our forebears could not have had any meaningful exposure to carbohydrates, except perhaps in the late summer when fruit ripened. Interestingly, this type of carbohydrate would have tended to increase fat creation and deposition so we could get through the winter when food and calories were less available. Now, however, we signal our bodies to store fat 365 days a year. And through science we are learning about the consequences.

The Framingham Heart Study, referenced in the first chapter and which identified a linear association between total cholesterol and cognitive performance, is just the tip of the iceberg. In the fall of 2012, a report in the *Journal of Alzheimer's Disease* published research from the Mayo Clinic revealing that older people who fill their plates with carbohydrates have nearly *four times* the risk of developing mild cognitive impairment (MCI), generally considered a precursor to Alzheimer's disease. Signs of MCI include problems with memory, language, thinking, and judgment. This particular study found that those whose diets were highest in healthy fats were 42 percent less likely to experience cognitive impairment; people who had the highest intake of protein from healthy sources like chicken, meat, and fish enjoyed a reduced risk of 21 percent.[5]

Earlier studies examining patterns in diet and risk for dementia revealed similar findings. One of the first studies to really compare the difference in fat content between an Alzheimer's brain and a healthy brain was published in 1998.[6] In this post-mortem study, researchers in the Netherlands found that the Alzheimer's patients had significantly reduced amounts of fats, notably cholesterol and free fatty acids, in their cerebrospinal fluid than did the controls. This was true regardless of whether the Alzheimer's patients had the defective gene—known as APoE ε4—that predisposes people to the disease.

In 2007, the journal *Neurology* published a study that looked at more than eight thousand participants who were sixty-five years or older and had totally normal brain function. The study followed them for up to four years, during which time some 280 people developed a form of dementia (most of the 280 were diagnosed with Alzheimer's).[7] The researchers aimed to identify patterns in their dietary habits, homing in on their consumption of fish, which contains lots of brain- and heart-healthy omega-3 fats. For people who never consumed fish, the risk of dementia and Alzheimer's disease during the four-year follow-up period was increased by 37 percent. In those individuals who consumed fish on a daily basis, risk for these diseases was reduced by 44 percent. Regular users of butter had no significant change in their risk for dementia or Alzheimer's, but people who regularly consumed omega-3-rich oils, such as olive, flaxseed, and walnut oils, were 60 percent less likely to develop dementia than those who did not regularly consume such oils. The researchers also found that people who regularly ate omega-6-rich oils — typical in the American diet — but not omega-3-rich oils or fish were twice as likely to develop dementia as people who didn't eat omega-6-rich oils. (See the box for a more in-depth explanation of these fats.) In 2016, an even larger study confirmed all these findings upon reviewing twenty-one cohort studies involving more than 181,000 people.[8] It was published in the *American Journal of Clinical Nutrition*, recommending "fishery products" for "lower risk of cognitive impairment."

Interestingly, many of these reports indicate that consumption of omega-3 oils can counterbalance the detrimental effect of omega-6 oils, and the researchers caution against eating omega-6 oils in the absence of omega-3s. I find results like these to be quite stunning, and informative.

THE OH-SO-MANY OMEGAS: WHICH ONES ARE GOOD?

We hear so much these days about omega-3 and omega-6 fats. Overall, omega-6 fats fall into the "bad fat" category; they are somewhat pro-inflammatory, and there is evidence that higher consumption of these fats is related to brain disorders. Unfortunately, the American diet is extremely high in omega-6 fats, which are found in many vegetable oils, including safflower oil, corn oil, canola oil, sunflower oil, and soybean oil; vegetable oil represents the number one source of fat in the American diet. According to anthropological research, our hunter-gatherer ancestors consumed omega-6 and omega-3 fats in a ratio of roughly 1:1.[9] Today we consume ten to twenty-five times more omega-6 fats than evolutionary norms, and we've dramatically reduced our intake of healthy, brain-boosting omega-3 fats (some experts believe our increased consumption of brain-healthy omega-3 fatty acids was responsible for the threefold increase in the size of the human brain). The following chart lists the omega-6 and omega-3 content of various oils.

Oil	Omega-6 Content	Omega-3 Content
canola	20%	9%
corn	61%	0%
cottonseed	50%	0%
flaxseed	14%	57%
peanut	32%	0%
safflower	75%	0%
sesame	42%	0%
soybean	51%	7%
sunflower	65%	0%
walnut	52%	10%

Note: Olive oil is not a vegetable oil (it comes from the olive, a fruit). It contains both omega-3s and omega-6s, but it owes its health benefits mostly to its monounsaturated fatty acids, mostly oleic acid. Coconut oil does not contain any omegas; it has what's called medium-chain fatty acids — more on this later.

Seafood is a wonderful source of omega-3 fatty acids, and even wild meat like beef, lamb, venison, and buffalo contain this fab fat. But a caveat to consider: If animals are fed grains (usually corn and soybeans), then they will not have adequate omega-3 in their diets and their meat will be deficient in these vital nutrients. Hence the call for consuming grass-fed beef and wild fish.

Beyond dementia, other neurological issues have been associated with low fat intake and cholesterol levels in particular. In a report published by the National Institutes of Health, researchers compared memory function in elderly individuals to cholesterol levels. They found that the people who did not suffer from dementia had much better memory function if they had higher levels of cholesterol. The conclusion of the report crisply stated: "High cholesterol is associated with better memory function." In the discussion that followed, the researchers asserted: "It is possible that individuals who survived beyond age eighty-five, especially those with high cholesterol, may be more robust."[10]

Parkinson's disease is also strongly related to lower levels of cholesterol. Researchers in the Netherlands writing in the *American Journal of Epidemiology* published a report in 2006 demonstrating that "higher serum levels of total cholesterol were associated with a significantly decreased risk of Parkinson's disease with evidence of a dose effect relation."[11] In fact, other research in 2008 published in the journal *Movement Disorders* showed that people with the lowest LDL cholesterol (the so-called bad cholesterol) were at increased risk for Parkinson's disease — by approximately 350 percent![12]

To understand how this could possibly be true, it helps to recall what I hinted at in the first chapter about LDL being a carrier protein that's not necessarily bad. The fundamental role of LDL in the brain is to capture life-giving cholesterol and transport it to the neuron, where it performs critically important functions. As we have now seen, when cholesterol levels are low, the brain simply doesn't work well, and individuals are at a significantly increased risk for neurological problems as a consequence. But a caveat: Once free radicals damage the LDL molecule, it's rendered much less capable of delivering cholesterol to the brain. In addition to oxidation destroying the LDL's function, sugar can also render it dysfunctional by binding to it and accelerating oxidation. And when that happens, LDL is no longer able to enter the astrocyte, a cell charged with nourishing neurons. In the last ten years, new research has shown that oxidized LDL is a key factor in the development of atherosclerosis. Hence, we should do everything we can to reduce the risk of LDL oxidation — not necessarily levels of LDL itself. A principal player in that risk of oxidation is higher levels of glucose; LDL is far more likely to become oxidized in the presence of sugar molecules that will bind to it and change its shape. Glycosylated proteins, which are the products of these reactions between proteins and sugar molecules, are associated with a fiftyfold increase in free radical formation as compared to non-glycosylated proteins. LDL is not the enemy. The problems occur when a higher-carbohydrate diet yields oxidized LDL and an increased risk of atherosclerosis. In addition, if and when LDL becomes a glycosylated molecule, it cannot present cholesterol to brain cells, and brain function suffers.

Somehow we have been led to believe that dietary fat will raise our cholesterol, which will in turn increase our risk for heart attacks and strokes. This notion continues to prevail despite research from more than two decades ago that proved otherwise. In 1994, the *Journal of the American Medical Association* published a trial that compared older adults with high cholesterol (levels above 240 mg/dL) to those with normal levels (below 200 mg/dL).[13] Over the course of four years, researchers at Yale University measured total cholesterol and high-density lipoprotein (HDL) in almost one thousand participants; they also tracked hospitalizations for heart attack and unstable angina and the rates of death from heart disease and from any other cause. No differences were found between the two groups. People with low total cholesterol had as many heart attacks and died just as frequently as those with high total cholesterol. And reviews of multiple large studies have routinely failed to find correlation between cholesterol levels and heart disease.[14] Mounting research like this prompted the late Dr. George Mann, once a researcher with the Framingham Heart Study, who died in 2013 at the age of ninety-five, to go on record back in the '70s stating:

> The diet-heart hypothesis that suggests that a high intake of fat or cholesterol causes heart disease has been repeatedly shown to be wrong, and yet, for complicated reasons of pride, profit, and prejudice, the hypothesis continues to be exploited by scientists, fund-raising enterprise, food companies, and even governmental agencies. The public is being deceived by the greatest health scam of the century.[15]

In addition to publishing over two hundred articles in medical journals, Dr. Mann expressed his views in several books, including his 1993 *Coronary Heart Disease: The Dietary Sense and Nonsense.*[16] Nothing could be further from the truth than the myth that if we lower our cholesterol levels, we might have a greater chance of living longer and healthier lives. Four years after Dr. Mann's book came out, a 1997 report appeared in the prestigious medical journal the *Lancet* that described researchers from the Netherlands who studied 724 elderly individuals whose average age was eighty-nine years and followed them for ten years.[17] What they found was truly extraordinary. During the study, 642 participants died. Each thirty-nine-point increase in total cholesterol corresponded to a 15 percent decrease in mortality risk. In the study, there was absolutely no difference in the risk of dying from coronary artery disease between the high- versus low-cholesterol groups, which is incredible when you consider the number of elderly folks who are taking powerful cholesterol-lowering drugs. Other common causes of death in the elderly were found to be dramatically associated with lower cholesterol. The authors reported: "Mortality from cancer and infection was significantly lower among the participants in the highest total cholesterol category than in the other categories, which largely explains the lower all-cause mortality in this category." In other words, people with the highest total cholesterol were less likely to die from cancer and infections — common fatal illnesses in older folks — than those with the lowest cholesterol levels. In fact, when you compare the lowest- and highest-cholesterol groups, the risk of dying during the study was reduced by a breathtaking 48 percent in those who had the highest cholesterol. High cholesterol can extend longevity.

Perhaps one of the most extraordinary studies performed on the positive impact of cholesterol on the entire neurological system is already a decade old. A 2008 report published in the journal *Neurology* describes high cholesterol as a protective factor in ALS.[18] There is no meaningful treatment for ALS, a devastating disease that I dealt with in my medical practice on a daily basis. ALS is a chronic degenerative disorder of the body's motor neurons that leads to death within two to five years of onset. (The FDA has approved one medication, Rilutek, that may extend life by approximately three months, at best. In 2017, the FDA approved Radicava to reduce the decline in daily functioning associated with the disease. Rilutek is very expensive and toxic to the liver; most patients refuse to take it. Radicava comes with side effects, most notably severe allergic reactions to its sulfite content.) In the 2008 study from French investigators, however, it was shown that those individuals with considerably higher cholesterol ratios lived, on average, one year longer than patients with lower levels, when compared with normal controls. As the authors stated: "Hyperlipidemia (high levels of cholesterol) is a significant prognostic factor for survival of patients with amyotrophic lateral sclerosis. This finding highlights the importance of nutritional intervention strategies on disease progression and claims our attention when treating these patients with lipid lowering drugs."

As the infomercials say, "But wait, there's more!" We can't limit our talk about fat to just brain health. Volumes have been written in the scientific literature about fat and heart health as well—but not in the context I know you're thinking about. In 2010, the *American Journal of Clinical Nutrition* published an astonishing study that revealed the truth behind urban legends about fat, especially the saturated kind, and heart disease.[19] The study was a retrospective evaluation of twenty-one previous medical reports involving more than 340,000 subjects followed from periods of five to twenty-three years. It concluded that "intake of saturated fat was not associated with an increased risk of coronary heart disease, stroke, or cardiovascular disease." In comparing the lowest to the highest consumption of saturated fat, the actual risk for coronary heart disease was 19 percent lower in the group consuming the highest amount of saturated fat. The authors also stated: "Our results suggested a publication bias, such that studies with significant associations tended to be received more favorably for publication." What the authors are implying is that when other studies presented conclusions that were more familiar to the mainstream (i.e., fat causes heart disease), not to mention more attractive to Big Pharma, they were more likely to get published. The truth is we thrive on saturated fats. In the words of Michael Gurr, PhD, author of *Lipid Biochemistry: An Introduction*, "Whatever causes coronary heart disease, it is not primarily a high intake of saturated fatty acids."[20]

In a subsequent report from the *American Journal of Clinical Nutrition*, a panel of leading researchers in the field of nutrition from around the globe clearly stated: "At present there is no clear relation of saturated fatty acid intake to these outcomes [of obesity, cardiovascular disease, incidence of cancer, and osteoporosis]." The researchers went on to say that research should be directed at "biological interactions between insulin resistance, reflected by obesity and physical inactivity, and carbohydrate quality and quantity."[21]

Before we look at more studies showing the benefits of fat, especially cholesterol-rich foods, let's consider how we got to the point where we reject the very foods that can feed our healthy brains and keep us supercharged for a long, vibrant life. This will require a short detour to the relationship between dietary fat and heart health, but the story ties directly into brain health.

A LITTLE HISTORY

If you're like most Americans, at some time in your life you've eaten more margarine than butter, felt like you were splurging when you polished off a plate of red meat, eggs, and cheese, and gravitated toward products that said "low-fat," "nonfat," or "cholesterol-free." I don't blame you for making these choices. We are all members of the same society that relies on "experts" to tell us what's good and, conversely, bad for us. We've lived through historic events in our understanding of human health over the past several generations, as well as momentous discoveries about what makes us sick and prone to disease. In fact, the turn of the twentieth century marked the very beginning of a huge shift in American life due to advances in technology and medicine. Within the span of a few decades, we had widespread access to antibiotics, vaccines, and public health services. Common childhood illnesses that once gravely lowered the average life span were vanishing, or at least coming under better control. More people moved into cities and left their agrarian lifestyles behind. We became more educated, better informed, and ever more sophisticated. But in a lot of ways, we also became more easily tantalized and deceived by information that wasn't fully deciphered and proven yet. You might not remember the days when doctors endorsed smoking cigarettes, for instance, but this same kind of ignorance has happened on a much subtler scale in the world of dieting. And sadly, much of it continues today.

In 1900, the typical city dweller consumed about 2,900 calories per day, with 40 percent of these calories coming from equal parts saturated and unsaturated fat. (Rural families living and working on farms probably ate more calories.) Theirs was a diet filled with butter, eggs, meats, grains, and seasonable fruits and vegetables. Few Americans were overweight, and the three most common causes of death were pneumonia, tuberculosis, and diarrhea and enteritis.

It was also around the turn of the twentieth century that the U.S. Department of Agriculture (USDA) began to keep track of food trends, noting a change in the consumption of the kind of fats Americans were eating. People were beginning to use vegetable oils instead of butter, which prompted food manufacturers to create hardened oils through the hydrogenated process so they resembled butter. By 1950 we had gone from eating about eighteen pounds of butter and a little under three pounds of vegetable oil each year to just over ten pounds of butter and more than ten pounds of vegetable oil. Margarine was rapidly gaining ground in our diets, too; at the turn of the century people consumed only two pounds per person per year, but by midcentury, people were eating around eight pounds.

Although the so-called lipid hypothesis had been around since the mid-nineteenth century, it wasn't until the mid-twentieth century that scientists tried to correlate a fatty diet with fatty arteries, as deaths from coronary artery disease (CAD) began to climb. According to the hypothesis, saturated animal fat raises blood cholesterol levels and leads to the deposition of cholesterol and other fats as plaques in the arteries. To bolster this theory, a University of Minnesota public health researcher named Ancel Keys showed a nearly direct correlation between calories from fat in the diet and deaths from heart disease among populations across seven countries. (He ignored countries that didn't fit this pattern, including many where people eat a lot of fat but don't get heart disease and others where the diets are low in fat yet their populations have a high incidence of fatal heart attacks.) The Japanese, whose diets have only 10 percent of calories coming from fat, showed the lowest CAD mortality—less than 1 in 1,000. The United States, on the other hand, had the highest CAD mortality—7 in 1,000—with 40 percent of its calories coming from fat.[22] On the surface, it would seem that these patterns point directly to the idea that fat is bad, and that fat causes heart disease. Little did scientists know then that these numbers weren't telling the whole story.

This erroneous thinking persisted, however, for the next several decades as researchers looked for more proof, which included the Framingham Heart Study, which found that people with higher cholesterol were more likely to be diagnosed with CAD and die from it. In 1956, the American Heart Association began pushing the "prudent diet," which called for replacing butter, lard, eggs, and beef with margarine, corn oil, chicken, and cold cereal. By the 1970s, the lipid hypothesis had become well established. At the heart of this hypothesis was the unyielding claim that cholesterol caused coronary artery disease.

This naturally motivated the government to do something, which led to the release of "Dietary Goals for the United States" by the Senate's Select Committee on Nutrition and Human Needs in 1977. As you can imagine, the goals aimed to lower fat intake and avoid foods high in cholesterol. "Artery-clogging" saturated fats were deemed especially bad. So down went meat, milk, eggs, butter, cheese, and tropical oils such as coconut and palm oil. This perspective also paved the way for the billion-dollar drug industry's focus on lipid-lowering medications. At the same time, health authorities began to advise people to replace these now-bad fats with carbohydrates and processed polyunsaturated vegetable oils, including soybean, corn, cottonseed, canola, peanut, safflower, and sunflower oils. Fast-food restaurants followed suit in the mid-1980s, switching from beef fat and palm oil to partially hydrogenated (trans fat) vegetable oil to fry their foods. Even though the USDA has since converted its food guide from a pyramid to a plate, it still communicates the idea that "fat is bad" and "carbs are good." In fact, the new "My Plate" doesn't feature fats at all, making it very confusing for consumers to know how fats fit into a healthy diet—and which kind.[23]

Dr. Donald W. Miller, retired cardiac surgeon and professor emeritus of surgery at the University of Washington, stated it perfectly in his 2010 essay entitled "Health Benefits of a Low-Carbohydrate, High-Saturated-Fat Diet": "The sixty-year reign of the low-fat, high-carbohydrate diet will end. This will happen when the health-destroying effects of excess carbohydrates in the diet become more widely recognized and the health benefits of saturated fats are better appreciated."[24] The lipid hypothesis has dominated cardiovascular circles for decades despite the fact that the number of contradictory studies exceeds those that are supportive. There hasn't been a published study in the last thirty years that has unequivocally demonstrated that lowering serum cholesterol by eating a low-fat, low-cholesterol diet prevents or reduces heart attack or death rates. And as Dr. Miller points out, population studies from around the world do not support the lipid hypothesis. We can even go as far back as 1968 to find studies that flatly dispel the notion of a low-fat diet as ideal. That year, the International Atherosclerosis Project examined twenty-two thousand corpses from fourteen nations and found that it didn't matter whether people ate large amounts of fatty animal products or followed a mostly vegetarian diet—the prevalence of arterial plaque was the same in all parts of the world, both in those with high rates of heart disease and in populations with little to no heart disease.[25] Which means that the thickening of the arterial wall could just be an unavoidable process of aging that doesn't necessarily correlate with clinical heart disease.

If eating saturated fat doesn't cause heart disease, then what does? Now let's look at these circumstances from the perspective of the brain, and then we'll circle back to matters of the heart. You'll soon be able to understand the root cause of both obesity and brain disease.

CARBS, DIABETES, AND BRAIN DISEASE

As I've already detailed, one of the ways in which grains and carbs set fire to the brain is through surges in blood sugar; this has direct negative effects on the brain that in turn start the inflammatory cascade. The science really comes down to your body's neurotransmitters. Neurotransmitters are your main mood and brain regulators, and when your blood sugar increases, there's an immediate depletion of the neurotransmitters serotonin, epinephrine, norepinephrine, GABA, and dopamine. At the same time, B-complex vitamins, which are needed to make those neurotransmitters (and a few hundred other things), get used up. Magnesium levels also diminish, and this handicaps both your nervous system and liver. In addition, high blood sugar triggers a reaction called "glycation," which we'll explore in detail in the next chapter. In simplest terms, glycation is the biological process whereby glucose, proteins, and certain fats become tangled together, causing tissues and cells to become stiff and inflexible, including those in the brain. More specifically, sugar molecules and brain proteins combine to create deadly new structures that contribute more than any other factor to the degeneration of the brain and its functioning. The brain is tremendously vulnerable to the glycating ravages of glucose, and this is made worse when powerful antigens like gluten accelerate the damage. In neurological terms, glycation can contribute to the shrinking of critical brain tissue.

Aside from sweetened beverages, grain-based foods are responsible for the bulk of carbohydrate calories in the American diet. Whether from pasta, cookies, cakes, bagels, or the seemingly healthful whole-grain bread, the carbohydrate load induced by our food choices ultimately doesn't serve us well when trying to enhance brain health and function. When you add to this list the potpourri of other high-carbohydrate foods like potatoes, corn, fruit, and rice, it's no wonder that Americans are now rightly called "carboholics." It's also not surprising that we have an epidemic of metabolic dysfunction and diabetes in our culture.

The data confirming the relationship between high carbohydrate consumption and diabetes is clear and profound. In 1992, the U.S. government endorsed a high-carb, low-fat diet. The American Heart Association and the American Diabetes Association followed suit in 1994, with the American Diabetes Association recommending that Americans consume 60 to 70 percent of their calories from carbohydrates. Between 1994 and 2015, the number of diabetes cases *tripled*.[26] Take a look in the following figure at the rapid upward slope from 1958 through 2015, during which the number of Americans diagnosed with diabetes went from a scant 1.58 million people to a colossal 23.35 million individuals.

This is significant since, as you already know, becoming diabetic doubles your risk of Alzheimer's disease. Even being prediabetic, when blood sugar issues are just beginning, is associated with a decline in brain function and shrinkage of the brain's memory center; it is also an independent risk factor for full-blown Alzheimer's disease.

Number and Percentage of U.S. Population with Diagnosed Diabetes, 1958–2015

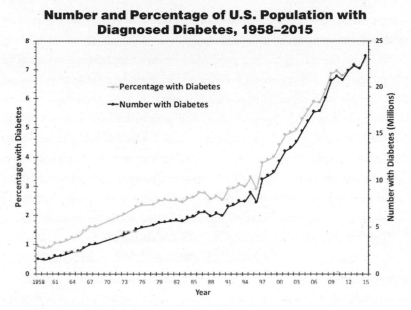

It's hard to believe that we couldn't have known about this connection between diabetes and dementia sooner, but it's taken us a long time to connect the dots and conduct the kind of longitudinal studies that such a conclusion requires. It's also taken us time to figure out the obvious question that stems from this link: How does diabetes contribute to dementia? I've already mentioned a few of the connections, but let me remind you. First, if you're insulin resistant, not only will you starve brain cells and spur their death, but your body may not be able to break down the amyloid protein that forms those infamous brain plaques associated with brain disease. Second, high blood sugar provokes menacing biological reactions that injure the body, by producing certain oxygen-containing molecules that damage cells and causing inflammation that can result in hardening and narrowing of the arteries in the brain (not to mention elsewhere in the body). This condition, known as atherosclerosis, can lead to vascular dementia, which occurs when blockages and strokes kill brain tissue. We tend to think about atherosclerosis in terms of the heart, but the brain can be equally affected by changes in its arteries' walls. Back in 2004, Australian researchers boldly stated in a review paper, "There is now a consensus that atherosclerosis represents a state of heightened oxidative stress characterized by lipid and protein oxidation in the vascular wall."[27] They also pointed out that such oxidation is a response to inflammation.

A most disturbing finding was made by Japanese researchers in 2011 when they looked at one thousand men and women over age sixty and found that "people with diabetes were twice as likely as the other study participants to develop Alzheimer's disease within fifteen years. They were also 1.75 times more likely to develop dementia of any kind."[28] This link remained true even after they took into account several factors associated with both diabetes and dementia risk, such as age, sex, blood pressure, and body mass index. As I've been highlighting throughout this book so far, newer research is now documenting how controlling blood sugar and reducing risk factors for type 2 diabetes can significantly reduce dementia risk.

I've had the pleasure of interviewing Melissa Schilling, professor of management at New York University (you can view the interview in its entirety at DrPerlmutter.com). Though she is not a medical researcher, her work and insights have gained her respect among established neurologists (me included); her interest in connecting diabetes to Alzheimer's has turned up an intriguing interpretation of the data. In 2016, she performed her own review of studies to reconcile a paradox: Elevated insulin, or hyperinsulinemia, significantly increases one's risk of Alzheimer's, but people with type 1 diabetes (who don't make insulin at all) are also thought to have a higher risk of the brain disease.[29] How could both be true? What Schilling hypothesizes is probably true and has been supported by known authorities on the subject. She theorizes that the culprit is the insulin-degrading enzyme, a product of insulin that breaks down both insulin and amyloid proteins in the brain. People who don't have enough insulin, such as those whose bodies' ability to produce insulin has been tapped out by diabetes, are not going to make enough of this enzyme to break up those brain clumps. Meanwhile, in people who use insulin to treat their diabetes and end up with a surplus of insulin, most of this enzyme gets used up breaking down that insulin, leaving not enough enzyme to address the amyloid brain clumps. According to Schilling, this can happen even in people who have prediabetes and probably don't know it yet.

I'd like to pause here for a moment to address a matter that frustrates me from a public service standpoint. We all know that diabetes management is important. But daily we are bombarded by commercials that push drugs to regulate blood sugar better and push down that A1C number, which you'll recall is a running average of blood sugar levels for the previous ninety days. This implies that getting the magic number of A1C below a specific level is the only important goal of diabetes management. *Absolutely nothing* could be further from the truth. Yes, we generally see overweight and obesity in association with type 2 diabetes, and the coexistence of these two issues is incredibly devastating for the brain. It is not enough to just manage blood sugar through drugs and stay overweight or obese. You can lower your A1C, balance your blood sugar, and eradicate diabetes *entirely through dietary change* — and the bonus is that you'll achieve an optimal weight, too. Dr. Sarah Hallberg, medical director at Virta Health and medical director and founder of the Indiana University–Arnett Health Medical Weight Loss Program, echoes this sentiment. When I interviewed her for my online program, *The Empowering Neurologist,* she vigorously underscored the power of dietary change in reversing diabetes and getting off management medications. In her words, "People are told they are 'stuck' with type 2 diabetes and they have to manage it with drugs in the hopes of slowing down the disease and avoiding its awful side effects (like limb amputations, blindness). I flatly reject that way of thinking. We have to start talking about disease reversal by managing lifestyle factors." I could not agree more.

The fact that we can lose our minds because we have "diabesity" should be enough of a motivator to change how we eat. But sometimes it takes a few visuals to see just how damaging the combination of excess weight and diabetes can be on a brain. A 2017 study that included researchers from South Korea, the University of Utah, and the Department of Internal Medicine at Brigham and Women's Hospital in Boston shows brain changes in both people who are overweight or obese with early stage type 2 diabetes and those of normal weight with early stage type 2 diabetes.[30] The changes were noted across a variety of parameters, such as brain thickness, cognitive performance, and C-reactive protein levels. The researchers measured much more severe and progressive abnormalities in brain structure and cognition in those who were overweight or obese with type 2 diabetes versus their normal-weight counterparts, as shown in the following graphics.

Type 2 Diabetics

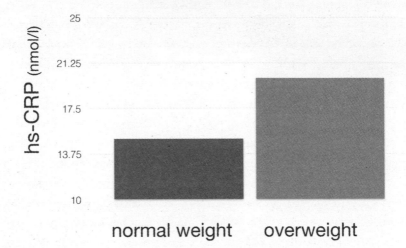

Type 2 Diabetics

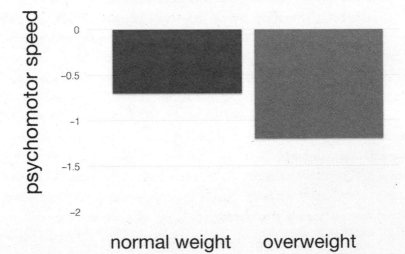

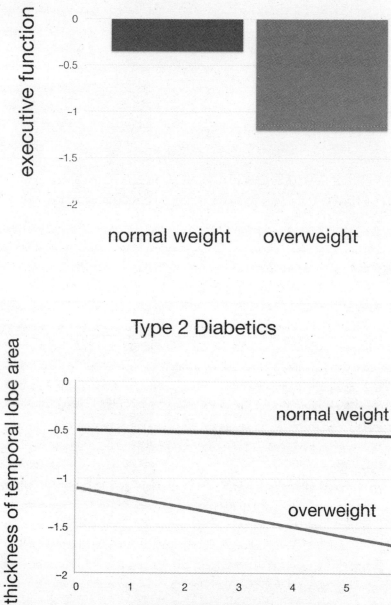

As a reminder, high-sensitivity C-reactive protein (hs-CRP) is a marker of inflammation, which we already know is a risk factor for brain damage and cognitive decline. "Executive function" is an umbrella term used to refer to the mental skills one has to have in order to perform basic tasks, manage oneself, and achieve certain goals. It's how we use information and solve problems. "Psychomotor speed" refers to how fast one can process information and act on it; it's one's fine motor skills that entail both thinking and movement. And your temporal lobes, which are just beneath your temples, are key to high-level auditory processing; they are what allow you to understand speech.

GET THE FACTS ON FAT: YOUR BRAIN'S BEST FRIEND

Manufacturers of processed foods continue to put the term "low-fat" on their labels to enhance sales, because so many people still buy into the notion that a low-fat diet is a good idea. But that is absolutely in direct contradiction with current science. A few pages ago I outlined studies done more than twenty years ago that documented higher mortality rates with carb consumption and, conversely, lower mortality rates with higher fat consumption (and lower risk for cardiovascular disease). I don't know why we are still talking about the relationship between fat and cholesterol and risk for a cardiovascular event. In a 2017 study in, once again, the highly regarded *Lancet* journal, researchers from multiple esteemed institutions around the world studied an incredibly large number of individuals aged thirty-five to seventy years (135,335), from eighteen countries, over an average of 7.4 years.[31] They carried out very specific assessments of the foods that these individuals ate and evaluated their food choices in terms of macronutrient composition (carbohydrates, protein, and fat), and specifically broke the fat consumption down to evaluate saturated fat, monounsaturated fat, and polyunsaturated fats. Further, they compared the diets to the risk of various endpoints including death, major cardiovascular event, stroke, and heart failure.

What the researchers discovered in this extensive study was quite compelling. They noted that higher carbohydrate consumption, comparing the highest consumers of carbohydrate with the lowest consumers of carbohydrate, was associated with risk of death increased by 28 percent. The amount of total fat, as well as each type of fat, was also dramatically associated with risk for death. Those consuming the highest level of total fat had a reduced risk of death during the study of 23 percent. Risk for death was reduced by 14 percent in those consuming the highest levels of saturated fat, while it was reduced by 19 percent in those consuming high levels of monounsaturated fat, and an incredible 20 percent in those who consumed the highest level of polyunsaturated fat. Higher consumption of the dreaded saturated fat was also associated with a 20 percent lower risk of stroke, comparing those who consumed the most with those who consumed the least. The authors concluded: "High carbohydrate intake was associated with higher risk of total mortality, whereas total fat and individual types of fat were related to lower total mortality. Total fat and types of fat were not associated with cardiovascular disease, myocardial infarction, or cardiovascular disease mortality, whereas saturated fat had an inverse association with stroke. Global dietary guidelines should be reconsidered in light of these findings."

A small pilot study in 2017 reported that Alzheimer's patients who followed the University of Kansas's ketogenic diet program for three months improved an average of four points on one of the most important cognitive assessments in dementia care, the Alzheimer's Disease Assessment Scale–cognitive domain (ADAS-cog).[32] The diet comprised 70 percent fat. In the words of Dr. Russell Swerdlow, who led the study and presented it at the Alzheimer's Association International Conference, "This is the most robust improvement in the ADAS-cog scale that I am aware of for an Alzheimer's interventional trial." Now here's the takeaway to remember: The diet improved cognition in Alzheimer's disease patients better than any anti-amyloid drug that has ever been tested. That clearly tells us something important about the power of diet, specifically carbs versus fats. In a much larger study published in 2015, a randomized clinical trial in an older population over the course of five years showed that a Mediterranean diet supplemented with olive oil or nuts is associated with improved cognitive function.[33] Later on, I'll suggest that one of the easiest ways to add good fat to your diet is to use lots of extra virgin olive oil. Studies show that this oil can not only lower risk of cognitive decline but also help protect against stroke and diabetes.[34] I don't know of any drugs on the market that can claim those benefits.

To fully grasp the bane of carbs and the benefits of fats, it helps to understand some basic biology. In the body, dietary carbohydrates, including sugars and starches, are converted to glucose, which you know by now tells the pancreas to release insulin into the blood. Insulin shuffles glucose into cells and stores glucose as glycogen in the liver and muscles. It's also the body's chief fat-building catalyst, converting glucose to body fat when the liver and muscles have no more room for glycogen. Carbohydrates—not dietary fats—are the primary cause of weight gain. (Think about it: Many farmers fatten animals destined for the butcher block with carbohydrates like corn and grain, not fats and proteins. You can see the difference just by comparing, for example, a cut of grain-fed New York strip steak and a grass-fed one: The grain-fed cut will contain a lot more fat.) This partly explains why one of the major health effects of a low-carbohydrate diet is weight loss. Moreover, a low-carb diet decreases blood sugar in diabetics and improves insulin sensitivity. In fact, replacing carbohydrates with fat is increasingly becoming the preferred method for treating type 2 diabetes.

When your diet is continuously rich in carbohydrates, which in effect keep your insulin pumps on, you severely limit (if not completely halt) the breakdown of your body fat for fuel. Your body gets addicted to that glucose. You may even use up your glucose but still suffer from a lockdown of available fat for fuel due to high volumes of insulin. In essence, the body becomes physically starved due to your carb-based diet. This is why many obese individuals cannot lose weight while continuing to eat carbs. Their insulin levels hold those fat stores hostage. (Gary Taubes explains this science beautifully in his writings, and you can view my interview with him on *The Empowering Neurologist*.)

Now let's turn to dietary fat. Fat is and always has been a fundamental pillar of our nutrition. Beyond the fact that the human brain consists of more than 70 percent fat, fat plays a pivotal role in regulating the immune system. Simply stated, good fats like omega-3s and monounsaturated fats reduce inflammation, while modified hydrogenated fats, so common in commercially prepared foods, dramatically increase inflammation. Certain vitamins, notably A, D, E, and K, require fat to get absorbed properly in the body, which is why dietary fat is necessary to transport these "fat-soluble" vitamins. Because these vitamins do not dissolve in water, they can be absorbed from your small intestine only in combination with fat. Deficiencies due to incomplete absorption of these vitally important vitamins are always serious, and any such deficiency can be linked to brain illness, among many other conditions. Without enough vitamin K, for instance, you won't be able to form blood clots upon injury and can even suffer from spontaneous bleeding (imagine that problem in the brain). Vitamin K also contributes to both brain and eye health, helping reduce the risk of age-related dementia and macular degeneration (and dietary fat from healthy sources such as those high in omega-3 fatty acids is good for preventing macular degeneration). Without adequate vitamin A, your brain won't develop properly; you will go blind and become exceptionally vulnerable to infections. A lack of vitamin D is known to be associated with increased susceptibility to several chronic diseases, including schizophrenia, Alzheimer's, Parkinson's, depression, seasonal affective disorders, and a number of autoimmune diseases such as type 1 diabetes.

If you follow today's conventional wisdom, you've been told that you're supposed to limit your total fat intake to no more than 20 percent of your calories (and when it comes to saturated fat, that percentage goes down to less than 10). You also know that this is difficult to achieve, but you can breathe a sigh of relief: It's misguided advice, and on my program you won't have to worry about counting fat grams or overall percentages. While the synthetic trans fats found in margarine and processed foods are poisonous, we know now that monounsaturated fats — such as the fat found in avocados, olives, and nuts — are healthy. We also know that the polyunsaturated omega-3 fatty acids in cold-water fish (such as salmon) and some plants (such as flaxseed oil) are good. But what about natural saturated fats such as those found in meat, egg yolks, cheese, and butter? As I've been detailing, saturated fat has gotten a bad rap. Most of us don't even question why these particular fats are unhealthy anymore; we just assume that the purported science is true. Or we erroneously place these fats in the same category as trans fats. But we need saturated fat, and our body has long been designed to handle the consumption of natural sources of it — even in high amounts.

Few people understand that saturated fat plays a pivotal role in a lot of biochemical equations that keep us healthy. If you were breast-fed as a baby, then saturated fats were your staple, as they make up 54 percent of the fat in breast milk. Every cell in your body requires saturated fats; they make up 50 percent of the cellular membrane. They also contribute to the structure and function of your lungs, heart, bones, liver, and immune system. In your lungs, one particular saturated fat, 16-palmitic acid, creates lung surfactant, reducing surface tension so that your alveoli—the tiny air sacs that capture oxygen from your inhalations and allow it to be absorbed into your bloodstream—are able to expand. Without surfactant, you would not be able to breathe because the wet surfaces of your lungs' alveoli would stick together and prevent your lungs from expanding. Having healthy lung surfactant prevents asthma and other breathing disorders.

Heart muscle cells prefer a type of saturated fat for nourishment, and bones require saturated fats to assimilate calcium effectively. With the help of saturated fats, your liver clears out fat and protects you from the adverse effects of toxins, including alcohol and compounds in medications. The white blood cells of your immune system partly owe their ability to recognize and destroy invading germs, as well as to fight tumors, to the fats found in butter and coconut oil. Even your endocrine system relies on saturated fatty acids to communicate the need to manufacture certain hormones, including insulin. And they help tell your brain when you are full so you can pull away from the table. I don't expect you to remember all this biology. I mention it as a way of emphatically expressing to you the biological necessity of saturated fat. For a complete list of where these good fats can be found (and where the bad fats lurk), see page 89.

THE CASE FOR CHOLESTEROL

If you've had your cholesterol levels tested, you've probably lumped HDL (high-density lipoprotein) and LDL (low-density lipoprotein) into two different categories—one "good" and one "bad." I've already mentioned these two labels for cholesterol in passing. But contrary to what you might think, they are not two different kinds of cholesterol. HDL and LDL reflect two different containers for cholesterol and fats, each of which serves a different role in the body. Several other lipoproteins also exist, such as VLDL (very low) and IDL (intermediate). And as I've already begun to outline, cholesterol—no matter which "kind"—is not as terrible as you've been taught to believe. Some of the most remarkable studies of late on the biological value of cholesterol—and for brain health in particular—clue us in on how the pieces to this puzzle fit together and tell a coherent story. As we've seen, science is only recently discovering that both fat and cholesterol are severely deficient in diseased brains and that high total cholesterol levels in late life are associated with increased longevity.[35] The brain holds only 2 percent of the body's mass but contains 25 percent of the total cholesterol, which supports brain function and development. One-fifth of the brain by weight is cholesterol!

Cholesterol forms membranes surrounding cells, keeps cell membranes permeable, and maintains cellular "waterproofing" so different chemical reactions can take place inside and outside the cell. We've actually determined that the ability to grow new synapses in the brain depends on the availability of cholesterol, which latches cell membranes together so that signals can easily jump across the synapse. It's also a crucial component in the myelin coating around the neuron, allowing quick transmission of information. A neuron that can't transmit messages is useless, and it only makes sense to cast it aside like junk—the debris of which is the hallmark of brain disease. In essence, cholesterol acts as a facilitator for the brain to communicate and function properly.

Moreover, cholesterol in the brain serves as a powerful antioxidant. It protects the brain against the damaging effects of free radicals. Cholesterol is a precursor for the steroid hormones like estrogen and the androgens, as well as for vitamin D, a critically important fat-soluble antioxidant. Vitamin D is also a powerful anti-inflammatory, helping rid the body of infectious agents that can lead to life-threatening diseases. Vitamin D is not really a vitamin; it acts more like a steroid in the body, or a hormone. Given that vitamin D is directly formed from cholesterol, you won't be surprised to hear that vitamin D levels are low in people with a variety of neurodegenerative diseases like Parkinson's, Alzheimer's, and multiple sclerosis. As we age, natural cholesterol levels generally increase in the body. This is good because as we age our production of free radicals increases. Cholesterol can offer a level of protection against these free radicals.

And beyond the brain, cholesterol plays other vital roles in human health and physiology. The bile salts secreted by the gallbladder, which are needed for the digestion of fat and, therefore, the absorption of fat-soluble vitamins like A, D, and K, are made of cholesterol. Having a low cholesterol level in the body would therefore compromise a person's ability to digest fat. It would also jeopardize the body's electrolyte balance since cholesterol helps manage that delicate equilibrium. In fact, cholesterol is regarded by the body as such an important collaborator that every cell has a way to make its own supply.

So what does this mean for dietary recommendations? For years we have been told to focus on low-cholesterol foods, but foods rich in cholesterol, such as eggs, are very helpful and should be considered "brain food." We have eaten cholesterol-rich foods for more than two million years. As you now know, the real culprits when it comes to decreased brain function and health are foods that are high on the glycemic index — basically, high in carbohydrates.

One of the most pervasive myths I'm constantly debunking is the notion that the brain prefers glucose for fuel. This also couldn't be further from the truth. The brain uses fat exceptionally well; it is considered a brain "super-fuel." This is why we use a fat-based diet as therapy for all manner of neuro-degenerative diseases (in chapter 7, I describe in detail how the brain accesses fat for fuel and what this means for health and for tailoring the perfect diet).

Part of the reason I am focusing on fats, and cholesterol in particular, is not only because these ingredients have everything to do with brain health, but also because we live in a society that continues to demonize them, and the powerful pharmaceutical industry preys on the public's misinformation and perpetuates falsehoods, many of which could physically destroy us. To really understand where I'm going with this, let's look at one problematic area: the statin epidemic.

THE STATIN EPIDEMIC AND THE LINK TO BRAIN DYSFUNCTION

Our understanding of how cholesterol is critical for brain health has brought me and many others in my field to believe that statins — the blockbuster drugs prescribed to millions of Americans to lower cholesterol—may cause or exacerbate brain disorders and disease.

Memory dysfunction is a known side effect of statins. The late Dr. Duane Graveline, who conducted pioneering research in space medicine with NASA and earned the nickname "Spacedoc," was a strong opponent of statins. He died in 2016 after suffering for years from a degenerative neuromuscular condition. Ever since he experienced total memory loss that he believed was caused by the statins he was taking at the time, he began collecting evidence of their side effects from people around the world. This led him to pen three books on the matter, the most famous of which is *Lipitor, Thief of Memory*.[36]

In February 2012, the FDA released a statement indicating that statin drugs could cause cognitive side effects such as memory lapses and confusion. One study performed by the American Medical Association and published in the *Archives of Internal Medicine* in January 2012 demonstrated an astounding 48 percent increased risk of diabetes among women taking statin medications.[37]

Risk of type 2 diabetes in women using statin drugs

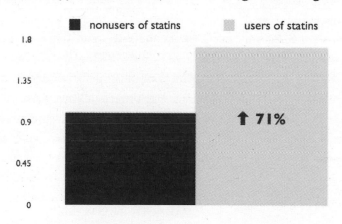

This study involved big numbers—more than 160,000 postmenopausal women—making it hard to ignore its significance and gravity. Recognizing that type 2 diabetes is a powerful risk factor for Alzheimer's disease, a relationship between statin drugs and cognitive decline or cognitive dysfunction is certainly understandable. Studies that have come out since then have also confirmed a connection, though risk percentages do vary and can depend on whether a person is already susceptible to developing diabetes.[38] This is an active area of study with differing opinions within the medical community. I've participated in many discussions about this topic, which does indeed get heated at times, with conflicting data. I invite you to go to my website and search for "statins"; there, you can access a roundtable discussion I had in 2013 with colleagues on the "Appropriate Clinical Use of Statins" and keep abreast of updates. While I continue to strongly advise against the use of statins, I do concede that there could be unique cases whereby their use's benefits outweigh the risks, and for reasons other than just "high cholesterol." But these cases are few and far between. It has to be individualized.

In 2009, Stephanie Seneff, a senior research scientist in the Computer Science and Artificial Intelligence Laboratory at MIT who became interested in the effects of drugs and diet on health and nutrition, wrote a compelling essay explaining why low-fat diets and statins may contribute to the development of Alzheimer's.[39] In it, she chronicles our knowledge of statins' side effects and paints a stunning portrait of how the brain suffers in their presence. She also synthesizes the latest science and input from other experts in the field. As Dr. Seneff explains, one of the main reasons statins promote brain disorder is that they handicap the liver's ability to make cholesterol. Consequently, the level of LDL in the blood drops significantly. As I've just detailed, cholesterol plays a vital role in the brain, enabling communication between neurons and encouraging the growth of new brain cells. In an ironic twist, the statin industry advertises its products by saying that they interfere with cholesterol production in the brain as well as in the liver.

Dr. Yeon-Kyun Shin, professor of biophysics at Iowa State University, is a noted authority on how cholesterol functions within neural networks to transmit messages. He put it bluntly in an interview for a *Science Daily* reporter:[40]

If you deprive cholesterol from the brain, then you directly affect the machinery that triggers the release of neurotransmitters. Neurotransmitters affect the data-processing and memory functions. In other words—how smart you are and how well you remember things. If you try to lower the cholesterol by taking medication that is attacking the machinery of cholesterol synthesis in the liver, that medicine goes to the brain too. And then it reduces the synthesis of cholesterol, which is necessary in the brain. Our study shows there is a direct link between cholesterol and the neurotransmitter release, and we know exactly the molecular mechanics of what happens in the cells. Cholesterol changes the shape of the proteins to stimulate thinking and memory.

In 2009, an updated review of two major studies completed in 2001 of statin medications used by more than twenty-six thousand individuals at risk for dementia and Alzheimer's disease showed that statins are not protective against Alzheimer's, which contradicted previous thinking. The lead author of the study, Bernadette McGuinness, was quoted by *Science Daily* as saying, "From these trials, which contained very large numbers and were the gold standard—it appears that statins given in late life to individuals at risk of vascular disease do not prevent against dementia."[41] When asked to comment on the results, UCLA researcher Beatrice Golomb said, "Regarding statins as preventive medicines, there are a number of individual cases in case reports and case series where cognition is clearly and reproducibly adversely affected by statins."[42] Golomb, who participated in that roundtable with me on the topic of statins, further added that various studies have demonstrated that statins either negatively affected cognition or were neutral, and that no trial has ever shown a positive outcome.

Besides statins' direct impact on cholesterol, they have an indirect effect on the supply of fatty acids and antioxidants. They not only reduce the amount of cholesterol contained in LDL particles, but also diminish the actual number of LDL particles. So in addition to depleting cholesterol, they limit the stash available to the brain of both fatty acids and antioxidants, which are also carried in the LDL particles. Proper brain functioning depends on all three of these substances[43] (and later on, you'll read about the importance of boosting the body's own natural production of antioxidants).

Another way in which statins may contribute to Alzheimer's, beautifully described by Dr. Seneff,[44] is by paralyzing cells' ability to make coenzyme Q10, a vitamin-like substance found throughout the body, where it serves an important role as an antioxidant and in producing energy for cells. Because coQ10 shares the same metabolic pathway as cholesterol, its synthesis is disrupted by statins, and the body and brain are deprived of it. Some of the side effects listed for statins, such as fatigue, shortness of breath, problems with mobility and balance, and muscular pain, weakness, and atrophy, are related to the loss of coQ10 in muscles and a reduced capacity for energy production. At the extreme, people who experience severe reactions to statins suffer from serious damage to their skeletal muscles. A deficiency in coQ10 also has been linked to heart failure, hypertension, and Parkinson's disease. Given all these effects, it's logical to see why coQ10 has been proposed as an actual treatment for Alzheimer's disease.

Finally, statins could have an indirect effect on vitamin D. The body makes vitamin D from cholesterol in the skin upon exposure to UV rays from the sun. If you were to look at the chemical formula for vitamin D, you'd have a hard time distinguishing it from cholesterol's formula; they look virtually identical. "If LDL levels are kept artificially low," writes Dr. Seneff, "then the body will be unable to resupply adequate amounts of cholesterol to replenish the stores in the skin once they have been depleted. This would lead to vitamin D deficiency, which is a widespread problem in America."[45] Vitamin D deficiency is not just about an increased risk for weak, soft bones and, at the extreme end, rickets; it's associated with many conditions that heighten one's risk for dementia, such as diabetes, depression, and cardiovascular disease. If the brain didn't demand vitamin D for proper development and function, then it wouldn't have widespread receptors for it.

The pros and cons of statins continue to be debated, and major studies have failed to show how they protect the body from illness. Although numerous studies do point to the positive effects statins have on reducing mortality rates in people with coronary artery disease, new research reveals that these outcomes have little to do with the cholesterol-lowering activity of these drugs and more likely reflect the fact that they reduce inflammation, a main-spring of the disease. But that doesn't mean that the trade-offs for taking a statin merit their seal of approval. For some, the risk of negative side effects is just too great. People with a low risk of heart disease but a high risk for other ailments would be putting themselves in harm's way if they chose to take a statin. If you are taking a statin because you are at high risk for a cardiovascular event, speak with your doctor about your particular risk-benefit profile. There are likely other ways to manage prevention without risking the downsides of statin treatment. When it comes to protecting your heart — and your brain — it's all about reducing carbs and, counterintuitively, upping dietary fat. And please stop worrying so much about cholesterol.

HOW CARBS — NOT CHOLESTEROL — CAUSE HIGH CHOLESTEROL

If you can limit carb intake to a range that is absolutely necessary (the details of which are in chapter 10) and make up the difference with delicious fats and protein, you can literally reprogram your genes back to the factory setting you had at birth. This is the setting that affords you the ability to be a mentally sharp, fat-burning machine.

It's important to understand that when you have a blood cholesterol test, the number that is represented is 75 to 80 percent derived from what your body manufactures and not necessarily what you've eaten. In fact, foods that are high in cholesterol actually decrease the body's production of cholesterol. We all make up to 2,000 milligrams of cholesterol every day because we desperately need it, and this is several times the amount found in our diets. But despite this amazing ability, it's critical to obtain cholesterol from dietary sources. Our bodies much prefer that we "spoon-feed" our cholesterol from the foods we eat rather than manufacture it internally, which is a complex multistep biological process that taxes the liver. Dietary cholesterol is so important that your body absorbs as much as it can for use.

What happens if you restrict your cholesterol intake, as so many people do today? The body sends out an alarm that indicates crisis (famine). Your liver senses this signal and begins to produce an enzyme called HMG-CoA reductase, which helps make up for the deficit by using carbohydrates in the diet to produce an excess supply of cholesterol. (This is the same enzyme that statins target.) As you can likely predict, it's a Molotov cocktail in the works: As you eat excessive carbohydrates while lowering your cholesterol intake, you incite a steady and punishing overproduction of cholesterol in the body. The only way to stop this internal pathway run amok is to consume an adequate amount of dietary cholesterol and back way off on carbs. Which explains why my "high-cholesterol" patients who go on my diet can safely return their levels to normal without drugs while enjoying cholesterol-rich foods.

IS THERE SUCH A THING AS DANGEROUSLY "HIGH CHOLESTEROL"?

Cholesterol is at most a minor player in coronary heart disease and represents an extremely poor predictor of heart attack risk. Over half of all patients hospitalized with a heart attack have cholesterol levels in the "normal" range. The idea that aggressively lowering cholesterol levels will somehow magically and dramatically reduce heart attack risk has now been fully and categorically refuted. The most important modifiable risk factors related to heart attack risk include smoking, excess alcohol consumption, lack of aerobic exercise, overweight, and a diet high in carbohydrates.

When I see patients with cholesterol levels of, say, 240 mg/dL or higher, it's almost a given that they will have received a prescription for a cholesterol-lowering medication from their general practitioners. This is wrong in thought and action. As discussed, cholesterol is one of the most critical chemicals in human physiology, especially as it relates to brain health. The best lab report to refer to in determining one's health status is hemoglobin A1C, not cholesterol levels. It is rarely, if ever, appropriate to consider high cholesterol alone to be a significant threat to health.

A good question: Who is deemed to have high cholesterol? Thirty years ago, the answer was anyone whose total cholesterol level was more than 240 mg/dL and who had other risk factors, such as being overweight and smoking. The definition changed after the Cholesterol Consensus Conference in 1984; then it became anyone with a total cholesterol level over 200, regardless of other risk factors. Today, many guidelines lower the threshold down to 180. And if you've had a heart attack, you're in a totally different category: No matter how low your cholesterol level is, you'll likely be prescribed a cholesterol-lowering medicine and told to maintain a low-fat diet. That is misguided advice in most cases.

SEX ED: IT'S ALL IN YOUR HEAD

Okay. So cholesterol is a good thing. But it's not just about your brain's wit, physical health, and future longevity. It's also about a very important part of your lifestyle that typically gets shoved under the carpet in serious health books. I'm talking about your sex life. How sparky is it?

Although I'm a neurologist, I encounter a fair share of people who suffer from sexual dysfunction and are either impotent and avoid sex altogether or who hoard bottles of pills to help them out. You know about these pills— the ones that get advertised like candy on the evening news and promise to transform your sex life. Past patients with sexual health woes obviously didn't come to me for that specifically, but it was a noted problem when I asked them about that part of their life in addition to any neurological issues I was addressing.

A quick anecdote: A seventy-five-year-old retired engineer once came to see me with a variety of complaints, including insomnia and depression. He had been taking sleeping pills for the past forty years, and his depression had worsened in the two to three months prior to his appointment. At the time I saw him, he was taking an antidepressant, a medication for anxiety, and Viagra for erectile dysfunction (ED). I first checked him for gluten sensitivity and discovered, to his surprise but not mine, a positive panel (this was back when I ordered such testing). He agreed to adopt a gluten-free, high-fat diet, and we communicated by telephone after about one month. That's when he had magnificent news: His depression had improved, and he no longer needed to take Viagra in order to have sex with his wife. He thanked me very much.

Most everyone can agree that sex has everything to do with what's going on in the brain. It's an act that's deeply tied to emotions, impulses, and thoughts. But it's also inexorably connected to hormones and blood chemistry. Without question, if you're depressed and not sleeping well, like my engineer patient, sex is the last thing on your mind. But one of the most common reasons for impotence is actually neither of these two conditions. It's what I've been talking about through much of this chapter: abysmally low cholesterol levels. And the studies to date have achieved proof of concept: Unless you have healthy testosterone levels (this goes for both men and women), you're not going to have a hot sex life, if any at all. And what makes testosterone? Cholesterol. What are millions of Americans doing today? Lowering their cholesterol levels through diet and/or taking statins. In the meanwhile, they are lowering their libido and ability to perform. Is it any wonder there's an epidemic of ED and demand for ED drugs today, not to mention (perhaps ironically) testosterone replacement therapy?

Plenty of studies have confirmed these connections.[46] Decreased libido is one of the most common complaints among those taking statins, and lab reports have repeatedly demonstrated low testosterone in statin consumers.[47] Those on statins are twice as likely to have low testosterone levels. Luckily, this condition is reversible by stopping the statin and increasing cholesterol intake. There are actually two ways that statins can lower testosterone. The first is by directly lowering levels of cholesterol. The second is by interfering with the enzymes that create active testosterone.

One study that came out in the United Kingdom in 2010 looked at 930 men with coronary heart disease and measured their testosterone levels.[48] Low testosterone was found in 24 percent of the patients, and the risk of dying was 12 percent in those with normal testosterone but 21 percent in those with low testosterone. The conclusion was staring them in the face: If you have coronary disease and low testosterone, you're at much greater risk of dying. So again we are giving statin medications to lower cholesterol, which lowers testosterone…and lower testosterone increases the risk of dying. Is this crazy or what?

I rest my case.

THE BELLY CONNECTION

After *Grain Brain* was first published, I turned to the role of the human microbiome on brain health—specifically, how the brain is intricately connected with the gut's microbial inhabitants, which are mostly bacteria. We now know that our lifestyle choices help shape and sustain our microbiome. We also know that the health of the microbiome factors into immune system function, inflammation levels, and risk for illnesses as diverse as depression, obesity, bowel disorders, diabetes, multiple sclerosis, asthma, autism, Alzheimer's, Parkinson's, and even cancer. They also help control gut permeability, an important concept we explored earlier that factors into the body's "set point" of inflammation. A break in the intestinal wall can cause food toxins such as gluten and pathogens to pass through and generate an immune response. This breach affects not only the gut, but also other organs and tissues, such as the skeletal system, the skin, the kidneys, the pancreas, the liver, and the brain.

Our microbial comrades do a lot of work on behalf of our physiology: They manufacture neurotransmitters and vitamins that we couldn't otherwise make, promote normal gastrointestinal function, provide protection from infection, regulate metabolism and the absorption of food, and help control blood sugar balance. They even affect whether we are overweight or lean, hungry or satiated. *Brain Maker* covered the science of the microbiome in depth, and I encourage you to go there to learn more about it.[49] The updated program in this book, however, will help you nourish and cultivate the best microbiome you can, which will help you achieve a brain that functions optimally. A great majority of the risk factors for an unhealthy intestinal microbiome are modifiable. These include things like diets high in refined carbohydrates, sugar, and processed foods, and dietary toxins such as gluten and processed vegetable oils.

THE SWEET TRUTH

I've covered a lot of ground in this chapter, mostly dealing with the role of fats on the brain. But we now have to ask ourselves the following: What happens when you inundate the brain with sugar instead? I started this chapter by addressing the ills of carbohydrates on our bodies, but I've saved the conversation about this particularly devastating carbohydrate for its own chapter. Thankfully, word has gotten out about the role of sugar in brain health. When I first wrote this book, this was a subject area that had remarkably little attention in the press. We all knew about the relationship between sugar and "diabesity," sugar and heart disease, sugar and fatty livers, sugar and metabolic syndrome, sugar and risk for cancer, etc., but sugar and brain dysfunction was unheard of until recently. And if you're not entirely sure about the connection, this next chapter is for you. It's time you got up close and personal with your brain on sugar.

CHAPTER 4

Not a Fruitful Union

This Is Your Brain on Sugar
(Natural or Not)

Evolutionarily, sugar was available to our ancestors as fruit for only a few months a year (at harvest time), or as honey, which was guarded by bees. But in recent years, sugar has been added to nearly all processed foods, limiting consumer choice. Nature made sugar hard to get; man made it easy.

— Dr. Robert Lustig et al.[1]

Sugar. Whether it's from a lollipop, Lucky Charms, or a slice of cinnamon-raisin bread, we all know that this particular carbohydrate is not the healthiest of ingredients, especially when it's consumed in excess or comes from refined or processed forms such as high-fructose corn syrup. We also know that sugar is partly to blame for challenges with our waistlines, appetites, blood sugar control, obesity, type 2 diabetes, and insulin resistance. But what about sugar and the brain?

In 2011, Gary Taubes, the author I mentioned in the previous chapter who wrote *Good Calories, Bad Calories* and *Why We Get Fat*,[2] penned an excellent piece for the *New York Times* titled "Is Sugar Toxic?"[3] In it, he chronicles not just the history of sugar in our lives and food products, but the evolving science behind understanding how sugar affects our bodies. This was followed by his next book, *The Case Against Sugar*, in late 2016, in which he lays out a compelling argument for sugar (both sucrose and high-fructose corn syrup) being the principal cause of the chronic diseases most likely to kill us all.[4] When I interviewed him, I asked him how he got into being such a trailblazer in this area of nutrition as an investigative science journalist. He told me that he was just following the data and that some of his friends in the physics community suggested that if he was interested in bad science (*Bad Science* being the title of an earlier work about cold fusion), he should look into what was going on in public health. That led him, not surprisingly, to more bad science.

In Taubes's 2011 book, he showcases the work of Robert Lustig, a specialist in pediatric hormone disorders and the leading expert in childhood obesity at the University of California, San Francisco, School of Medicine, who makes a case for sugar being a "toxin" or a "poison." It is the main villain in his bestselling 2012 book *Fat Chance* and a topic I discussed at length with him in a recent interview.[5] Lustig doesn't harp so much on the consumption of these "empty calories"; his issue with sugar is that it has unique characteristics, specifically in the way the various kinds of sugar are metabolized by the human body. Dr. Lustig has been one of the pioneers in raising awareness as to the addictive issues surrounding sugar as well as its profoundly detrimental effects on human health.

Lustig likes to use the phrase "isocaloric but not isometabolic" when he describes the difference between pure glucose, the simplest form of sugar, and table sugar, which is a combination of glucose and fructose. (Fructose, which I'll get to in a moment, is a type of naturally occurring sugar found exclusively in fruit and honey.) When we eat 100 calories of glucose from a potato, for instance, our bodies metabolize it differently—and experience different effects—than if we eat 100 calories of sugar comprising half glucose and half fructose. Here's why.

Your liver takes care of the fructose component of sugar. Glucose from other carbs and starches, on the other hand, is processed by every cell in the body. So consuming both types of sugar (fructose and glucose) at the same time means your liver has to work harder than if you ate the same number of calories from glucose alone. And your liver will also be taxed if it's hit with liquid forms of these sugars, those found in soda or fruit juices. Drinking liquid sugar is not the same as eating, say, an equivalent dose of sugar in whole apples. Fructose, by the way, is the sweetest of all naturally occurring carbohydrates, which probably explains why we love it so much. But contrary to what you might think, it has the lowest glycemic index of all the natural sugars. The reason is simple: Because the liver metabolizes most of the fructose, it has no immediate effect on our blood sugar and insulin levels, unlike sugar or high-fructose corn syrup, whose glucose ends up in general circulation and raises blood sugar levels. Don't let that fact fool you, however. While fructose may not have an immediate effect, it has more long-term effects when it's consumed in sufficient quantities from unnatural sources. And the science is well documented: Consuming fructose is associated with impaired glucose tolerance, insulin resistance, high blood fats, and hypertension. And because it does not trigger the production of insulin and leptin, two key hormones in regulating our metabolism, diets high in fructose lead to obesity and its metabolic repercussions. (I will clarify later what this means for those who enjoy eating lots of fruit. Fortunately, for the most part, you can consume some fruit. The quantity of fructose in most whole fruit pales in comparison to the levels of fructose in processed foods.)

We hear about sugar and its effects on virtually every other part of the body *except for the brain*. This, again, is a subject area that's gotten remarkably little attention in the press. The questions to ask, and the ones I'll answer in this chapter, are:

- What does excess sugar consumption do to the brain?
- Can the brain distinguish between different types of sugar? Does it "metabolize" sugar differently depending on where it's coming from?

If I were you, I'd put down that biscuit or biscotti you're having with your caffè mocha and buckle up. After reading this chapter, you'll never look at a sugary treat or beverage in quite the same way.

SUGAR AND CARBS 101

Let me begin by defining a few terms. What, exactly, is the difference between table sugar, fruit sugar, high-fructose corn syrup, and the like?

Good question. As I've said, fructose is a type of sugar naturally found in fruit and honey. It's a monosaccharide just like glucose, whereas table sugar (sucrose)—the white granulated stuff we sprinkle in coffee or dump into a bowl of cookie batter—is a combination of glucose and fructose, thus making it a disaccharide (two molecules linked together). The majority of the fructose we consume is not in its natural form (that is, as part of sucrose) or source (whole fruit). The average American consumes 163 grams of refined sugars (652 calories) per day, and of this, roughly 76 grams (302 calories) are from the highly processed form of fructose, derived from high-fructose corn syrup.[6] High-fructose corn syrup, which is what we find in our sodas, juices, and many processed foods, is yet another combination of molecules dominated by fructose—it's about 55 percent fructose, 42 percent glucose, and 3 percent other carbohydrates. I use the word "about" because some studies have shown that high-fructose corn syrup can contain much more free fructose than labeled. Dr. Michael Goran, director of the Childhood Obesity Research Center and professor of preventive medicine at the University of Southern California, identified levels of free fructose as high as 65 percent in soda purchased in the Los Angeles area.[7]

High-fructose corn syrup was introduced in 1978 as a cheap replacement for table sugar in beverages and food products. No doubt you've heard about it in the media, which has attacked this artificially manufactured ingredient for being the root cause of our obesity epidemic. But this misses the point. While it's true we can blame our bulging waistlines and diagnoses of related conditions such as obesity and diabetes on our consumption of high-fructose corn syrup, we can also point to all other sugars as well since they are all carbohydrates, a class of biomolecules that share similar characteristics. Carbohydrates are simply long chains of sugar molecules, as distinguished from fat (chains of fatty acids), proteins (chains of amino acids), and DNA. But you already know that not all carbohydrates are created equal. And not all carbohydrates are treated equally by the body. The differentiating feature is how much a certain carbohydrate will raise blood sugar and, in effect, insulin. Meals that are higher in carbohydrates, and especially those that are higher in simple glucose, cause the pancreas to increase its insulin output in order to store the blood sugar in cells. During the course of digestion, carbohydrates are broken down and sugar is liberated into the bloodstream, again causing the pancreas to increase its output of insulin so glucose can penetrate cells. Over time, higher levels of blood sugar will cause increased production of insulin output from the pancreas.

The carbs that trigger the biggest surge in blood sugar are typically the most fattening for that very reason. They include anything made with refined flour (breads, cereals, pastas); starches such as rice, potatoes, and corn; and liquid carbs like soda, beer, and fruit juice. They all get digested quickly because they flood the bloodstream with glucose and stimulate a surge in insulin, which then packs away the excess calories as fat. What about the carbs in vegetables? Those carbs, especially the ones in leafy green vegetables such as broccoli and spinach, are tied up with indigestible fiber, so they take longer to break down. The fiber essentially slows down the process, causing a slower funneling of glucose into the bloodstream. In addition, vegetables contain more water relative to their weight than starches, and this further dampens the blood sugar response. When we eat whole fruits, which obviously contain fruit sugar, the water and fiber will also "dilute" the blood sugar effect. If you take, for instance, a peach and a baked potato of equal weight, the potato will have a much bigger effect on blood sugar than the watery, fibrous peach. However, that's not to say that the peach—or any other fruit for that matter—won't cause problems.[8]

Our caveman ancestors did in fact eat fruit, but not every day of the year. We haven't yet evolved to be able to handle the copious amounts of fructose we consume today—especially when we get our fructose from manufactured sources. Natural fruit has relatively little sugar when compared to, say, a can of regular soda, which has a massive amount. A medium-size apple contains about 44 calories of sugar in a fiber-rich blend thanks to the naturally occurring soluble pectin fiber in the apple and the insoluble fiber in the skin; conversely, a 12-ounce can of Coke or Pepsi contains nearly twice that—80 calories of sugar. If you juice several apples and concentrate the liquid down to a 12-ounce beverage (thereby losing the fiber), lo and behold you get a blast of 85 sugar calories that could just as well have come from a soda. When that fructose hits the liver, most of it gets converted to fat and sent to our fat cells. No wonder fructose was called the most fattening carbohydrate more than forty years ago by biochemists. And when our bodies get used to performing this simple conversion with every meal, we can fall into a trap in which even our muscle tissue becomes resistant to insulin. Gary Taubes describes this domino effect brilliantly in *Why We Get Fat*: "So, even though fructose has no immediate effect on blood sugar and insulin, over time—maybe a few years—it is a likely cause of insulin resistance and thus the increased storage of calories as fat. The needle on our fuel-partitioning gauge will point toward fat storage, even if it didn't start out that way."[9]

The most disturbing fact about our addiction to sugar is that when we combine fructose and glucose (which we often do when we eat foods made with table sugar), the fructose might not do much to our blood sugar right away, but the accompanying glucose takes care of that—stimulating insulin secretion and alerting the fat cells to prepare for more storage. The more sugars we eat, the more we tell our bodies to transfer them to fat. This happens not only in the liver, leading to a condition called fatty liver disease, but elsewhere in the body as well. Hello, love handles, muffin tops, beer bellies, and the worst kind of fat of all—invisible visceral fat that hugs our vital organs.

I love how Taubes draws a parallel between the cause-and-effect relationship uniting carbohydrates and obesity, and the link between smoking and cancer: If the world had never invented cigarettes, lung cancer would be a rare disease. Likewise, if we didn't eat such high-carb diets, obesity would be a rare condition.[10] I'd bet that other related conditions would be uncommon as well, including diabetes, heart disease, dementia, and cancer. And if I had to name the kingpin here in terms of avoiding all manner of disease, I'd say "diabetes." That is to say, don't become diabetic.

THE DEATH KNELL IN DIABETES

I cannot reiterate enough the importance of avoiding the path to diabetes, and if diabetes is already a card you're playing with, then keeping blood sugars balanced is key. In the United States there are close to 11 million adults sixty-five years or older with type 2 diabetes, which speaks volumes to the magnitude of the potential catastrophe on our hands if all these individuals—plus the 23.1 million adults (48.3 percent) aged sixty-five or older who have prediabetes—develop Alzheimer's.[11] The data that supports the relationship between diabetes and Alzheimer's disease is profound, but it's important to understand that diabetes is a powerful risk factor for simple cognitive decline. This is especially true in individuals whose diabetes is under poor control. Case in point: In June 2012, the *Archives of Neurology* published an analysis of 3,069 elderly adults to determine if diabetes increased the risk of cognitive decline and if poor blood sugar control was related to worse cognitive performance.[12] When first evaluated, about 23 percent of the participants actually had diabetes, while the remaining 77 percent did not (the researchers intentionally chose a "diverse group of well-functioning older adults"). A small percentage, however, of that 77 percent went on to develop diabetes during the nine-year study. At the beginning of the study a panel of cognitive tests was performed, and over the next nine years these tests were repeated.

The conclusion stated the following: "Among well-functioning older adults, DM [diabetes mellitus] and poor glucose control among those with DM are associated with worse cognitive function and greater decline. This suggests that severity of DM may contribute to accelerated cognitive aging." The researchers demonstrated a fairly dramatic difference in the rate of mental decline among those with diabetes as compared to the non-diabetics. More interesting still, they also noted that even at the start of the study, baseline cognitive scores of the diabetics were already lower than those of the controls. The study also found a direct relationship between the rate of cognitive decline and higher levels of hemoglobin A1C, a marker of blood glucose control. The authors stated, "Hyperglycemia (elevated blood sugar) has been proposed as a mechanism that may contribute to the association between diabetes and reduced cognitive function." They went on to state that "hyperglycemia may contribute to cognitive impairment through such mechanisms as the formation of advanced glycation end products, inflammation, and microvascular disease."

Before I get to explaining what advanced glycation end products are and how they are formed, let's turn to one more study done earlier, in 2008. This one, from the Mayo Clinic and published in the *Archives of Neurology,* looked at the effects of the duration of diabetes. In other words, does how long one has diabetes play into the severity of cognitive decline? You bet. The numbers are eye-popping: According to the Mayo's findings, if diabetes began before a person was sixty-five years old, the risk for mild cognitive impairment was increased by a whopping 220 percent. And the risk of mild cognitive impairment in individuals who had diabetes for ten years or longer was increased by 176 percent. If people were taking insulin, their risk was increased by 200 percent. The authors described a proposed mechanism to explain the connection between persistent high blood sugar and Alzheimer's disease: "increased production of advanced glycation end products."[13] Just what are these glycation end products cropping up in the medical literature in reference to cognitive decline and accelerated aging? I mentioned them briefly in the previous chapter, and I will explain their significance in the next section.

ONE MAD COW AND MANY CLUES TO NEUROLOGICAL DISORDERS

I remember the hysteria that swept the globe in the mid-1990s when fears of mad cow disease spread quickly as people in Britain began to document evidence of transmission of the disease from cattle to humans. In the summer of 1996, Peter Hall, a twenty-year-old vegetarian, died of the human form of mad cow, called variant Creutzfeldt-Jakob disease. He'd contracted it from eating beef burgers as a child. Soon thereafter, other cases were confirmed, and countries, including the United States, started banning beef imports from Britain. Even McDonald's stopped serving burgers momentarily in some areas until scientists could ferret out the origins of the outbreak and measures were taken to eradicate the problem. Mad cow disease, also called bovine spongiform encephalopathy, is a rare bovine disorder that infects cattle; the nickname comes from the odd behavior sick cows express when infected. Both forms are types of prion diseases, which are caused by deviant proteins that inflict damage as they spread aggressively from cell to cell.

While mad cow disease isn't usually classified with classic neurodegenerative diseases such as Alzheimer's, Parkinson's, and Lou Gehrig's disease, all the conditions have a similar deformation in the structure of proteins needed for normal, healthy functioning. Granted, Alzheimer's, Parkinson's, and Lou Gehrig's disease are not transmissible to people the way mad cow is, but they nevertheless result in similar features that scientists are just beginning to understand. And it all boils down to deformed proteins.

Much in the way we now know that dozens of degenerative diseases are linked by inflammation, we also know that dozens of those same diseases — including type 2 diabetes, cataracts, atherosclerosis, emphysema, and dementia — are linked to deformed proteins. What makes prion diseases so unique is the ability of those abnormal proteins to confiscate the health of other cells, turning normal cells into misfits that lead to brain damage and dementia. It's similar to cancer in that one cell hijacks the normal regulation of another cell and creates a new tribe of cells that don't act like healthy ones. Working in laboratories with mice, scientists are finally collecting evidence to show that major neurodegenerative conditions follow parallel patterns.[14]

Proteins are among the most important structures in the body — they practically form and shape the entire body itself, carrying out functions and acting like master switches to our operating manual. Our genetic material, or DNA, codes for our proteins, which are then produced as a string of amino acids. They need to achieve a three-dimensional shape to carry out their tasks, such as regulating the body's processes and guarding against infection. Proteins gain their shape through a special folding technique; in the end, each protein achieves a distinctive shape that helps determine its unique function.

Obviously, deformed proteins cannot serve their function well or at all, and unfortunately, mutant proteins cannot be fixed. If they fail to fold properly into their correct shape, at best they are inactive and at worst, toxic. Usually cells have built-in technology to extinguish deformed proteins, but aging and other factors can interfere with this process. When a toxic protein is capable of inducing other cells to create misfolded proteins, the result can be disastrous. Which is why the goal for many scientists today is to find a way to stop the cell-to-cell spread of misshapen proteins and literally halt these diseases in their tracks.

Stanley Prusiner, the director of the Institute for Neurodegenerative Diseases at the University of California, San Francisco, discovered prions, which earned him the Nobel Prize in 1997. In 2012, he was part of a team of researchers who authored a landmark paper presented in the *Proceedings of the National Academy of Sciences* that showed that amyloid-beta protein associated with Alzheimer's shares prion-like characteristics.[15] In their experiment, they were able to follow the progression of disease by injecting amyloid-beta protein into one side of mice's brains and observing its effects. Using a light-generating molecule, they could see the marauding proteins collect as the mice's brains lit up— a toxic chain of events that's similar to what happens in the Alzheimer's brain.

This discovery holds clues to more than brain disease. Scientists who focus on other areas of the body have also been looking at the impact of shape-shifting proteins. In fact, "mad" proteins may play a role in a range of diseases. Type 2 diabetes, for example, can be seen from this perspective when we consider the fact that people with diabetes have demented proteins in their pancreas that can negatively affect insulin production (which raises the question: Does chronic high blood sugar cause the deformation?). In atherosclerosis, the cholesterol buildup typical of the disease could be caused by protein misfolding. People with cataracts have rogue proteins that collect in the eye lens. Cystic fibrosis, a hereditary disorder caused by a defect on the DNA, is characterized by improper folding of the CFTR protein. And even a type of genetically caused emphysema owes its devastation to the buildup of certain proteins made in the liver that are supposed to reach the lungs to protect them. Instead, those proteins accumulate in the liver and leave the lungs vulnerable to disease even in the absence of tobacco smoke exposure.

Okay, so now that we've established that wayward proteins play a role in disease and especially neurological degeneration, the next question is: *What causes the proteins to misfold?* With a condition like cystic fibrosis, the answer is more clear-cut because we have identified a specific genetic defect. But what about other ailments that have mysterious origins, or that don't manifest until later in life? Let's turn to those glycation end products.

Glycation is the biochemical term for the bonding of sugar molecules to proteins, fats, and amino acids; the spontaneous reaction that causes the sugar molecule to attach itself is sometimes referred to as the Maillard reaction. Louis Camille Maillard first described this process in the early 1900s.[16] Although he predicted that this reaction could have an important impact on medicine, not until 1980 did medical scientists turn to it when trying to understand diabetic complications and aging.

This process forms advanced glycation end products (AGEs), which cause protein fibers to become misshapen and inflexible. To get a glimpse of AGEs in action, simply look at someone who is prematurely aging—someone with a lot of wrinkles, sagginess, discolored skin, and a loss of radiance for their age. What you're seeing is the physical effect of proteins hooking up with renegade sugars, which explains why AGEs are now considered key players in skin aging.[17] Or check out a chain-smoker: The yellowing of the skin is another hallmark of glycation. Smokers have fewer antioxidants in their skin, and the smoking itself increases oxidation in their bodies and skin. So they cannot combat the by-products of normal processes like glycation because their bodies' antioxidant potential is severely weakened and, frankly, overpowered by the volume of oxidation. For most of us, the external signs of glycation show up in our thirties, when we've accumulated enough hormonal changes and environmental oxidative stress, including sun damage.

Glycation is an inevitable fact of life, just like inflammation and free radical production to some degree. It's a product of our normal metabolism and fundamental in the aging process. We can even measure glycation using technology that illuminates the bonds formed between sugars and proteins. In fact, dermatologists are well versed in this process. With high-tech cameras, they can capture the difference between youth and age just by taking a fluorescent image of children and comparing it to the faces of older adults. The children's faces will come out very dark, indicating a lack of AGEs, whereas the adults' will beam brightly as all those glycation bonds light up.

Clearly, the goal is to limit or slow down the glycation process. Many anti-aging schemes are now focused on how to reduce glycation and even break those toxic bonds. But this cannot happen when we consume a high-carb diet, which speeds up the glycation process. Sugars in particular are rapid stimulators of glycation, as they easily attach themselves to proteins in the body (and here's a good bit of trivia: High-fructose corn syrup, the number one source of dietary calories in America, increases the rate of glycation by a factor of ten).

When proteins become glycated, at least two important things happen. First, they become much less functional. Second, once proteins become bonded to sugar, they tend to attach themselves to other similarly damaged proteins and form cross-linkages that further inhibit their ability to function. But perhaps far more important is that once a protein is glycated, it becomes the source of a dramatic increase in the production of free radicals. This leads to the destruction of tissues, damaging fat, other proteins, and even DNA. Again, glycation of proteins is a normal part of our metabolism. But when it's excessive, many problems arise. High levels of glycation have been associated with not only cognitive decline, but also kidney disease, diabetes, vascular disease, and, as mentioned, the actual process of aging itself.[18] Keep in mind that any protein in the body is subject to being damaged by glycation and can become an AGE. Because of the significance of this process, medical researchers around the world are hard at work trying to develop various pharmaceutical ways to reduce AGE formation. But clearly, the best way to keep AGEs from forming is to reduce the availability of sugar in the first place.

Beyond just causing inflammation and free radical–mediated damage, AGEs are associated with damage to blood vessels and are thought to explain the connection between diabetes and vascular issues. As I noted in the previous chapter, the risk of coronary artery disease is dramatically increased in diabetics, as is the risk of stroke. Many individuals with diabetes have significant damage to the blood vessels supplying the brain, and while they may not have Alzheimer's, they may suffer from dementia caused by this blood supply issue.

Earlier I explained that LDL—the so-called bad cholesterol—is an important carrier protein bringing vital cholesterol to brain cells. Only when it becomes oxidized does it wreak havoc on blood vessels. And we now understand that when LDL becomes *glycated* (it's a protein, after all), this dramatically increases its oxidation.

The link between oxidative stress and sugar cannot be overstated. When proteins are glycated, the amount of free radicals formed is increased fiftyfold; this leads to loss of cellular function and eventually cell death.

This calls our attention to the powerful relationship between free radical production, oxidative stress, and cognitive decline. We know that oxidative stress is directly related to brain degeneration.[19] Studies show that damage to lipids, proteins, DNA, and RNA by free radicals happens early in the journey to cognitive impairment, and long before signs of serious neurological disorders such as Alzheimer's, Parkinson's, and Lou Gehrig's disease show up. Sadly, by the time a diagnosis is made, the damage is already done. The bottom line is that if you want to reduce oxidative stress and the action of free radicals harming your brain, you have to reduce the glycation of proteins. Which is to say, you have to diminish the availability of sugar. Pure and simple.

Most doctors employ a measurement of one glycated protein routinely in their medical practice. I've already mentioned it: hemoglobin A1C. This is the same standard laboratory measurement used to measure blood sugar control in diabetics. So, while your doctor may be measuring your hemoglobin A1C from time to time to get an understanding of your blood sugar control, the fact that it's glycated protein has vast and extremely important implications for your brain health. But hemoglobin A1C represents more than just a simple measurement of average blood sugar control over a 90- to 120-day period.

Hemoglobin A1C is the protein found in the red blood cell that carries oxygen and binds to blood sugar, and this binding is increased when blood sugar is elevated. While hemoglobin A1C doesn't give a moment-to-moment indication of what the blood sugar is, it is extremely useful in that it shows what the "average" blood sugar has been over the previous ninety days. This is why hemoglobin A1C is frequently used in studies that try to correlate blood sugar control to various disease processes like Alzheimer's, mild cognitive impairment, and coronary artery disease. Let's not forget the more recent study I spotlighted in the previous chapter that came out in 2017 in which a large group of researchers set out to "uncouple the effects of overweight/obesity from those of type 2 diabetes on brain structures and cognition."[20] They wanted to document the effects of overweight and obesity on the brains of people with early stage type 2 diabetes. In addition to finding that "overweight/obese participants with type 2 diabetes had more severe and progressive abnormalities in brain structures and cognition during early stage type 2 diabetes compared with normal-weight participants," they also measured A1C levels in their subjects. Not surprisingly, the overweight/obese group showed much higher levels.

It's well documented that glycated hemoglobin is a risk factor for diabetes, but it's also been correlated with risk for stroke, coronary heart disease, and death from other illnesses. These correlations have been shown to be strongest with any measurement of hemoglobin A1C above 6.0 percent.

We now have evidence to show that elevated hemoglobin A1C is associated with changes in brain size. In one particularly eye-opening study, published in the journal *Neurology*, researchers looking at MRIs to determine which lab test correlated best with brain atrophy found that the hemoglobin A1C demonstrated the most powerful relationship.[21] When comparing the degree of brain tissue loss in those individuals with the lowest hemoglobin A1C (4.4 to 5.2) to those having the highest hemoglobin A1C (5.9 to 9.0), the brain loss in those individuals with the highest hemoglobin A1C was almost doubled during a six-year period. So hemoglobin A1C is far more than just a marker of blood sugar balance—and it's absolutely under your control!

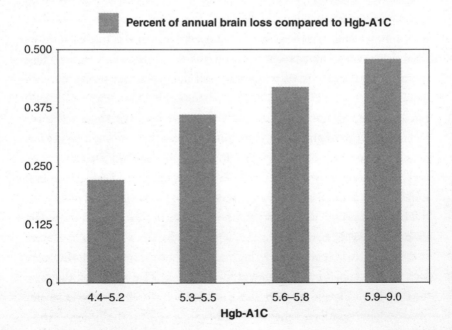

An ideal hemoglobin A1C would be in the 4.8 to 5.4 range. Keep in mind that reducing carbohydrate ingestion, weight loss, and physical exercise will ultimately improve insulin sensitivity and lead to a reduction of hemoglobin A1C.

You also should know that there's now documented evidence proving a direct relationship between hemoglobin A1C and the future risk of depression. One study that looked at more than four thousand men and women whose average age was sixty-three showed a direct correlation between hemoglobin A1C and "depressive symptoms."[22] Poor glucose metabolism was described as a risk factor for the development of depression in these adults. The bottom line: The glycation of proteins is bad news for the brain.

EARLY ACTION

As I've already described, having normal blood sugar levels may mean that the pancreas is working overtime to keep that blood sugar normal. Based upon this understanding, you can see that high insulin levels will happen long before blood sugar rises and a person becomes diabetic. That's why it's so important to check not only your fasting blood sugar, but also your fasting insulin level. An elevated fasting insulin level is an indicator that your pancreas is trying hard to normalize your blood sugar. It's also a clear signal that you are consuming too much carbohydrate. And make no mistake about it: Even being insulin resistant is a powerful risk factor for brain degeneration and cognitive impairment. It's not good enough to look at the diabetes data as it relates to brain disease and be confident that your risk has been ameliorated because you are not diabetic. And if your blood sugar happens to be normal, the only way you will know if you are insulin resistant is to have your fasting blood insulin level checked. Period.

Need more evidence? Consider an Italian study done back in 2005 that looked at 523 people aged seventy to ninety years who did not have diabetes or even elevated blood sugar.[23] Many of them were insulin resistant, however, as determined by their fasting insulin levels. The study revealed that those individuals who were insulin resistant had a dramatically increased risk of cognitive impairment compared to those within the normal range.

Overall, the lower the insulin level, the better. The average insulin level in the United States is about 8.8 µIU/mL for adult men and 8.4 for women. But with the degree of obesity and carbohydrate abuse in America, it's safe to say that these "average" values are likely much higher than what should be considered ideal. Patients who are being very careful about their carbohydrate intake might have insulin levels indicated on their lab report as less than 2.0. This is an ideal situation—a sign that the individual's pancreas is not being overworked, blood sugars are under excellent control, there is very low risk for diabetes, and there is no evidence of insulin resistance. The important point is that if your fasting insulin level is elevated—anything over 5.0 should be considered elevated—it can improve, and I will show you how to do that in chapter 10.

Before we move on, let me update you on more recent science showing just how bad high blood sugar is on the brain. I know I have already been emphasizing this point, but I want to reiterate it so you don't forget: The impact of blood glucose on the brain is not exclusive to type 2 diabetes. Blood glucose levels *even in the normal range* can have a significant impact on total brain and gray matter atrophy. Translation: Sugar in the blood means shrinkage in the brain. This conclusion came from that 2018 review paper I've already mentioned from a group of Australian researchers who conducted follow-up studies from previous ones.[24] It covered numerous other studies done worldwide to show the strong correlation between blood glucose levels, which again is a factor of carbohydrate consumption, and brain decline and atrophy—despite the presence of diabetes. Which means that the association between blood glucose and brain atrophy and risk for dementia is important even in healthy individuals. In fact, even mild elevations of blood sugar have now been demonstrated to reduce the functionality of various brain regions that are typically involved in Alzheimer's disease. You see, "normal" is poorly defined, and even if your doctor tells you that you're within the "normal" range, you could be on the high end of that range, teetering on the cusp of being diabetic. So it's no surprise that going on a low-carb diet will help control blood sugar and reduce risk for dementia, and this is now fact backed by science. For people who already have type 2 diabetes, the science shows that "the effectiveness of the [low-carbohydrate] diet may be comparable to that of insulin therapy."[25] Also keep in mind that from age sixty onward, the average adult brain atrophies 0.5 percent per year. While this may seem small, it adds up. And now we'll see that brain volume can also be a factor of body fat.

THE FATTER YOUR BODY, THE SMALLER YOUR BRAIN

Most everyone has a pretty good idea that carrying around extra weight is unhealthy. But if you needed just one more reason to drop the excess pounds, perhaps the fear of losing your mind—physically and literally—will help motivate you.

When I was studying to be a doctor, the prevailing wisdom was that fat cells were primarily storage bins where unwanted masses of excess could hang out benignly on the sidelines. But that was a grossly misguided perspective. Today we know that fat cells do more than simply store calories; they are far more involved in human physiology. Masses of body fat form complex, sophisticated hormonal organs that are anything but passive. You read that right: Fat is an *organ*.[26] And it could very well be one of the body's most industrious organs, serving a lot of functions beyond keeping us warm and insulated. This is especially true of visceral fat—the fat wrapped around our internal, "visceral" organs such as the liver, kidneys, pancreas, heart, and intestines. Visceral fat has also gotten a lot of press lately: We know now that this type of fat is the most devastating to our health. We may lament our thunder thighs, under-arm curtains, cellulite, and big butts, but the worst kind of fat is the kind many of us cannot even see, feel, or touch. In extreme cases we do see it in the bulging bellies and muffin tops that are the outward signs of fat-enveloped internal organs belowdecks. (For this very reason, waist circumference is often a measurement of "health," as it predicts future health challenges and mortality; the higher your waist circumference, the higher your risk for disease and death.[27])

It's well documented that visceral fat is uniquely capable of triggering inflammatory pathways in the body as well as signaling molecules that disrupt the body's normal course of hormonal actions.[28] This, in turn, keeps the cascade of negative effects from visceral fat going. In addition, visceral fat does more than just generate inflammation down the road through a chain of biological events; visceral fat itself becomes inflamed. This kind of fat houses tribes of inflammatory white blood cells. In fact, the hormonal and inflammatory molecules produced by visceral fat get dumped directly into the liver, which, as you can imagine, responds with another round of ammunition (i.e., inflammatory reactions and hormone-disrupting substances). Long story short: More than merely a predator lurking behind a tree, visceral fat is an enemy that is armed and dangerous. The number of health conditions now linked to visceral fat is tremendous, from the obvious ones such as obesity and metabolic syndrome to the not-so-obvious—cancer, autoimmune disorders, and brain disease.

The dots connecting excessive body fat, obesity, and brain dysfunction are not hard to follow given the information you've already learned in this book. Excessive body fat increases not only insulin resistance, but also the production of inflammatory chemicals that play directly into brain degeneration.

In a 2005 study, the waist-to-hip ratios of more than one hundred individuals were compared to structural changes in their brains.[29] The study also looked at brain changes in relation to fasting blood sugar and insulin levels. What the authors wanted to determine was whether or not a relationship existed between the brain's structure and the size of a person's belly. And the results were striking. Essentially, the larger a person's waist-to-hip ratio (i.e., the bigger the belly), the smaller the brain's memory center, the hippocampus. The hippocampus plays a critical role in memory, and its function is absolutely dependent upon its size. As your hippocampus shrinks, your memory declines. More striking still, the researchers found that the higher the waist-to-hip ratio, the higher the risk for small strokes in the brain, also known to be associated with declining brain function. The authors stated: "These results are consistent with a growing body of evidence that links obesity, vascular disease, and inflammation to cognitive decline and dementia." Other studies since then have confirmed the finding: For every excess pound put on the body—especially central obesity, as defined by a high waist-to-hip ratio—the brain gets a little smaller. How ironic that the bigger the body gets, the smaller the brain gets.

In a joint research project between UCLA and the University of Pittsburgh, neuroscientists examined brain images of ninety-four people in their seventies who had participated in an earlier study of cardiovascular health and cognition.[30] None of the participants had dementia or other cognitive impairments, and they were followed for five years. What these researchers found was that the brains of obese people—defined by having a body mass index above 30—looked sixteen years older than their healthy counterparts of normal weight. And those who were overweight—defined by having a body mass index between 25 and 30—looked eight years older than their leaner counterparts. More specifically, the clinically obese people had 8 percent less brain tissue, while the overweight had 4 percent less brain tissue compared to normal-weight individuals. Much of the tissue was lost in the frontal and temporal lobe regions of the brain, the place from which we make decisions and store memories, among other things. The authors of the study rightfully pointed out that their findings could have serious implications for aging, overweight, or obese individuals, including a heightened risk for Alzheimer's disease.

Without a doubt, vicious cycles are at play here, each of which is contributing to the other. Genetics could affect one's propensity to overeat and gain weight, and this then factors into activity levels, insulin resistance, and risk for diabetes. Diabetes then affects weight control and blood sugar balance. Once a person becomes diabetic and sedentary, it's inevitable that a breakdown in tissues and organs occurs, and not just in the brain. What's more, once the brain begins to degenerate and physically shrink, it begins to lose its ability to function properly. That is to say, the brain's appetite and weight-control centers won't be firing on all cylinders and could actually be misfiring, and this again feeds the vicious cycle.

It is important to understand that weight loss needs to happen right now, as changes take place as soon as an individual begins to carry excess body fat. To some degree, we can predict whose brain will suffer thirty years from now simply by measuring body fat. In a 2008 report, California scientists combed through the records of more than 6,500 people who were evaluated in the mid-1960s to 1970s.[31] They wanted to know: Who got dementia? When these folks were first evaluated an average of thirty-six years earlier, various measurements were made of their bodies to determine how much fat they had. These included the size of the belly, thigh circumference, and height and weight. Roughly three decades later, those individuals who had more body fat had a dramatically increased risk for dementia. Of the original group, 1,049 were diagnosed as having dementia. When the scientists compared the group with the least body fat to the group with the highest body fat, they found that those in the highest body fat group had an almost twofold increased risk of dementia. The authors reported, "As is the case for diabetes and cardiovascular disease, central obesity [belly fat] is also a risk factor for dementia." I should also note that being overweight in midlife and then losing the weight can still have consequences, which makes a stronger case for avoiding excess weight to begin with. In 2018, a paper out of the UK had some unfortunate findings after following more than ten thousand people over twenty-eight years.[32] Obesity at fifty years old but not at sixty or seventy years old was still associated with risk for dementia. While the conclusions were ominous ("The current obesity epidemic may affect future dementia rates"), my hope is that we can use this data to inspire change today.

A True GB Story

Grain Brain was one of the first books I read when diagnosed with deadly brain cancer, and I truly believe it saved my life. I was diagnosed with "terminal" highly malignant brain cancer in 2013. I embarked on a highly therapeutic ketogenic diet to starve my cancer and boost the mitochondria of my healthy cells, with special help from my own "farm"-acy. Today, three years later, not only am I alive, but thriving as my scans show no cancerous processes at all. An added benefit has been the complete reversal/elimination of polycystic ovary syndrome, Hashimoto's thyroiditis, breast fibroids, joint pain/arthritis, and seasonal allergies, and a very healthy amount of weight loss. My blood work shows massive reductions in inflammation markers, as well as blood sugar! ~ Alison G.

THE POWER OF WEIGHT LOSS (BESIDES WHAT YOU ALREADY KNOW)

As study after study has proven, weight loss through dieting alone or in combination with exercise can have a dramatic effect on insulin signaling and insulin sensitivity.[33]

The take-home lesson is clear: You can improve insulin sensitivity and reduce your risk of diabetes (not to mention all manner of brain diseases) simply by making lifestyle changes that melt away that fat. And if you add exercise to the dieting, you'll stand to gain even bigger benefits. By now you should know that I'm going to prescribe a low-carb diet rich in healthy fats, including cholesterol. And don't take my word for it. Just turn to the latest studies proving the power of this type of diet. In 2012 the *Journal of the American Medical Association* published the effects of three popular diets on a group of overweight or obese young adults.[34] Each of the participants tried each of the diets for a month—one was low-fat (60 percent of the calories came from carbohydrate, 20 percent from fat, and 20 percent from protein), one was low-glycemic (40 percent of the calories came from carbohydrate, 40 percent from fat, and 20 percent from protein), and the third was a very low-carbohydrate diet (10 percent of the calories came from carbohydrates, 60 percent from fat, and 30 percent from protein). All the diets provided the same number of calories, but those on the low-carb, high-fat diet burned the most calories. The study also looked at insulin sensitivity during the four-week period on each diet, finding that the low-carb diet triggered the biggest improvement in insulin sensitivity—almost twice that of the low-fat diet. Triglycerides, a powerful cardiovascular risk marker, averaged 66 in the low-carb group and 107 in the low-fat group. (As an aside, elevated triglyceride levels are also a hallmark of too many carbs in the diet.) The authors pointed out that the lab results they measured in the low-fat diet showed changes in people's blood chemistry that left them vulnerable to weight gain. Clearly, the best diet for maintaining weight loss is a low-carbohydrate, high-fat one.

Many other studies performed since then have arrived at the same conclusion: A low-carb, high-fat diet will outperform a low-fat, high-carb diet any day, and by virtually every measure in the body, from internal chemistry to external waistline. And when we consider all the parameters that affect health, and specifically brain health, such as weight loss, insulin sensitivity, blood sugar control, and even C-reactive protein, a low-carbohydrate diet is substantially more effective than any other diet. Those other diets will result in outcomes that heighten your risk for a multitude of brain dysfunctions, from daily nuisances like headaches to chronic migraines, anxiety disorders, ADHD, and depression. And if the thought of being as sharp as a whip until your last breath on earth isn't enough to motivate you, then consider all the benefits that your heart (and virtually every organ in your body) will gain by ditching a low-fat diet. In March 2013, the *New England Journal of Medicine* published a large landmark study showing that people aged fifty-five to eighty who ate a Mediterranean diet were at lower risk of heart disease and stroke—by as much as 30 percent—than those on a typical low-fat diet.[35] The results were so profound that scientists halted the study early because the low-fat diet proved too damaging for the people eating lots of commercially baked goods rather than sources of healthy fats. The Mediterranean diet is famous for being rich in olive oil, nuts, beans, fish, fruits and vegetables, and even wine with meals. Although it does allow room for grains, it's very similar to my dietary protocol. In fact, if you modify the traditional Mediterranean diet by removing all gluten-containing foods and limiting sugary fruits and non-gluten carbs, you have yourself the perfect grain-brain-free diet. (Note: In 2018, the authors of the original 2013 study published in the *New England Journal of Medicine* retracted their original paper and republished a reanalysis of their data in the same journal following criticism about their methodology.[36] Although there were flaws in their original study, mainly due to the limitations of conducting studies on diet outcomes and controlling for factors the researchers can't really control, the conclusions remained the same.)

The idea of "what's good for the heart is good for the brain" is now fact-backed science. In 2017, the Mediterranean-style diet was again endorsed for brain health when a study was published in *Neurology* showing that older people who adhered closely to the diet enjoyed greater brain volume.[37] The UK-based researchers measured brain volume using magnetic resonance imaging in 401 people when they were seventy-three years old and again when they were seventy-six. Even after adjusting for other factors that could explain the difference in brain volume, such as diabetes, hypertension, and even education, the researchers' conclusions were clear: Lower adherence to a Mediterranean-style diet is predictive of brain atrophy over a three-year period. Interestingly, the participants with the strongest adherence averaged 10 milliliters greater total brain volume than those with the lowest.

DON'T BE FOOLED BY SUGAR SUBSTITUTES

When this book was first published, I did not sound the alarm about sugar substitutes because the studies had yet to emerge. Although we used to think that sugar substitutes like saccharin, sucralose, and aspartame didn't have a metabolic impact because they don't raise insulin, it turns out that they can indeed wreak tremendous metabolic havoc and cause the same metabolic disorders as real sugar. How so? They do this by changing the microbiome in ways that favor bacterial imbalances (dysbiosis), blood sugar imbalances, and an overall unhealthy metabolism. And yes, the food and beverage industry has had a splitting headache over this latest study, which was published in 2014 in the journal *Nature* and has since been replicated in other studies, including ones that show just how bad artificial sweeteners can be: Consuming artificially sweetened "diet" drinks can heighten risk for diabetes, with some studies showing a doubling of the risk for people who drink two diet beverages a day.[38] And you know what that means in terms of risk for Alzheimer's disease. In 2017, the journal *Stroke* also released a bombshell paper when it reported on the risk for stroke, Alzheimer's, and dementia in general among those who drank artificially sweetened drinks. What they found was those who drank one or more artificially sweetened drinks per day had almost a threefold increased risk for stroke, threefold increased risk for Alzheimer's disease, and 2.5 times the risk for developing dementia.[39]

Artificially sweetened soft drinks and dementia risk

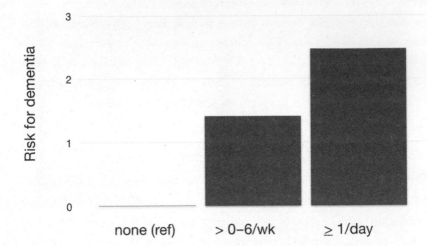

Artificially sweetened soft drinks and Alzheimer's risk

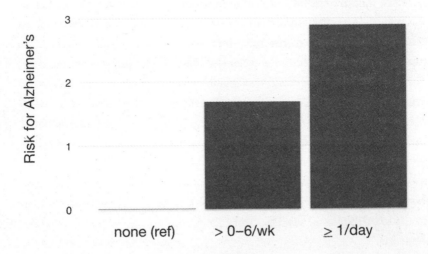

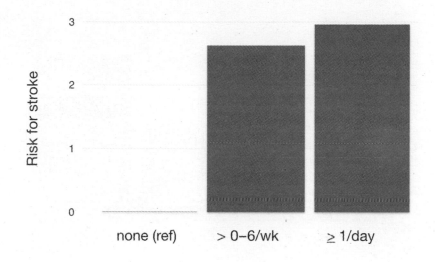

AN APPLE A DAY?

No, an apple a day may not keep the doctor away. Now that I've held so many of your favorite foods in contempt, I can hear the uncertainty: "How can the body live on fat and never get fat?" Ah, it's an excellent question. I'm going to tackle that very conundrum shortly and settle any confusion about how you can live—and thrive—on fats. It sounds absurd to think we can live on virtually no carbs but copious amounts of fat and cholesterol in our diet. But we can, and we should if we're going to protect our genome. Despite what food marketers would have you believe, we've had a fat-based diet shaping our genome for the past 2.6 million years. Why change that? As you've already read, when we did we got *fat*.

The story of reversing this trend and gaining back the lean, toned, lithe bodies we're designed to have, and a sharp brain to boot, starts with a look at the brain's fundamental properties.

CHAPTER 5

The Gift of Neurogenesis and Controlling Master Switches

How to Change Your Genetic Destiny

The brain is a far more open system than we ever imagined, and nature has gone very far to help us perceive and take in the world around us. It has given us a brain that survives in a changing world by changing itself.

— Dr. Norman Doidge (The Brain That Changes Itself)

WE ARE DESIGNED to be smart people our entire lives. The brain is supposed to work well until our last breath. But most of us assume, wrongly, that with age comes cognitive decline. We think it's an inevitable part of aging, much like hearing loss or wrinkles. This impression is a pernicious fallacy. The truth is that we're living a life that's not suited to what we're genetically supposed to do. Period. The diseases we see nowadays are largely brought on by our lifestyle not being in harmony with our genetic predisposition. But we can change this and return our DNA to its original programming. Better yet, we can reprogram some of our DNA to function even more advantageously. And this isn't science fiction.

How often do we hear people say things like, "I'll probably get [insert disease here] because it runs in my family." No doubt our genetic heritage does play a role in determining our risk for various health conditions. But what leading-edge medical research now understands is that we have the power to change our genetic destiny.

One of the hottest areas of research today is epigenetics, the study of particular sections of your DNA (called "marks") that essentially tell your genes when and how strongly to express themselves. Like conductors of an orchestra, these epigenetic marks direct not only your health and longevity but also how you pass on your genes to future generations. Our day-to-day lifestyle choices have a profound effect on the activity of our genes. And this is empowering. We now know that the food choices we make, the stress we experience or avoid, the exercise we get or neglect, the quality of our sleep, and even the relationships we choose actually choreograph to a significant degree which of our genes are active and which remain suppressed. Here's what is most compelling: We can change the expression of more than 70 percent of the genes that have a direct bearing on our health and longevity.

This chapter explains how we can enhance the expression of our "healthy genes" while turning off those genes that trigger such detrimental events as inflammation and the production of free radicals. The genes involved in causing inflammation and free radical production are strongly influenced by fat and carbohydrate dietary choices, and this information will further support the recommendations made in the upcoming chapters.

THE STORY OF NEUROGENESIS

Does every cocktail you drink really kill thousands of brain cells? As it turns out, we are not stuck with the number of neurons we're born with, or even those that develop in early childhood. We can grow new neurons throughout our entire lives. We can also fortify existing brain circuits and create entirely new and elaborate connections, too, with new brain cells. I've been lucky enough to participate in this discovery that has overturned generations of conventional wisdom in neuroscience, though many people still believe otherwise. During my college years I was given the opportunity to explore the brain using technology that was just in its infancy. It was in the early 1970s, and the Swiss had begun developing microscopes that could be used by neurosurgeons performing delicate brain procedures. While this technology was evolving and surgeons in the United States were eager to adopt this new approach to brain surgery, a problem soon became evident.

While learning to actually use the operating microscope was relatively easy, the neurosurgeons found that they were becoming somewhat lost in terms of understanding the anatomy of the brain from this new microscopic perspective. I was nineteen years old and just starting my junior year in college when I received a phone call from Dr. Albert Rhoton, a pioneering neurosurgeon and researcher who became internationally known. (After a storied career spanning five decades at the University of Florida College of Medicine, he passed away in 2016.) At the time he called me, Dr. Rhoton was leading the way for expansion of the use of the operating microscope in the United States and wanted to create the first anatomy text of the brain as seen through the microscope. He invited me to spend the following summer studying and mapping the brain, and it was from this research that we eventually published a series of research papers and book chapters that gave neurosurgeons the needed road map to more carefully operate on the brain.

In addition to anatomy, we also had the opportunity to explore and develop other aspects of microneurosurgery, including innovative instruments and procedures. Spending so much time behind the microscope, I had become quite adept at manipulating and repairing extremely small blood vessels that, prior to the use of the microscope, would have been destroyed during brain operations, often with dire consequences. Our lab had gained international recognition for its achievements in this new and exciting field and often attracted visiting professors from around the world. And it was soon after a delegation of Spanish neurosurgeons had visited that I found myself accepting an invitation to continue my research at the prestigious Centro Ramón y Cajal in Madrid, Spain. Their microneurosurgery program was in its infancy, but their team was dedicated, and I felt honored to be assisting them in their groundwork efforts, especially those dealing with understanding the brain's blood supply. The hospital was named in honor of Dr. Santiago Ramón y Cajal, a Spanish pathologist and neuroscientist working at the turn of the twentieth century, who is still regarded as the father of modern neurology; images of him on the walls were numerous, and there was clearly a deep sense of pride among my Spanish colleagues that they could claim such an influential scientist as their own. In 1906 he won the Nobel Prize in medicine for his pioneering investigations of the microscopic structure of the brain. Today, hundreds of his handmade drawings are still used for educational purposes.

During my visit to Madrid I was compelled to learn more about Dr. Ramón y Cajal and came to deeply respect his explorations of human brain anatomy and function. One of his major tenets held that brain neurons were unique compared to other cells of the body, not only because of their function, but also because they lacked the ability to regenerate. The liver, for example, perpetually regenerates by growing new liver cells, and similar regeneration of cells occurs in virtually all other tissues, including skin, blood, bone, and intestines.

I admit that I was pretty well sold on this theory that brain cells do not regenerate, but I did wonder back then why it wouldn't make sense for the brain to retain the ability to regenerate—to have the ability to grow new brain neurons. After all, researchers at the Massachusetts Institute of Technology had shown previously that neurogenesis, the growth of new brain neurons, occurred in rats throughout their entire lifetime. And so much about the human body is regeneration; it relies on continuous self-renewal to survive. For example, certain blood cells turn over every few hours, taste receptor cells get replaced every ten days, skin cells turn over every month, and muscle cells take about fifteen years to completely renew themselves. In the last decade, scientists have proven that the heart muscle—an organ that we long thought was "fixed" since birth—does in fact experience cellular turnover as well.[1] When we're twenty-five years old, about 1 percent of our heart muscle cells are replaced every year; but by the age of seventy-five, that rate has fallen to less than half a percent per year. If you reach the age of eighty, your heart will have renewed itself—been *replaced*—four times. Put another way, you don't die with the same heart you were born with. Hard to believe that we've only recently come to identify and understand this phenomenon in the body's blood-pumping machine. And now we've finally decoded the brain and discovered its self-renewing qualities.

Dr. Ramón y Cajal couldn't possibly have known just how malleable and "plastic" the brain could be given the technology he was working with. At that time, DNA hadn't been decoded yet and there was little understanding of the impact genes could have on functionality. In his seminal 1928 book *Degeneration and Regeneration of the Nervous System*, Ramón y Cajal stated: "In adult centers the nerve paths are something fixed, ended, immutable. Everything may die, nothing may be regenerated."[2] If I could change his statement to reflect what we know today, I'd swap out the words *fixed, ended,* and *immutable* for the absolute opposite: *pliable, open-ended,* and *alterable.* I'd also say that brain cells may die, but they most certainly *can* be regenerated. Indeed, Ramón y Cajal made great contributions to our knowledge of the brain and how neurons work; he was even ahead of his time in trying to understand the pathology of inflammation. But his belief that the brain was somehow stuck with its bill of goods is one that pervaded for most of human history—until modern science in the late twentieth century proved just how flexible the brain could be.

In an earlier book, *Power Up Your Brain: The Neuroscience of Enlightenment,* Dr. Alberto Villoldo and I told the story of how science has come to understand the gift of neurogenesis in humans. Although scientists have long proven neurogenesis in various other animals, it wasn't until the 1990s that scientists began focusing exclusively on trying to demonstrate neurogenesis in humans.[3] In 1998, the journal *Nature Medicine* published a report by Swedish neurologist Peter Eriksson in which he claimed that within our brains exists a population of neural stem cells that are continually replenished and can differentiate into brain neurons.[4] And indeed, he was right: We all experience brain "stem cell therapy" every minute of our lives. This has led to a new science called neuroplasticity.

The revelation that neurogenesis occurs in humans throughout our lifetimes has provided neuroscientists around the world with an exciting new reference point, with implications spanning virtually the entire array of brain disorders.[5] It also has instilled hope among those searching for clues to stopping, reversing, or even curing progressive brain disease. The idea of regenerating brain neurons has established a new level of excitement in scientists dedicated to studying neurodegenerative disorders. It's also paved the way for novel treatments, transforming the lives of people who have suffered from serious brain injuries or disease. Look no further than Norman Doidge's works *The Brain That Changes Itself: Stories of Personal Triumph from the Frontiers of Brain Science* and *The Brain's Way of Healing: Remarkable Discoveries and Recoveries from the Frontiers of Neuroplasticity* to hear of real-life tales that prove just how pliable our brains—and our human potential— are.[6] If stroke victims can learn to speak again and people born with partial brains can train their brains to rewire themselves to work as a whole, imagine the possibilities for those of us who just hope to preserve our mental faculties.

The burning question: How can we grow new brain neurons? In other words, what influences neurogenesis? And what can we do to enhance this natural process?

The process, as one might expect, is controlled by our DNA. Specifically, a gene located on chromosome 11 codes for the production of a protein called "brain-derived neurotrophic factor," or BDNF. BDNF plays a key role in creating new neurons. But beyond its role in neurogenesis, BDNF protects existing neurons, ensuring their survivability while encouraging synapse formation, the connection of one neuron to another—a process vital for thinking, learning, and higher levels of brain function. Studies have demonstrated decreased levels of BDNF in Alzheimer's patients, which, based on an understanding of how BDNF works, should not come as a surprise.[7] One year after *Grain Brain* was first published, in a seminal study published in the *Journal of the American Medical Association*, researchers at Boston University found that in a group of more than 2,100 elder people followed for ten years, 140 of them developed dementia.[8] Those with the highest levels of BDNF in their blood had less than half the risk for dementia as compared to those who had the lowest levels of BDNF. In comparing those who had the lowest level of BDNF at the beginning of the study with those who had the highest level, those at the highest range of BDNF had as much as a 50 percent reduced risk of developing dementia. So powerful is the relationship between BDNF and Alzheimer's disease that it is now looked upon as representing a "biomarker" to predict the ability of a person to resist cognitive decline with Alzheimer's disease.[9] Levels of BDNF are not just linked to risk for Alzheimer's; it's associated with a variety of neurological conditions, including epilepsy, anorexia nervosa, depression, schizophrenia, and obsessive-compulsive disorder. Newer research has even shown that low levels in women can equate with greater risk for suicide:[10]

The following conditions and behaviors have been scientifically linked to low levels of BDNF:[11]

Alzheimer's disease	Alcohol addiction
Schizophrenia	Neurodevelopmental
Major depressive disorder	disorders
Bipolar disorder	Eating disorders
Anxiety-related disorders	Sleep disorders
Stimulant addiction	History of suicide attempt(s)
Opiate addiction	Obesity

We now have a firm understanding of the factors that influence our DNA to produce BDNF. And fortunately, these factors are mostly under our direct control. The gene that turns on BDNF is activated by a variety of lifestyle habits, including physical exercise, caloric restriction, following a ketogenic diet, and the addition of certain nutrients like curcumin and the omega-3 fat DHA.

This is an empowering lesson because all these factors are within our grasp, representing choices we can make to flip the switch that spurs the growth of new brain cells. Let's explore them individually.

THIS IS YOUR (NEW) BRAIN ON EXERCISE

I'm going to save the bulk of this conversation for chapter 8, which explores in great depth the role of exercise in preventing cognitive decline. The science is stunning. In the 2014 JAMA study I referenced above, the researchers stated, in reference to their results showing the power of BDNF in protecting against cognitive decline: "This is of particular interest because serum BDNF levels can be elevated through simple lifestyle measures such as increased physical activity."[12] Indeed, physical exercise is a like a button on the BDNF-making switch. It's also one of the most potent ways of changing your genes; put simply, when you exercise, you literally exercise your genes. Aerobic exercise in particular not only turns on genes linked to longevity, but also targets the BDNF gene, the brain's "growth hormone." More specifically, aerobic exercise has been shown to increase BDNF, reverse memory decline in elderly humans, and actually increase growth of new brain cells in the brain's memory center. Exercise isn't just for trim looks and a strong heart; perhaps its most powerful effects are going on silently in the upstairs room where our brains reside. The emerging scientific view of human evolution and role of physical activity gives a whole new meaning to the phrase "jog your memory." A million years ago, we triumphed over long distances because we could outrun and outwalk most other animals. This ultimately helped make us the clever human beings we are today. The more we moved, the fitter our brain became. And even today our brain's healthy functioning requires regular physical activity despite the passage of time and ills of the aging process.

CALORIC RESTRICTION

Another epigenetic factor that turns on the gene for BDNF production is calorie restriction. Extensive studies have clearly demonstrated that when animals are on a reduced-calorie diet (typically reduced by around 30 per cent), their brain production of BDNF shoots up and they show dramatic improvements in memory and other cognitive functions. But it's one thing to read experimental research studies involving rats in a controlled environment and quite another to make recommendations to people based upon animal research. Fortunately, we finally have ample human studies demonstrating the powerful effect of reducing caloric intake on brain function, and many of these studies have been published in our most well-respected medical journals.[13]

In January 2009, for example, the *Proceedings of the National Academy of Science* published a study in which German researchers compared two groups of elderly individuals—one that reduced their calories by 30 percent and another that was allowed to eat whatever they wanted. The researchers were interested in whether changes could be measured between the two groups' memory function. At the conclusion of the three-month study, those who were free to eat without restriction experienced a small but clearly defined decline in memory function, while memory function in the group on the reduced-calorie diet actually increased, and significantly so. Knowing that current pharmaceutical approaches to brain health are very limited, the authors concluded, "The present findings may help to develop new prevention and treatment strategies for maintaining cognitive health into old age."[14]

Further evidence supporting the role of calorie restriction in strengthening the brain and providing more resistance to degenerative disease comes from Dr. Mark P. Mattson, chief of the Laboratory of Neurosciences at the National Institute on Aging (NIA). He reported:

> Epidemiological data suggest that individuals with a low calorie intake may have a reduced risk of stroke and neurodegenerative disorders. There is a strong correlation between per capita food consumption and risk for Alzheimer's disease and stroke. Data from population-based case control studies showed that individuals with the lowest daily calorie intakes had the lowest risk of Alzheimer's disease and Parkinson's disease.[15]

Mattson was referring to a population-based longitudinal prospective study of Nigerian families, in which some members moved to the United States. Many people believe that Alzheimer's disease is something you "get" from your DNA, but this particular study told a different story. It was shown that the incidence of Alzheimer's disease among Nigerian immigrants living in the United States was increased compared to their relatives who remained in Nigeria. Genetically, the Nigerians who moved to America were the same as their relatives who remained in Nigeria.[16] All that changed was their environment—specifically, their caloric intake. The research clearly focused on the detrimental effects that a higher caloric consumption has on brain health. In a 2016 study published in *Johns Hopkins Health Review*, Mattson again emphasized the value of caloric restriction in warding off neurodegenerative diseases while at the same time improving memory and mood.[17] One way to do that is through intermittent fasting, which we'll fully explore in chapter 7. Another way, obviously, is to trim back your daily consumption.

If the prospect of reducing your calorie intake by 30 percent seems daunting, consider the following: On average, we consume 23 percent more calories a day than we did in 1970.[18] Based on data from the Food and Agriculture Organization of the United Nations, the average American adult consumes more than 3,600 calories daily.[19] Most would consider "normal" calorie consumption to be around 2,000 calories daily for women and 2,500 for men (with higher requirements depending on level of activity/ exercise). A 30 percent cut of calories from an average of 3,600 per day equals 1,080 calories.

We owe a lot of our increased calorie consumption to sugar. Remember, the average American consumes roughly 163 grams (652 calories) of refined sugars a day—reflecting upward of a 30 percent hike in just the last three decades.[20] And of that amount, about 76 grams (302 calories) are from high-fructose corn syrup. So focusing on just reducing sugar intake may go a long way toward achieving a meaningful reduction in calorie intake, and this would obviously help with weight loss. Indeed, obesity is associated with reduced levels of BDNF, as is elevation of blood sugar. Remember, too, that increasing BDNF provides the added benefit of actually reducing appetite. I call that a double bonus.

But if the figures above still aren't enough to motivate you toward a diet destined to help your brain, in many respects, the same pathway that turns on BDNF production can be activated by intermittent fasting (which, again, I'll detail in chapter 7).

The beneficial effects in treating neurologic conditions using caloric restriction actually aren't news for modern science, though; they have been recognized since antiquity. Calorie restriction was the first effective treatment in medical history for epileptic seizures. But now we know how and why it's so effective: It confers neuroprotection, increases the growth of new brain cells, and allows existing neural networks to expand their sphere of influence (i.e., neuroplasticity).

While low caloric intake is well documented in relation to promoting longevity in a variety of species—including roundworms, rodents, and monkeys—research has also demonstrated that lower caloric intake is associated with a decreased incidence of Alzheimer's and Parkinson's disease. And the mechanisms by which we think this happens are via improved mitochondrial function and controlling gene expression.

Consuming fewer calories decreases the generation of free radicals while at the same time enhancing energy production from the mitochondria, the tiny organelles in our cells that generate chemical energy in the form of ATP (adenosine triphosphate). Mitochondria have their own DNA, and we know now that they play a key role in degenerative diseases such as Alzheimer's and cancer. Caloric restriction also has a dramatic effect on reducing apoptosis, the process by which cells undergo self-destruction. Apoptosis happens when genetic mechanisms within cells are turned on that culminate in the death of that cell. While it may seem puzzling at first as to why this should be looked upon as a positive event, apoptosis is a critical cellular function for life as we know it. Pre-programmed cell death is a normal and vital part of all living tissues, but a balance must be struck between effective and destructive apoptosis. In addition, caloric restriction triggers a decrease in inflammatory factors and an increase in neuroprotective factors, specifically BDNF. It also has been demonstrated to increase the body's natural antioxidant defenses by boosting enzymes and molecules that are important in quenching excessive free radicals.

In 2008, Dr. Veronica Araya of the University of Chile in Santiago reported on a study she performed during which she placed overweight and obese subjects on a three-month calorie-restricted diet, with a total reduction of 25 percent of calories.[21] She and her colleagues measured an exceptional increase in BDNF production, which led to notable reductions in appetite. It's also been shown that the opposite occurs: BDNF production is decreased in animals on a diet high in sugar.[22] Findings like this have since been replicated.

One of the most well-studied molecules associated with caloric restriction and the growth of new brain cells is sirtuin-1 (SIRT1), an enzyme that regulates gene expression. In monkeys, increased SIRT1 activation enhances an enzyme that degrades amyloid—the starch-like protein whose accumulation is the hallmark of diseases like Alzheimer's.[23] In addition, SIRT1 activation changes certain receptors on cells, leading to reactions that have the overall effect of reducing inflammation. Perhaps most important, activation of the sirtuin pathway by caloric restriction enhances BDNF. BDNF not only increases the number of brain cells, but also enhances their differentiation into functional neurons (again, because of caloric restriction). For this reason, we say that BDNF enhances learning and memory.[24]

THE BENEFITS OF A KETOGENIC DIET

While caloric restriction is able to activate these diverse pathways, which are not only protective of the brain but enhance the growth of new neuronal networks, the same pathway can be activated by the consumption of special fats called ketones. By far the most important fat for brain energy utilization is beta-hydroxybutyrate (beta-HBA), and we'll explore this unique fat in more detail in the next chapter. This is why the so-called ketogenic diet has been a treatment for epilepsy since the early 1920s and is now being reevaluated as a therapeutic option in the treatment of Parkinson's disease, Alzheimer's disease, ALS, depression, and even cancer and autism.[25] It's also showing promise for weight loss and ending type 2 diabetes. In mice models, the diet rescues hippocampal memory deficits, and extends healthy lifespan.

Google the term "ketogenic diet" and well over a million results pop up. Between 2015 and 2017, Google searches for the term "keto" increased ninefold. But the studies demonstrating a ketogenic diet's power date back further. In one 2005 study, for example, Parkinson's patients actually had a notable improvement in symptoms that rivaled medications and even brain surgery after being on a ketogenic diet for just twenty-eight days.[26] Specifically, consuming ketogenic fats (i.e., medium-chain triglycerides, or MCT oil) has been shown to impart significant improvement in cognitive function in Alzheimer's patients.[27] Coconut oil, from which we derive MCTs, is a rich source of an important precursor molecule for beta-hydroxybutyrate and is a helpful approach to treating Alzheimer's disease.[28] A ketogenic diet has also been shown to reduce amyloid in the brain,[29] and it increases gluta-thione, the body's natural brain-protective antioxidant, in the hippocam-pus.[30] What's more, it stimulates the growth of mitochondria and thus increases metabolic efficiency.[31]

Dominic D'Agostino is a researcher in neuroscience, molecular pharma-cology, and physiology at the University of South Florida. He has written extensively on the benefits of a ketogenic diet, and in my *Empowering Neu-rologist* interview with him he stated: "Research shows that ketones are pow-erful energy substrates for the brain and protect the brain by enhancing antioxidant defenses while suppressing inflammation. No doubt, this is why nutritional ketosis is something pharmaceutical companies are aggressively trying to replicate." I have also done a lot of homework in understanding the brain benefits of ketosis—a metabolic state whereby the body burns fat for energy and creates ketones in the process. Put simply, your body is in a state of ketosis when it's creating ketones for fuel instead of relying on glucose. And the brain loves it.

While science typically has looked at the liver as the main source of ketone production in human physiology, it is now recognized that the brain can also produce ketones in special cells called astrocytes. These ketone bodies are profoundly neuroprotective. They decrease free radical produc-tion in the brain, increase mitochondrial biogenesis, and stimulate produc-tion of brain-related antioxidants. Furthermore, ketones block the apoptotic pathway that would otherwise lead to self-destruction of brain cells.

Unfortunately, ketones have gotten a bad rap. I remember in my intern-ship being awakened by a nurse to treat a patient in "diabetic ketoacidosis." Physicians, medical students, and interns become fearful when challenged by a patient in such a state, and with good reason. It happens in insulin-dependent type 1 diabetics when not enough insulin is available to metabo-lize glucose for fuel. The body turns to fat, which produces these ketones in dangerously high quantities that become toxic as they accumulate in the blood. At the same time, there is a profound loss of bicarbonate, and this leads to significant lowering of the pH (acidosis). Typically, as a result, patients lose a lot of water due to their elevated blood sugars, and a medical emergency develops.

This condition is exceedingly rare, and again, it occurs in type 1 diabetics who fail to regulate their insulin levels. Our normal physiology has evolved to handle some level of ketones in the blood; in fact, we are fairly unique in this ability among our comrades in the animal kingdom, possibly because of our large brain-to-body weight ratio and the high energy requirements of our brain. At rest, 20 percent of our oxygen consumption is used by the brain, which represents only 2 percent of the human body. In evolutionary terms, the ability to use ketones as fuel when blood sugar was exhausted and liver glycogen was no longer available (during starvation) became mandatory if we were to survive and continue hunting and gathering. Ketosis proved to be a critical step in human evolution, allowing us to persevere during times of food scarcity. To quote Gary Taubes, "In fact, we can define this mild ketosis as the normal state of human metabolism when we're not eating the carbohydrates that didn't exist in our diets for 99.9 percent of human history. As such, ketosis is arguably not just a natural condition but even a particularly healthful one."[32]

There is a relationship between ketosis and calorie restriction, and the two can pack a powerful punch in terms of enhancing brain health. When you restrict calories (and carbs in particular) while upping fat intake, you trigger ketosis and increase levels of ketones in the blood. In 2012, when researchers at the University of Cincinnati randomly assigned twenty-three older adults with mild cognitive impairment to either a high-carbohydrate or very low-carbohydrate diet for six weeks, they documented remarkable changes in the low-carb group.[33] They observed not only improved verbal memory performance but also reductions in weight, waist circumference, fasting glucose, and fasting insulin. Now here's the important point: "Ketone levels were positively correlated with memory performance."

German researchers back in 2009 demonstrated in fifty healthy, normal to overweight elderly individuals that when calories were restricted along with a 20 percent increase in dietary fat, there was a measurable increase in verbal memory scores.[34] Another small study, yes, but their findings were published in the respected *Proceedings of the National Academy of Sciences* and spurred further research like that of the 2012 experiment. These individuals, compared to those who did not restrict calories, demonstrated improvements in their insulin levels and decline in their C-reactive protein, the infamous marker of inflammation. As expected, the most pronounced improvements were in people who adhered the most to the dietary challenge.

Research and interest in ketosis have exploded in recent years and will continue. The key to achieving ketosis, as we'll see later in detail, is to severely cut carbs and increase dietary fat. It's that simple. You have to be carb restricted if you want to reach this brain-blissful state.

CURCUMIN AND DHA

Curcumin, the main active ingredient in the spice turmeric, is currently the subject of intense scientific inquiry, especially as it relates to the brain. It has been used in traditional Chinese and Indian (ayurvedic) medicine for thousands of years. Although it is well known for its antioxidant, anti-inflammatory, antifungal, and antibacterial activities, its ability to increase BDNF in particular has attracted the interest of neuroscientists around the world, especially epidemiologists searching for clues to explain why the prevalence of dementia is markedly reduced in communities where turmeric is used in abundance. In 2018, a study conducted by researchers at UCLA hit the media for its stunning results: People with mild memory problems who took 90 milligrams of curcumin twice daily for eighteen months experienced significant improvements in their memory and attention abilities.[35] They also had a boost in mood. This was a well-designed, double-blind and placebo-controlled study that involved forty adults between fifty and ninety years old. Thirty of the volunteers underwent positron emission tomography (PET) scans to determine the levels of amyloid and tau in their brains at the start of the study and after eighteen months. (Tau proteins are a microscopic component of brain cells that are essential to neuronal survival. But when they undergo chemical changes, they can become damaged or altered and thus harmful.) After the trial, the brain scans showed significantly less amyloid and tau signals in regions of the brain that control memory and emotional functions than those who took placebos. The researchers are embarking on a follow-up study with a larger number of participants. (More on curcumin in chapter 7.)

Perhaps no other brain-boosting molecule is receiving as much attention lately as is docosahexaenoic acid (DHA). For the past several decades, scientists have been aggressively studying this critical brain fat for at least three reasons. First, more than two-thirds of the dry weight of the human brain is fat, and of that fat, one-quarter is DHA. Structurally, DHA is an important building block for the membranes surrounding brain cells, particularly the synapses, which lie at the heart of efficient brain function. Numerous studies have shown a correlation between DHA levels and brain volume, including one from 2014 that assessed more than 1,100 postmenopausal women enrolled in the Women's Health Initiative Memory Study.[36] As with many of these studies, the researchers used MRI brain scans to measure brain volume at the beginning of the study and eight years later. Higher levels of DHA equated with a bigger brain, specifically with regard to hippocampal volume. A previous study, in 2012, found the same results upon examining more than 1,500 men and women who were part of the Framingham Study.[37] This is good news for those of us who want to offset the brain's natural shrinkage with age, because we can take action to consume more DHA.

Second, DHA is an important regulator of inflammation. It naturally reduces the activity of the COX-2 enzyme, which turns on the production of damaging inflammatory chemicals. DHA also acts like a warrior in many ways when it enters hostile territory brought on by poor diet. It can fight back inflammation when a war ensues within the intestinal lining of a gut that is gluten sensitive. And it can block the damaging effects of a diet high in sugar, especially fructose, and help prevent metabolic dysfunctions in the brain that can result from too many carbs in the diet. In 2016, the *American Journal of Clinical Nutrition* reported that DHA beats out another popular omega-3 fatty acid, eicosapentaenoic acid (EPA) in terms of its anti-inflammatory properties. In the researchers' words: "DHA is more effective than EPA in modulating specific markers of inflammation as well as blood lipids."[38]

The third, and arguably most exciting, activity of DHA is its role in regulating gene expression for the production of BDNF. Put simply, DHA helps orchestrate the production, connectivity, and viability of brain cells while at the same time enhancing function.

THE WHOLE GRAIN TRUTH

In a completed double-blind interventional trial, now known by its acronym MIDAS (Memory Improvement with DHA Study), a group of 485 individuals whose average age was seventy and who had mild memory problems were given either a supplement containing DHA from marine algae or a placebo for six months.[39] At the end of the study, not only did blood DHA levels double in the group receiving the DHA, but the effects upon brain function were outstanding. Lead researcher of the study, Dr. Karin Yurko-Mauro, commented: "In our study, healthy people with memory complaints who took algal DHA capsules for six months had almost double the reduction in errors on a test that measures learning and memory performance versus those who took a placebo.... The benefit is roughly equivalent to having the learning and memory skills of someone three years younger."

Another study done of 815 individuals aged sixty-five to ninety-four years found that those who consumed the highest amount of DHA had a breathtaking 60 percent reduction in risk for developing Alzheimer's disease.[40] This level of protection beats other popular fatty acids such as EPA and linolenic acid. The Framingham Heart Study pointed to a magnificent protective effect, too. When researchers compared blood levels of DHA in 899 men and women over a nearly ten-year period, during which some people developed dementia and Alzheimer's, they calculated a 47 percent lower risk for such diagnoses in those who maintained the highest levels of DHA in their blood.[41] The researchers also found that consuming more than two servings of fish per week was associated with a 59 percent reduction in the occurrence of Alzheimer's disease.

When parents ask me how they can address their kids' behavioral problems, I often mention DHA. Because of DHA's role in triggering BDNF, it is important in utero, as well as during infancy and childhood. But many kids today aren't getting enough DHA, and this is partly why we are seeing so many cases of attention deficit hyperactivity disorder (ADHD). I can't tell you how many times I've "cured" ADHD just by recommending a DHA supplement. In chapter 10, I'll give you my dosage recommendations for this important supplement.

How can we increase our DHA? Our bodies can manufacture small amounts of DHA, and we are able to synthesize it from a common dietary omega-3 fat, alpha-linolenic acid. But it's hard to get all the DHA we need from the food we eat, and we can't rely on our body's natural production of it, either. We need at least 200 to 300 milligrams daily, but most Americans consume less than 25 percent of this target and would do well to go beyond this bare minimum. In chapter 10, I'll offer my prescription for ensuring you're getting enough, and show you how to do so easily through dietary and supplementary sources.

INTELLECTUAL STIMULATION BOLSTERS NEW NETWORKS

If common knowledge didn't tell us that keeping the brain intellectually stimulated was a good thing for brain health, then crossword puzzles, continuing education courses, museum hunting, and even reading wouldn't be so popular. And, as it turns out, we know that challenging the mind fortifies new neural networks. Much in the way our muscles gain strength and functionality when physically challenged through exercise, the brain similarly rises to the challenges of intellectual stimulation. The brain becomes not only faster and more efficient in its processing capacity, but also better able to store more information. Again, Dr. Mattson's summary of the proof from the literature is informative: "In regards to aging and age-related neurodegenerative disorders, the available data suggest that those behaviors that enhance dendritic complexity and synaptic plasticity also promote successful aging and decrease risk of neurodegenerative disorders."[42] He goes on to offer several examples. He notes that people with more education have a lower risk for Alzheimer's disease, and that protection from age-related neurodegenerative disorders in general likely begins during the first several decades of life. To this end, Dr. Mattson points to studies that show how individuals with the best linguistic abilities as young adults have a reduced risk for dementia. And he writes that "data from animal studies suggest that increased activity in neural circuits that results from intellectual activity stimulates the expression of genes that play a role in its neuroprotective effects."

THE POWER OF MEDITATION

Meditating is far from a passive activity. Studies show that people who meditate are at much less risk of developing brain disease, among other maladies.[43] Learning to meditate takes time and practice, but it has multiple proven benefits, all of which play into our longevity. Visit my website at DrPerlmutter.com for resources on how to learn this technique.

THE ANTIOXIDANT HOAX[44]

Advertisements proclaiming the virtues of an exotic fruit juice or extract that has the highest antioxidant content on earth are ubiquitous. You may wonder: Why all the hype? What is the benefit of ingesting an antioxidant? As you know by now, antioxidants help control marauding free radicals, and the brain generates tremendous amounts of free radicals but lacks the level of antioxidant protection found elsewhere in the body. Fortunately, we now understand how to compensate for this harmful disparity, but we can't do this by consuming antioxidants themselves. Our DNA can actually turn on the production of protective antioxidants in the presence of specific signals, and this internal antioxidant system is far more powerful than any nutritional supplement. So if you're eating exotic berries or downing vitamins E and C in a bid to outrun those free radicals, consider the following.

In 1956, Dr. Denham Harman demonstrated that free radicals are "quenched" by antioxidants, and the whole antioxidant industry was born.[45] His theories became more refined in 1972 when he recognized that the mitochondria, the actual source of free radicals, are themselves most at risk of free radical damage, and that when mitochondrial function is compromised because of such damage, aging results.[46]

Understanding the powerfully damaging effects of free radicals, especially as they relate to the brain, has encouraged researchers to seek out better antioxidants to provide the brain with a measure of protection in an attempt to not only stave off disease but also enhance function. For example, the relationship between mild cognitive impairment and free radicals was well described in a 2007 report from the late Dr. William Markesbery, then director of the University of Kentucky Sanders-Brown Center on Aging. In this report, Dr. Markesbery and colleagues demonstrated that cognitive function begins to decline early on—well before a brain disease is diagnosed. He also noted that elevated markers for oxidative damage to fat, protein, and even DNA correlate directly to the degree of mental impairment. Markesbery states, "These studies establish oxidative damage as an early event in the pathogenesis of Alzheimer's disease that can serve as a therapeutic target to slow the progression or perhaps the onset of the disease."[47]

The authors continue, "Better antioxidants and agents used in combination to up-regulate defense mechanisms against oxidation will be required to neutralize the oxidative component of the pathogenesis of Alzheimer's disease. It is most likely that to optimize these neuroprotective agents, they will have to be used in the pre-symptomatic phase of the disease." In layman's terms: We need to stimulate our body's innate defense against free radicals long before the signs and symptoms of cognitive decline surface. And when we recognize that if we live to be eighty-five years or older, our risk for Alzheimer's is 50 percent, there are a lot of people who should consider that they are "pre-symptomatic" right now.

If our brain tissue is being assaulted by free radicals, does it make sense to load up on antioxidants? To answer the question, we need to consider our cells' energy suppliers, the mitochondria. In the normal process of producing energy, each mitochondrion produces hundreds if not thousands of free radical molecules each day. Multiply that by the ten million billion mitochondria that we each possess and you come up with an unfathomable number, ten followed by eighteen zeros. One might ask, how effective would, say, a vitamin E capsule or a tablet of vitamin C be when confronted by this onslaught of free radicals? Common antioxidants work by sacrificing themselves to become oxidized when faced with free radicals. Thus, one molecule of vitamin C is oxidized by one free radical. (This one-to-one chemistry is called a stoichiometric reaction by chemists.) Can you imagine how much vitamin C or other oral antioxidant it would take to neutralize the untold number of free radicals generated by the body on a daily basis?

Fortunately, and as one would expect, human physiology has developed its own biochemistry to create more protective antioxidants during times of high oxidative stress. Far from being entirely dependent on external food sources of antioxidants, our cells have their own innate ability to generate antioxidant enzymes on demand. High levels of free radicals turn on a specific protein in the nucleus called Nrf2, which essentially opens the door for the production of a vast array of not only our body's most important antioxidants, but also detoxification enzymes. If excessive free radicals induce better antioxidant production through this pathway, then the next obvious question is, what else activates Nrf2?

Now this is where the story gets really exciting. New research has identified a variety of modifiable factors that can turn on the Nrf2 switch, activating genes that can produce powerful antioxidants and detoxification enzymes. Pharmacologist Dr. Ling Gao has found that when the omega-3 fats EPA and DHA are oxidized, they significantly activate the Nrf2 pathway. For years researchers have noted decreased levels of free radical damage in individuals who consume fish oil (the source of EPA and DHA), but with this new research, the relationship between fish oil and antioxidant protection is now clear. As Dr. Gao reported, "Our data support the hypothesis that the formation of... compounds generated from oxidation of EPA and DHA in vivo can reach concentrations high enough to induce Nrf2-based antioxidant and... detoxification defense systems."[48]

DETOXIFICATION: WHAT IT MEANS FOR BRAIN HEALTH

The human body produces an impressive array of enzymes that serve to combat the large number of toxins to which we are exposed in our external environments as well as those that are generated internally through the course of our normal metabolism. These enzymes are produced under the direction of our DNA and have evolved over hundreds of thousands of years.

Glutathione is regarded as one of the most important detoxification agents in the human brain. A fairly simple chemical, glutathione is a tripeptide, meaning it consists of only three amino acids. But despite its simplicity, glutathione has far-reaching roles in brain health. First, it serves as a major antioxidant in cellular physiology, not only helping protect the cell from free radical damage, but also protecting the delicate and life-sustaining mitochondria. Glutathione is so important as an antioxidant that scientists often measure cellular glutathione levels as an overall indicator of cellular health. Glutathione is a powerful factor in detoxification chemistry as well, binding to various toxins to render them less noxious. Most important, glutathione serves as a substrate for the enzyme glutathione S-transferase, which is involved in transforming a multitude of toxins, making them more water soluble and thus more easily excreted. Deficiencies in the function of this enzyme are associated with a wide range of medical problems, including melanoma, diabetes, asthma, breast cancer, Alzheimer's disease, glaucoma, lung cancer, Lou Gehrig's disease, Parkinson's disease, and migraine headaches, to name a few. With this understanding of the cardinal roles of glutathione as both an antioxidant and a major player in detoxification, it makes sense to do everything possible to maintain and even enhance glutathione levels, which is exactly what my protocol will help you to achieve.

Not surprisingly, calorie restriction has also been demonstrated in a variety of laboratory models to induce Nrf2 activation. When calories are reduced in the diets of laboratory animals, they not only live longer (likely as a result of increased antioxidant protection), but also become remarkably resistant to the development of several cancers. And it is this attribute that further supports the fasting program described in the next chapter.

Several natural compounds that turn on antioxidant and detoxification pathways through activation of the Nrf2 system have been identified. Among these are curcumin from turmeric, green tea extract, silymarin (milk thistle), bacopa extract, DHA, sulforaphane (contained in broccoli), and ashwagandha. Each of these substances is effective in turning on the body's innate production of key antioxidants, including glutathione. And if none of these compounds sounds like something you're used to having daily in your diet, then you'll be happy to know that coffee is one of the most powerful Nrf2 activators in nature. Several molecules in coffee, some of which are partly present in the raw material while others are generated during the roasting process, are responsible for this positive effect.[49]

Aside from antioxidant function, activation of the Nrf2 pathway turns on the genes to produce a vast array of protective chemicals that further support the body's detoxification pathways while dampening inflammation—all good things for brain health.

THE "ALZHEIMER'S GENE"

Since decoding the entire human genome more than fifteen years ago, we've managed to accumulate a great deal of evidence about which genes map to which outcomes, good or bad. If you were paying attention to the news in the early to mid-1990s, you probably learned that science had discovered an "Alzheimer's gene," an association between a particular gene and the risk for Alzheimer's disease. And you likely wondered, *Do I have it?*

First, a quick lesson in biochemistry, courtesy of the National Institute on Aging (part of the National Institutes of Health). Genetic mutations, or permanent changes in one or more specific genes, do not always cause disease. But some do, and if you inherit a disease-causing mutation, then you will likely develop the disease. Sickle cell anemia, Huntington's disease, and cystic fibrosis are examples of inherited genetic disorders. Sometimes, a genetic *variant* can occur, whereby changes in a gene can lead to a disease, but not always. More often, the variant simply increases or decreases one's risk of developing a certain disease or condition. If a variant is known to increase risk but not necessarily trigger disease, it's called a genetic risk factor.[50]

To be clear, scientists have not identified a specific gene that causes Alzheimer's disease. But one genetic risk factor that appears to increase one's risk of developing the disease is associated with the apolipoprotein E (ApoE) gene on chromosome 19. It encodes the instructions for making a protein that helps transport cholesterol and other types of fat in the bloodstream. It comes in several different forms, or alleles. The three main forms are ApoE ε2, ApoE ε3, and ApoE ε4.

ApoE ε2 is relatively rare, but if you inherit this allele, you're more likely to develop Alzheimer's disease later in life. ApoE ε3 is the most common allele, but it's believed to neither increase nor decrease your risk. ApoE ε4, however, is the one typically mentioned in the media and feared the most. In the general population, it's present in about 25 to 30 percent of people, and about 40 percent of all people with Alzheimer's carry this allele. So again, you're probably wondering if you carry this risk factor and what it can mean for you and your future.

Unfortunately, we don't know how this allele increases one's risk for Alzheimer's disease. The mechanism is poorly understood. People who are born with the ApoE ε4 allele are more likely to develop the disease at an earlier age than those who do not carry it. It's important to remember that inheriting an ApoE ε4 allele does not mean that your fate is sealed. You won't necessarily be stricken with Alzheimer's. Some people whose DNA contains the ApoE ε4 allele never suffer from any cognitive decline. And there are plenty of people who develop Alzheimer's but lack any of these genetic risk factors.

A simple DNA screening test can determine if you have this gene, but even if you do, there's something you can do about it. My protocol is all about taking charge of your brain's destiny, despite your DNA. I can't reiterate this enough: The fate of your health — and peace of mind, as the next chapter shows — is largely in your hands.

CHAPTER 6

Brain Drain

*How Gluten Robs Your—and Your
Children's—Peace of Mind*

*As a rule, what is out of sight disturbs men's minds more seriously than
what they see.*

— JULIUS CAESAR

IF SUGARS AND GLUTEN-FILLED CARBS, including your daily whole-grain breads and favorite comfort foods, are slowly impinging on your brain's long-term health and functionality, what else can these ingredients do on a more short-term basis? Can they trigger changes in behavior, seize control of focus and concentration, and underlie some tic disorders and mood conditions like depression? Can they be the culprit in chronic headaches and even migraines?

Yes, they can. The facts of "grain brain" go far beyond just hampering neurogenesis and increasing your risk for cognitive challenges that will progress stealthily over time. As I've already hinted at throughout the previous chapters, a diet heavy in inflammatory carbs and low in healthy fats messes with the mind in more ways than one—affecting risk not just for dementia but for common neurological ailments such as ADHD, anxiety disorder, Tourette's syndrome, mental illness, migraines, and even autism.

Up until now, I've focused primarily on cognitive decline and dementia. Now, let's turn to gluten's destructive effects on the brain from the perspective of these common behavioral and psychological disorders. I'll start with the afflictions that are often diagnosed in young children, and then move on to cover a wider array of issues that are found in people of every age. One thing will be clear: The removal of gluten from the diet and the adoption of a grain-brain-free way of life is often the surest ticket to relief for these brain ailments that plague millions, and this simple "prescription" can often trump drug therapy.

A True GB Story that Transformed an Entire Family

I was diagnosed with hypothyroidism in the fall of 2013 and my doctor prescribed levothyroxine. I saw some improvement of my symptoms initially but as time went by, they all returned. I became very frustrated and turned to the Internet for information and advice. I learned that gluten can damage the thyroid and asked my doctor if he thought I should go gluten-free. His response: "It's a gimmick." So, I continued to take my medication and feel miserable. The next spring, I decided to give up carbohydrate-filled snacks for Lent. Within forty-eight hours, I felt better than I had in a long time. It made me think about my diet, so I did some more research about gluten and decided to give it up to see if that helped. I jumped in headfirst and implemented this into my diet and life. I was able to get off the thyroid medication and my bloodwork has been great ever since.

My youngest son has always been sick. He has battled chronic asthma and a myriad of other maladies since birth. During the spring of 2014, his health took a turn for the worse. I removed the gluten from his diet, but he still missed the last two months of school due to illness. Toward the end of that school year, he received the diagnosis of reflex neurovascular dystrophy. We were able to rehab him with a lot of physical therapy in the form of hiking. He was doing fairly well at the beginning of the 2015 school year, but his diet slipped a bit from strict gluten-free. The next thing we knew, he was getting sickness after sickness again, and becoming overweight. He wound up missing the last two months of that school year as well. I knew I had to force him to adapt to the low-carb, gluten-free way of eating. It was not easy with a thirteen-year-old child. There were many diffi-cult times as we navigated through what he could and could not have. I also found a functional medicine doctor, who helped us reach a diagnosis of Candida and a very low-functioning immune system. Thanks to his new lifestyle, he has lost an astounding 18 pounds in about nine months! He has continued to thrive and his immune sys-tem has never been better.

My husband has also adapted to this way of eating. He concluded a couple of years before I had my issues that he had Candida and tried different strategies, including a calorie-restrictive diet. When he saw how much the *Grain Brain* protocol helped me, he gave it a try and has seen a big difference in the way he feels. If he goes off the track, he notices it right away.

My daughter has had headaches, chronic sinus infections, and stomachaches for years. She thought I was crazy when I was so excited about *Grain Brain* and was making so many changes in the house. I did not force her, but I spoke ad nauseam about the benefits of this lifestyle. I knew that she would not acquiesce unless it was her decision and under her terms. She came to her own conclusion a year ago to go gluten-free and realized what a huge difference it made in her life. I convinced her to get rid of all grains about two months ago and we are currently working on her sugar intake as she still eats more fruit than she should.

Grain Brain has tremendously helped each member of our family. This book opened my eyes to all that is wrong with our food supply, not to mention the way doctors are trained in medical school. I am so incredibly thankful for this information and I will be grain-free for the rest of my life. ~ Wendy S.

GLUTEN'S ROLE IN BEHAVIORAL AND MOVEMENT DISORDERS

I first saw Stuart when he had just turned four years old. He was brought to my center by his mother, Nancy, whom I had known for several years; she was a physical therapist who had treated many of our patients. Nancy began by describing her concerns about Stuart and reported that although she really hadn't noticed anything wrong with her son, his preschool teacher felt he was unusually "active" and felt it would be a good idea to have him evaluated. I was not the first doctor to see him because of this concern. The week before visiting us, Stuart's mom had taken him to their pediatrician, who proclaimed that Stuart "was ADHD" and had written a prescription for Ritalin.

Nancy was rightfully concerned about placing her son on the drug, and this prompted her to look into other options. She began by explaining that her son had frequent anger outbursts and that he "shook uncontrollably when frustrated." She described how the preschool teacher complained that Stuart was unable to "stay on task," making me wonder exactly what tasks require undivided focus in a four-year-old.

Stuart's past medical history was revealing. He had suffered lots of ear infections and had been on countless rounds of antibiotics. At the time I evaluated him, he was on a six-month course of prophylactic antibiotics in hopes of reducing his risk for continued ear infections. But beyond the ear problems, Stuart persistently complained of joint pain, so much so that he was now also taking Naprosyn, a powerful anti-inflammatory, on a regular basis. I assumed Stuart hadn't been breast-fed and learned that my assumption was correct.

Three things of importance were noted during his examination. First, he was a mouth-breather, a sure indication of ongoing inflammation in the nasal passages. Second, his face demonstrated classic "allergic shiners," dark circles under the eyes that correlate with allergies. And third, he was indeed very active. He couldn't sit still for more than ten seconds, getting up to explore every inch of the exam room and tearing up the crinkly paper that adorns most doctors' examination tables.

Rather than reach for a drug to treat symptoms, we decided instead to target the cause of this child's issues, namely, inflammation. Inflammation was playing a central role in virtually everything going on in this young boy's physiology, including his ear problems, joint issues, and inability to compose himself.

I explained to Nancy that we had to go gluten-free. And to help rebuild a healthy gut after his extensive antibiotic exposure, we needed to add some beneficial bacteria, probiotics, to his regimen. Finally, the omega-3 fat DHA was added to the list.

What happened next couldn't have been scripted any better. After two and a half weeks, Stuart's parents received a phone call from his preschool teacher thanking them for deciding to put him on medication as he had "vastly improved" in his demeanor. And his parents noted that he had become calm and more interactive, and was sleeping better. But his transformation wasn't due to medication. It was purely through diet that he was able to realize "vast" improvements in his health and attitude.

I received a note from Nancy two and a half years later stating: "We have been able to start him in school as the youngest student in the class. He has been able to excel in reading and math, and we do not anticipate any further problems with him being hyperactive. He has been growing so fast that he is one of the tallest kids in his class."

Attention deficit hyperactivity disorder (ADHD) is one of the most frequent diagnoses offered in the pediatrician's office. Parents of hyperactive children are led to believe that their children have some form of a disease that will limit their ability to learn. The medical establishment too often convinces parents that medication is the best "quick fix." The whole notion that ADHD is a specific disease easily remedied by a pill is convenient but alarming. In some schools across the United States, as many as 25 percent of students are routinely receiving powerful, mind-altering medications, the long-term consequences of which have never been studied!

Although the American Psychiatric Association states in its *Diagnostic and Statistical Manual of Mental Disorders* that roughly 5 percent of school-aged children have ADHD, studies have estimated higher rates in community samples, and data from surveys of parents collected by the Centers for Disease Control and Prevention (CDC) paint a different picture.[1] According to the latest data from the CDC, which came out in 2016, approximately 9.4 percent of children aged two to seventeen years have been diagnosed with ADHD. That translates to an estimated 6.1 million children; Kentucky ranks the highest with a staggering 18.7 percent of children diagnosed.[2] As reported by the *New York Times*, "About two-thirds of those with a current diagnosis receive prescriptions for stimulants like Ritalin or Adderall, which can drastically improve the lives of those with ADHD but can also lead to addiction, anxiety, and occasionally psychosis."[3] This has prompted the American Psychiatric Association to consider changing its definition of ADHD so more people are diagnosed — and treated with drugs. Dr. Thomas R. Frieden, the former director of the CDC, has said that the rising rates of stimulant prescriptions among children are like the overuse of pain medications and antibiotics in adults, and I agree. In the words of Dr. Jerome Groopman, a professor of medicine at Harvard Medical School and prolific writer, who was interviewed for the *Times,* "There's a tremendous push where if the kid's behavior is thought to be quote-unquote abnormal — if they're not sitting quietly at their desk — that's pathological, instead of just childhood."[4] So what does it mean when our definition of childhood gets trampled by fuzzy diagnoses like ADHD? I also find it interesting that the U.S. significantly outpaces the rest of the world in its consumption of stimulant drugs (e.g., Adderall and Ritalin) used to treat the symptoms of ADHD. Although children are still the primary users of these drugs, the number of adults using them has been increasing at a much faster pace lately. I am saddened by the fact that the billion-dollar psychotropic pharmaceutical industry is predicated on the idea that people will take a pill to treat symptoms, while the underlying disorder is ignored.

Aside from the dramatic rise in the use of medications to treat ADHD over the past decade, the use of psychiatric drugs has soared: One in six Americans now takes a psychiatric drug to treat psychological and behavioral disorders. These include antidepressants, anxiety relievers, and antipsychotics. Interestingly, women are far more likely to take a drug for a mental health condition than men: 21 percent compared with 12 percent.[5] (Harvard researchers theorize that this could be due to hormonal changes in women that are linked to puberty, pregnancy, and menopause. Although depression can affect men and women equally, women are typically more likely to seek medical help.) The CDC reports a fivefold increase in the number of children under age eighteen on psychostimulants from the period 1988 to 1994 to the period 2007 to 2010, with the most recent rate of 4.2

percent published in 2014. The rate of antipsychotic prescriptions for children has increased sixfold over these two periods, according to a study of office visits within the National Ambulatory Medical Care Survey.[6]

Eleven percent of Americans over age twelve take antidepressants, but the percentage skyrockets when you look at the number of women in their forties and fifties who have been prescribed antidepressants—a whopping 23 percent.

Given the soaring rates of mental and behavioral disorders for which powerful drugs are increasingly used, why isn't anyone drawing attention to the underlying reasons for this trend? And how can we propose solutions that don't entail hazardous pharmaceuticals? At the root of the problem? That sticky wheat protein, gluten. Although the jury is still out on the connections between gluten sensitivity and behavioral or psychological issues, we do know a few facts:

- People with undiagnosed and untreated celiac disease may be at increased risk for developmental delay, learning difficulties, tic disorders, and ADHD.[7]

- Depression and anxiety are often severe in patients with gluten sensitivity.[8] This is primarily due to the cytokines that block production of critical brain neurotransmitters like serotonin, which is essential in regulating mood. With the elimination of gluten and often dairy, many patients have been freed from not just their mood disorders but other conditions caused by an overactive immune system, like allergies and arthritis.

- As many as 45 percent of people with autism spectrum disorders (ASD) have gastrointestinal problems.[9] Although not all gastrointestinal symptoms in ASD result from celiac disease, data shows an increased prevalence of celiac in pediatric cases of autism, compared to the general pediatric population.

The good news is that we can reverse many of the symptoms of neurological, psychological, and behavioral disorders just by going gluten-free and adding supplements like DHA and probiotics to our diet. And to illustrate the impact of such a simple, drug-free prescription, consider the story of KJ, whom I met more than a decade ago. She was five years old at the time and had been diagnosed with Tourette's syndrome, a type of tic spectrum disorder characterized by sudden, repetitive, nonrhythmic movements (motor tics) and verbal utterances that involve discrete muscle groups. Science says that the exact cause of this neurological anomaly is unknown, but we do know that, like many neuropsychiatric disorders, it has genetic roots that can be worsened by environmental factors. I think future research will bear out the truth behind many cases of Tourette's and show gluten sensitivity at play

At KJ's initial office visit, her mother explained that in the previous year her daughter had developed involuntary contractions of her neck muscles for unknown reasons. She had received various types of massage therapy, which provided some improvement, but the problem would come and go. It eventually worsened to the point that KJ had aggressive movements in her jaw, face, and neck. She also persistently cleared her throat and produced various grunting noises. Her primary doctor had diagnosed Tourette's syndrome.

When taking her history I noted that three years prior to the onset of her serious neurological symptoms, she'd begun to have bouts of diarrhea and chronic abdominal pain that were still with her. Two days after starting a gluten-free diet, *all* of the abnormal movements, throat clearing, grunting sounds, and even abdominal pain had vanished. To this day, KJ is symptom-free and can no longer be considered a person with Tourette's syndrome. So compelling was her response that I often use this case when lecturing to health-care professionals.

Warning: Drugs used to treat ADHD have resulted in cases of permanent Tourette's syndrome. Science has been documenting this since the early 1980s.[10] Now that we have the research to prove the powerful effect of going gluten-free, it's time we change—no, *make*—history.

Another case I'd like to share brings us back to ADHD. The parents of KM, a sweet nine-year-old girl, brought her to me because of classic signs of ADHD and "poor memory." What was interesting about her history was that her parents described her difficulties with thinking and focusing as "lasting for days," after which she would remain "fine" for several days. Academic evaluations indicated she was functioning at a mid-third-grade level. She seemed very composed and engaged, and when I reviewed her various achievement tests, I confirmed that she was indeed functioning at a level typical for her age.

Lab work identified two potential culprits in her challenges: gluten sensitivity and below-normal blood levels of DHA. I prescribed a strict gluten-free diet and 400 milligrams of supplemental DHA daily, and asked her to stop consuming aspartame, or NutraSweet, as she drank several diet sodas a day. Three months later, her mom and dad were thrilled with her progress, and even KM was smiling ear to ear. New academic testing had her math calculation skills at the early fifth-grade level, overall academic skills at the mid-fourth-grade level, and story recall ability at the mid-eighth-grade level.

To quote a letter I received from her mother:

> [KM] is completing third grade this year. Prior to removing gluten from her diet, academics, especially math, were difficult. As you can see, she is now soaring in math. Based upon this test, entering the fourth grade next year she would be at the top of her class. The teacher indicated if she skipped fourth grade and went to fifth grade, she would be in the middle of the class. What an accomplishment!

Stories like this are commonplace in my practice. I've known about the "achievement effect" from going gluten-free for a long time, but thankfully the scientific proof is finally catching up to the anecdotal evidence. One study that really stood out for me was published in 2006; it documented a very revealing "before and after" story of people with ADHD who went gluten-free for six months. What I love about this particular study is that it examined a broad spectrum of individuals—from the age of three to fifty-seven years—and it employed a well-respected behavioral scale for ADHD called the Conners Comprehensive Behavior Rating Scale. After six months, the improvements were significant:[11]

"No close attention to details" was reduced by 36 percent.

"Difficulty sustaining attention" was reduced by 12 percent.

"Fails to finish work" diminished by 30 percent.

"Easily distracted" diminished by 46 percent.

"Often blurts out answers and quotes" diminished by 11 percent.

The overall "average score" for those studied was lowered by 27 percent. My hope is that more people will join my crusade and take action to make us all healthier—and smarter.

HOW C-SECTIONS INCREASE RISK OF ADHD

Babies who are born via cesarean section have a higher risk of developing ADHD, but why? Understanding the links in the chain gives credence to the importance of healthy gut bacteria to sustain intestinal health and overall wellness. When a baby passes through the birth canal naturally, billions of beneficial bacteria wash over the child, thereby inoculating the newborn with appropriate probiotics, whose pro-health effects remain for life. If a child is born via C-section, however, he or she misses out on this shower of sorts, and this sets the stage for bowel inflammation and, therefore, an increased risk of sensitivity to gluten and ADHD later in life.[12]

New research is also giving moms another reason to breast-feed, as babies who are regularly breast-fed when they are first introduced to foods containing gluten have been shown to cut their risk of developing celiac disease by 52 percent, compared with those who are not being breast-fed.[13] One of the reasons for this might be that breast-feeding cuts the number of gastrointestinal infections, lowering the risk of a compromised lining of the bowel. It may also curb the immune response to gluten.

CAN AUTISM BE TREATED WITH A GLUTEN-FREE DIET?

I get a lot of questions about the possible relationship between gluten and autism. As many as 1 in 150 children born today will develop a form of the condition across a wide spectrum; in 2015, a new government survey of parents reported that one in forty-five children aged three to seventeen— more than a million children—has been diagnosed with autism spectrum disorder (ASD).[14] This is notably higher than the official government estimate of one in sixty-eight American children with autism, by the Centers for Disease Control and Prevention.[15] A neurological disorder that usually appears by the time a child is three years old, autism affects the development of social and communication skills. Scientists are trying to figure out the exact causes of autism, which is likely rooted in both genetic and environmental origins. A number of risk factors are being studied, including genetic, infectious, metabolic, nutritional, and environmental, but less than 10 to 12 percent of cases have specific causes that can be identified.

We know there is no magic-bullet cure for autism, just as there isn't for schizophrenia or bipolar disorder. These brain maladies are uniquely different, but they all share one underlying characteristic: inflammation, some of which could simply be the result of sensitivity to dietary choices. While it remains a topic of debate, some people who suffer from autism respond positively to the removal of gluten, sugar, and sometimes dairy from their diets. In one particularly dramatic case, a five-year-old diagnosed with severe autism was also found to have serious celiac disease that prevented him from absorbing nutrients. His autistic symptoms abated once he went gluten-free, prompting his doctors to recommend that all children with neurodevelopmental problems be assessed for nutritional deficiencies and malabsorption syndromes like celiac. In some cases, nutritional deficiencies that affect the nervous system may be the root cause of developmental delays that mirror autism.[16]

I'll admit that we lack the kind of gold-standard scientific research that we need to draw any conclusive connections, but it's worth taking a sweeping view of the topic and considering some logical inferences.

Let me begin by pointing out a parallel trend in the rise of autism and celiac disease. That is not to say the two are categorically linked, but it's interesting to note a similar pattern in sheer numbers. What these two conditions do indeed have in common, however, is the same fundamental feature: inflammation. As much as celiac is an inflammatory disorder of the gut, autism is an inflammatory disorder of the brain. It's well documented that autistic individuals have a higher level of inflammatory cytokines in their system. For this reason alone, it's worthwhile to ponder the effectiveness of reducing all antibody–antigen interactions in the body, including those involving gluten.

One early study from the United Kingdom published in 1999 showed that when twenty-two autistic children on a gluten-free diet were monitored over a five-month period, a number of behavioral improvements were recorded. Most alarming, when the children accidentally ingested gluten after they'd started their gluten-free diet, "the speed with which behavior changed as a result…was dramatic and noticed by many parents."[17] The study also noted that it took at least three months for the children to show an improvement in their behavior. For any parent regulating a child's diet, it's important to not lose hope early on if behavioral changes don't occur right away. Stay the course for three to six months before expecting any noticeable improvement.

Some experts have questioned whether those morphine-like compounds I defined earlier—exorphins—are partly to blame. When gluten-containing foods and milk proteins cause exorphins to be released, they may stimulate various receptors in the brain and raise the risk not just for autism but for schizophrenia as well.[18] More research is needed to flesh out these theories, but we can potentially reduce the risks of developing these conditions and better manage them.

Despite the lack of research, it is clear that the immune system plays a role in the development of autism, and that the same immune system connects gluten sensitivity to the brain. There's also something to be said for the "layering effect," where one biological issue ushers in another down a chain of events. If a child is acutely sensitive to gluten, for instance, the immune response in the gut can lead to behavioral and psychological symptoms, and in autism this can lead to an "exacerbation of effects," as one team of researchers put it.[19]

DOWN AND OUT

It's a heartbreaking fact I called out earlier. Depression is the leading cause of disability worldwide. It's also the fourth leading contributor to the global burden of disease. The World Health Organization has estimated that by the year 2020, depression will become the second largest cause of suffering — next only to heart disease. In many developed countries, such as the United States, depression is already among the top causes of mortality.[20]

What's even more disquieting is the white elephant sitting in the medicine cabinets of many depressed people: the bottles of so-called antidepressants. Drugs like Prozac, Paxil, Zoloft, and countless others are by far the most common treatments for depression in the United States, despite the fact that they have been shown in many cases to be no more effective than a placebo and in some cases can be exceedingly dangerous and even lead to suicides. New science is starting to show just how murderous these drugs can be. To wit: When researchers in Boston looked at more than 136,000 women between the ages of fifty and seventy-nine, they discovered an undeniable link between those who were using antidepressants and their risk for strokes and death in general. Women on antidepressants were 45 percent more likely to experience strokes and had a 32 percent higher risk of death from all causes.[21] The findings, published in the *Archives of Internal Medicine*, came out of the Women's Health Initiative, a major public health investigation focusing on women in the United States. And it didn't matter whether people were using newer forms of antidepressants, known as selective serotonin reuptake inhibitors (SSRIs), or older forms known as tricyclic antidepressants, such as Elavil. SSRIs are typically used as antidepressants, but they can be prescribed to treat anxiety disorders and some personality disorders. They work by preventing the brain from reabsorbing the neurotransmitter serotonin. By changing the balance of serotonin in the brain, neurons send and receive chemical messages better, which in turn boosts mood.

Unsettling studies have reached a tipping point, and some Big Pharma companies are backing away from antidepressant drug development (though they still make a lot of money in this department—to the tune of more than 15 billion dollars a year globally). As reported in the *Journal of the American Medical Association*, "The magnitude of benefit of antidepressant medication compared with placebo increases with severity of depression symptoms and may be minimal or nonexistent, on average, in patients with mild or moderate symptoms."[22]

This isn't to say that certain medications aren't helpful in some severe cases, but the implications are huge. Let's briefly review some other intriguing findings that will inspire anyone thinking of taking an antidepressant to try another route to happiness.

Low Mood and Low Cholesterol

I've already made my case for cholesterol in nourishing the brain's health. As it turns out, innumerable studies have demonstrated that depression runs much higher in people who have low cholesterol.[23] And people who start taking cholesterol-lowering medication (statins) can become much more depressed.[24] I've witnessed this myself in my own practice. It's unclear if the depression is a direct result of the drug itself, or if it simply reflects a consequence of a lowered cholesterol level—or a combination thereof, which is the explanation I favor.

Studies dating back to the 1990s show a connection between low total cholesterol and depression, not to mention impulsive behaviors including suicide and violence. Dr. James M. Greenblatt, a dually certified child and adult psychiatrist and author of *The Breakthrough Depression Solution*, wrote a beautiful article for *Psychology Today* in 2011 in which he summarized the evidence.[25] In 1993, elderly men with low cholesterol were found to have a 300 percent higher risk of depression than their counterparts with higher cholesterol.[26] A 1997 Swedish study identified a similar pattern: Among three hundred otherwise healthy women aged thirty-one to sixty-five, those in the bottom tenth percentile for cholesterol levels experienced significantly

more depressive symptoms than the others in the study with higher cholesterol levels.[27] In 2000, scientists in the Netherlands reported that men with
long-term low total cholesterol levels experienced more depressive symptoms than those with higher cholesterol levels.[28] According to a 2008 report
published in the *Journal of Clinical Psychiatry*, "Low serum cholesterol may
be associated with suicide attempt history."[29] The researchers looked at a
group of 417 patients who had attempted suicide — 138 men and 279
women — and compared them with 155 psychiatric patients who had not
attempted suicide, as well as 358 healthy control patients. The study defined
low serum cholesterol as less than 160. The results were quite dramatic. It
showed that individuals in the low-cholesterol category were 200 percent
more likely to have attempted suicide. And in 2009, the *Journal of Psychiatric
Research* published a study that followed nearly 4,500 U.S. veterans for fifteen years.[30] Depressed men with low total cholesterol levels faced a seven-
fold increased risk of dying prematurely from unnatural causes such as
suicide and accidents than the others in the study. As noted earlier, suicide
attempts have long been shown to run higher in people who have low total
cholesterol.

I could go on and on showcasing studies from all around the world that
arrive at the same conclusion for both men and women: If you've got low
cholesterol, you've got a much higher risk of developing depression. And the
lower you go, the closer you are to harboring thoughts of suicide. I don't
mean to say this in a casual manner, but we have documented proof now
from many respected institutions of just how serious this cause-and-effect
relationship is. This relationship is also well documented in the field of bipolar disorder.[31] Those who are bipolar are much more likely to attempt suicide
if they have low cholesterol.

The Gluten Blues

Science has long observed an overlap between celiac disease and depression,
much like the overlap between celiac and ADHD and other behavioral disorders. Reports of depression among celiac disease patients began appearing
in the 1980s. In 1982 Swedish researchers reported that "depressive psycho-

pathology is a feature of adult celiac disease."[32] A 1998 study determined that about one-third of those with celiac disease also have depression.[33] More recently, in a 2015 review paper, a large group of researchers from both Europe and Argentina underscored the psychological burden of celiac disease, calling on health-care professionals to pay attention to these patients in particular.[34]

Let's go back to some of these important studies. In one particularly large study published in 2007, Swedish researchers again evaluated close to fourteen thousand celiac patients and compared them to more than sixty-six thousand healthy controls.[35] They wanted to know the risk of being depressed if you have celiac disease as well as the risk of having celiac disease if you are depressed. It turned out that celiac patients had an 80 percent higher risk of depression, and the risk of actually being diagnosed with celiac disease in individuals who were depressed was increased 230 percent. In 2011, another study from Sweden found that the risk of suicide among people with celiac disease was increased by 55 percent.[36] Yet another study done by a team of Italian researchers found that celiac disease ups one's risk of major depression by a stunning 270 percent.[37]

A logical question: How does depression relate to a damaged intestine? Once the lining of the gut is injured by celiac disease, it is ineffective at absorbing essential nutrients, many of which keep the brain healthy, such as zinc, tryptophan, and the B vitamins. What's more, these nutrients are necessary ingredients in the production of neurological chemicals such as serotonin. Also, the vast majority of feel-good hormones and chemicals are produced around your intestines by what scientists now call your "second brain."[38] The nerve cells in your gut are not only regulating muscles, immune cells, and hormones, but also manufacturing an estimated 80 to 90 percent of your body's serotonin. In fact, your intestinal brain makes more serotonin than the brain that rests in your skull.

Some of the more critical nutritional deficiencies that have been linked to depression include vitamin D and zinc. You already know the importance of vitamin D in a multitude of physiological processes, including mood regulation. Zinc similarly is a jack-of-all-trades in the body's mechanics. In addition to aiding the immune system and keeping memory sharp, zinc is required in the production and use of those mood-friendly neurotransmitters. This helps explain why supplemental zinc has been shown to enhance the effects of antidepressants in people with major depression. (Case in point: A 2009 study found that people who hadn't been helped by antidepressants in the past finally reported improvements once they started to supplement with zinc.[39]) Dr. James M. Greenblatt, whom I mentioned a few pages ago, has written extensively on this topic and, like me, sees a lot of patients whose antidepressants have failed them. Once these patients avoid foods containing gluten, their psychological symptoms resolve. In another article for *Psychology Today*, Greenblatt writes: "Undiagnosed celiac disease can exacerbate symptoms of depression or may even be the underlying cause. Patients with depression should be tested for nutritional deficiencies. Who knows, celiac disease may be the correct diagnosis and not depression."[40] Many physicians ignore nutritional deficiencies and don't think about testing for gluten sensitivity because they are so used to (and comfortable with) writing prescriptions for medication.

It's important to note that a common thread in many of these studies is the length of time needed to turn things around in the brain. As with other behavioral disorders, such as ADHD and anxiety disorder, it can take at least three months for individuals to feel a total sense of relief. It's critical to stay the course once embarking on a gluten-free diet. Don't lose hope if you don't have significant improvements right away. But do realize that you're likely to experience a dramatic improvement in more ways than one. I once treated a professional tennis instructor who was crippled by depression and not improving despite the use of multiple antidepressant medications prescribed by other doctors. When I diagnosed his sensitivity to gluten and he adopted a gluten-free diet, he was transformed. His depressive symptoms evaporated, and he returned to peak performance on the court.

When it comes to the link between gluten and brain-related disorders like depression, we also can't forget about the role of inflammation. One of the facts that have come to light in the scientific literature more recently is that depression is now considered an inflammatory disorder. We now understand that inflammatory markers, the same that we see elevated in heart disease, are also elevated in the depressed patient. This is actually not "new" information, but if you were to ask someone on the street about depression, you'd be likely to hear something along the lines of "It's a chemical imbalance in the brain." The role of inflammation in mental illness—from depression to schizophrenia—has been documented over the past twenty years.[41] The field of psychiatry has known about the role of the immune system in the onset of depression for the better part of the last century. But only recently have we begun to understand the connection, thanks to better technology and longitudinal studies.[42] Higher levels of inflammation dramatically increase the risk of developing depression. And the higher the levels of inflammatory markers, the worse the depression. This places depression right in line with other inflammatory disorders such as Parkinson's disease, multiple sclerosis, and Alzheimer's disease.

Some of the studies have been downright eye-opening. For example, when scientists give healthy people with no signs of depression an infusion of a substance to trigger inflammation, classic depressive symptoms develop almost instantly. Similarly, it's been shown that when people are given interferon for the treatment of hepatitis C, which increases inflammatory cytokines, a quarter of those individuals develop major depression.[43] Interferons are a group of naturally occurring proteins that form an integral part of the immune system, but they can be made and given as a drug to treat certain viral infections. What's even more compelling is new research demonstrating that antidepressant medications may work in some people by virtue of their ability to decrease inflammatory chemicals. Put another way, the actual mechanism for modern antidepressants may have nothing at all to do with their effect on brain chemicals and everything to do with decreasing inflammation.

MENTAL STABILITY THROUGH DIET

All this talk about gluten's insidious connection to common psychological disorders no doubt raises questions about gluten's role in virtually every ailment that involves the mind, from the most common mental disorder in America—anxiety, which affects approximately forty million adults—to complex afflictions such as schizophrenia and bipolar disorder.

What does the science say about gluten and our more perplexing mental illnesses such as schizophrenia and bipolar disorder? These are complicated maladies for which genetic and environmental factors are in play, but study after study demonstrates that people with these diagnoses often show gluten sensitivity as well. And if they have a history of celiac disease, they are at much higher risk of developing these psychiatric disorders than anyone else. What's more, we now have documented evidence that mothers who are sensitive to gluten give birth to children who are nearly 50 percent more likely to develop schizophrenia later in life.

The 2012 study, published in the *American Journal of Psychiatry,* adds to a growing body of evidence that many diseases that show up later in life originate before and shortly after birth. The authors of the study, who hail from Johns Hopkins and Sweden's Karolinska Institute, one of Europe's largest and most prestigious medical universities, stated the facts beautifully: "Lifestyle and genes are not the only factors that shape disease risk, and factors and exposures before, during, and after birth can help pre-program much of our adult health. Our study is an illustrative example suggesting that a dietary sensitivity before birth could be a catalyst in the development of schizophrenia or a similar condition twenty-five years later."[44]

If you're wondering how in the world they managed to make this connection, look no further than the details of their analyses, which entailed a look at birth records and neonatal blood samples of children born between 1975 and 1985 in Sweden. About 211 of the 764 kids examined developed mental disorders later in life characterized by a significant derangement of their personality and a loss of touch with reality. The team measured levels of IgG antibodies to milk and wheat in the blood samples to figure out that the "children born to mothers with abnormally high levels of antibodies to the wheat protein gluten were nearly 50 percent more likely to develop schizophrenia later in life than children born to mothers with normal levels of gluten antibodies."[45] This association remained true even after the scientists ruled out other factors known to increase the risk of developing schizophrenia, such as the mother's age during pregnancy and whether the child was born via C-section (by and large, genetic factors and environmental impacts in utero weigh much more heavily into one's risk for schizophrenia than environmental factors encountered later in life). But children born to mothers with abnormally high levels of antibodies to milk protein didn't appear to be at an increased risk for psychiatric disorders.

The authors added a fascinating historical note to their paper as well. It wasn't until World War II that a suspicion about the connection between psychiatric disorders and maternal food sensitivity started to surface. U.S. Army researcher Dr. F. Curtis Dohan was among the first scientists to notice a relationship between postwar Europe's food scarcity (and, consequently, a lack of wheat in the diet) and considerably fewer hospitalizations for schizophrenia. Although the observation couldn't prove the association at the time, since then we've had the benefits of long-term studies and modern technologies to verify the case against gluten.

The significance of prenatal programming has become a huge field of study over the past several decades, exploding more recently with new ways to study how early life events program offspring for a host of adverse health outcome. This burgeoning area even has a distinguished center of gravity called the DOHaD Society—the International Society for Developmental Origins of Health and Disease. Researchers worldwide continue to document profound relationships between prenatal environments and exposures and later onset of disease, from mental illness to cardiovascular disease and diabetes. In a 2015 paper entitled "Prenatal Programming of Mental Illness," the authors write, "The womb may be as important as the home."[46] This quote paid homage to British epidemiologist Dr. David J. Barker, who introduced the concept that the "the womb may be more important than the home" in 1990.[47]

Studies have also shown that a low-carb, high-fat diet just like the one I outline in chapter 7 can improve symptoms of not only depression but also schizophrenia. One woman who has been chronicled in the literature, known by the initials CD, had a complete resolution of her schizophrenia symptoms when she adopted a gluten-free, low-carb diet.[48] She was first diagnosed at the age of seventeen, and experienced paranoia, disorganized speech, and daily hallucinations throughout her life. Before adopting a low-carb diet at the age of seventy, she'd been hospitalized multiple times for suicide attempts and increased psychotic symptoms. Medication failed to improve her symptoms. Within the first week on the new diet, CD reported feeling better and having more energy. And within three weeks, she was no longer hearing voices or "seeing skeletons."

A FIX FOR THE COMMON HEADACHE?

I can't imagine what it would be like to suffer from daily headaches, but I've treated many patients who've shouldered the weight of that kind of suffering throughout their lives. Take, for example, a sixty-six-year-old gentleman whom I first saw in January 2012. I'll call him Cliff.

Cliff had endured thirty long years with pretty much the same unrelenting headache, and he wins a gold medal for trying his best to extinguish the pain. His attempts included a litany of drugs from those designed for migraines, like Imitrex, to narcotic painkillers such as Vicodin, prescribed after consultations with top headache clinics—all to no avail. Aside from being ineffective, he found that many of these medications slowed him down significantly. Although Cliff mentioned that he thought his headaches were related to foods, he couldn't say this was always the case. Nothing in his medical history jumped out at me, but when we discussed his family history, he said that his sister also experienced ongoing headaches and had significant food intolerances. This bit of information led me to probe a little further. I learned that Cliff had a twenty-year history of muscle stiffness, and that his sister carried a specific antibody related to gluten sensitivity that is also associated with what is called "stiff-person syndrome."

When I checked Cliff's blood work, several things stood out. He was highly reactive to eleven proteins related to gluten. Like his sister, he showed a strong reaction with respect to the antibody associated with stiff-person syndrome. I also noted that he was quite sensitive to cow's milk. As with so many of my patients, I placed him on a diet that restricted gluten and dairy. After three months, he told me that he hadn't needed to use Vicodin at all the previous month, and on a scale from 1 to 10 his worst headache was now a manageable 5 rather than a screaming 9. Best of all, his headaches no longer lingered all day; they lasted only three or four hours. While Cliff was not totally cured, his relief was substantial and, for him, very gratifying. In fact, he was so pleased with his outcome that he has allowed me to use his photograph when I present his case, now published, to health-care practitioners.

I've had plenty more patients come through my doors and leave with a pain-free head, thanks to the adoption of a gluten-free diet. One woman with a similar experience had been to countless doctors, tried innumerable prescription drugs, and undergone high-tech brain scans. Nothing worked until she met me and my prescription pad for a gluten sensitivity test. And lo and behold her villain—and cure—were identified.

Headaches are one of our most common maladies, and migraines in particular are the third most prevalent illness in the world.[49] In the United States alone, more than 39 million men, women, and children suffer from migraines, and millions more suffer from chronic headaches.[50] Incredibly, twenty-first-century medicine remains focused on treating *symptoms* for what is often a fully preventable problem. If you're a chronic headache sufferer, why not try a gluten-free diet? What have you got to lose?

Big Headaches in Brief

For the purposes of this discussion, I include all types of headaches in one category. So whether you're dealing with tension headaches, cluster headaches, sinus headaches, or migraines, for the most part I refer to headaches as a collective basket of conditions that share the same characteristic: pain in the head due to physical and biochemical changes in the brain. For the record, migraines tend to be the most painful kind and are often accompanied by nausea, vomiting, and sensitivity to light. But a headache is a headache, and if you've got one, your top priority is finding a solution. Once in a while, however, I will specifically refer to migraines.

An untold number of things can trigger a headache, from a bad night's sleep or changes in the weather to chemicals in foods, sinus congestion, head trauma, brain tumors, or too much alcohol. The exact biochemistry of headaches, especially migraines, is under active study. But we know a lot more today than we ever did before. And for those sufferers who can't nail down a reason (and thus a likely solution) for their headaches, my bet is that nine times out of ten that reason could be undiagnosed gluten sensitivity.

In 2012, researchers at Columbia University Medical Center in New York finished a yearlong study that documented chronic headaches among 56 percent of people who were gluten sensitive and 30 percent of those with celiac disease (the ones labeled as gluten sensitive had not tested positive for celiac disease but reported symptoms when they ate foods with wheat; again, whether or not you feel symptoms of gluten sensitivity, assume you are impacted by this ingredient).[51] They also found that 23 percent of those with inflammatory bowel disease had chronic headaches as well. When the researchers teased out the prevalence of migraines, they found much higher percentages of sufferers among the celiac group (21 percent) and the inflammatory bowel disease group (14 percent) than in the control group (6 percent). When asked to explain the connection, the lead researcher, Dr. Alexandra Dimitrova, alluded to the ultimate perpetrator of all: inflammation. To quote Dr. Dimitrova:

It's possible the patients with [inflammatory bowel disease] have a generalized inflammatory response, and this may be similar in celiac disease patients, where the whole body, including the brain, is affected by inflammation.... The other possibility is that there are antibodies in celiac disease that may...attack the brain cells and membranes covering the nervous system and somehow cause headaches. What we know for sure is that there is a higher prevalence of headache of any kind, including migraine headaches, compared to healthy controls.

She went on to say that many of her patients report major improvements in the frequency and severity of their headaches once they adopt a gluten-free diet; for some, headaches completely vanish.

Dr. Marios Hadjivassiliou, whom I've referenced throughout this book, has done extensive studies on headaches and gluten sensitivity.[52] Among his most astonishing work are the brain MRI scans that show profound changes in the white matter of headache patients with gluten sensitivity. The abnormalities are indicative of the inflammatory process. Most of these patients were resistant to normal drug treatments for their headaches, yet once they adopted a gluten-free diet, they were relieved of their suffering.

Dr. Alessio Fasano, who heads the Center for Celiac Research and Treatment at Massachusetts General Hospital, is a world-renowned pediatric gastroenterologist and a leading researcher in the area of gluten sensitivity.[53] I mentioned him early on in the book. When I met with him at a national conference where we both were speaking, he told me that it's no longer news to him that gluten-sensitive patients, including those with diagnosed celiac disease, frequently suffer from headaches. We lamented together how unfortunate it is that this type of gluten-triggered headache is misunderstood by the general public. It has such an easy fix, yet few of the afflicted know that they are sensitive to gluten.

When Italian researchers conducted a gluten-free trial experiment on eighty-eight children with celiac disease and chronic headaches, they found that 77.3 percent of them experienced significant improvement in headaches when they maintained a gluten-free diet, and 27.3 percent of those who improved actually became headache-free. The study also found that 5 percent of the kids with headaches who were not previously diagnosed with celiac were indeed found to have celiac disease; this was a much larger percentage than the 0.6 percent researchers had documented in the general pediatric population studied. Thus the risk of headache in the celiac group was increased by 833 percent. The authors concluded, "We recorded—in our geographical area—a high frequency of headaches in patients with CD [celiac disease] and vice versa with a beneficial effect of a gluten-free diet. Screening for CD could be advised in the diagnostic workup of patients with headache."[54]

Is it coincidence that so many kids with chronic headaches also have a strong sensitivity to gluten? And is it fortuity that the removal of gluten from their diets magically ushers their headaches away? No. And no. Unfortunately, many children with chronic headaches are never tested for gluten sensitivity, and they are placed instead on powerful drugs. The standard approach to

The prevalence of migraine headache in the pediatric population is increasing. Prior to the onset of puberty, migraine affects girls and boys equally. Thereafter, females outnumber males by about three to one. Children with migraines have a 50 to 75 percent risk of becoming adult migraine sufferers, and the disease is inherited in 80 percent of cases. Childhood migraines represent the third leading cause of school absence.[55]

treating headaches in kids includes the use of nonsteroidal anti-inflammatory medications, aspirin-containing compounds, triptans, ergot alkaloids, and dopamine antagonists. To prevent headaches, some of the drugs used include tricyclic antidepressants; various anticonvulsants including divalproex sodium; and more recently, topiramate, antiserotonergic agents, beta blockers, and calcium channel blockers. Topiramate, which is used to treat epilepsy, comes with awful side effects that would alarm any parent and be distressing to a child: weight loss, anorexia, abdominal pain, difficulty concentrating, sedation, and paresthesia (the feeling of "pins and needles" or of a limb "falling asleep").[56] I don't know about you, but I wouldn't want my kid to experience these side effects, even if they are temporary, to manage a headache that has nothing to do with what the drug was designed for. Numerous studies have emerged to show that, for the most part, anticonvulsants don't alleviate headaches in kids any better than a placebo.[57] In fact, leading researchers in headaches have been pressing for more studies to be done on children because few drugs have been proven effective and safe to use. The focus on drugs rather than dietary choices and nutritional supplementation sadly keeps us from addressing the underlying cause of the headache.

Big Bellies Make for Big Headaches

You already know that belly fat raises your risk for a medley of health problems (heart disease, diabetes, dementia, to name a few). But people don't think about their increased risk for headaches just by virtue of their waist circumference. Surprise: Waist circumference is a better predictor of migraine activity than general obesity in both men and women up until age fifty-five. Only in the last decade have we been able to scientifically show how strong this link is, thanks in part to researchers from Philadelphia's Drexel University College of Medicine, who mined data amassed from more than twenty-two thousand participants in the ongoing National Health and Nutrition Examination Survey (NHANES).[58] The data included a wealth of valuable information to examine, from calculations of abdominal obesity (as measured by waist circumference) and overall obesity (as determined by body mass index) to people's reports on how often they experienced headaches and migraines. Even after controlling for overall obesity, the researchers determined that for both men and women between the ages of twenty and fifty-five — the age bracket when migraine is most common — excess belly fat was affiliated with a significant increase in migraine activity. Women carrying extra fat around their belly were 30 percent more likely to suffer from migraines than women without excess belly fat. This held true even when the researchers accounted for overall obesity, risk factors for heart disease, and demographic characteristics.

Plenty of other studies show the inexorable bond between obesity and risk for chronic headaches.[59] One particularly large study looked at more than thirty thousand people and found that chronic daily headaches were 28 percent higher in the obese group than in the healthy controls of normal weight. Those who were morbidly obese had a 74 percent increased risk of having a chronic daily headache. When the researchers took a closer look at those who suffered from migraines in particular, overweight people had a 40 percent increased risk, and the obese had a 70 percent increased risk.[60]

By this point in the book you know that fat is a hugely powerful hormonal organ and system that can generate pro-inflammatory compounds. Fat cells secrete an enormous amount of cytokines, which trigger inflammatory pathways. Headaches are, at their root, manifestations of inflammation, just like most of the other brain-related ailments we've been covering.

It makes sense, then, that studies examining the relationship between lifestyle factors (e.g., overweight, low physical activity, and smoking) and recurrent headaches connect belly fat and chronic headaches. In 2010, researchers in Norway interviewed 5,847 adolescent students about their headaches and had them complete a comprehensive questionnaire about their lifestyle habits in addition to a clinical examination.[61] Those who said they regularly engaged in physical activity and were not smokers were classified as having a good lifestyle status. These students were compared to those who were deemed to be less healthy due to one or more of the negative lifestyle habits.

The results? The kids who were overweight were 40 percent more likely to suffer from headaches; the risk was 20 percent higher in those who didn't exercise much; and the smokers had a 50 percent increased risk. These percentages, however, were compounded when a student checked off more than one risk factor. If a student was overweight and smoked and didn't exercise, he or she carried a much higher risk for chronic headaches. And again, the study pointed to the effects of inflammation in fueling the firestorm.

The bigger your belly, the more at risk you are for headaches. Seldom do we think about our lifestyle and diet when we get a headache. Instead, we turn to drugs and await the next pound in the head. All the studies to date, however, show how important lifestyle is when it comes to managing, treating, and permanently curing headaches. If you can reduce sources of inflammation (lose the extra weight, eliminate gluten, go low-carb and high good fat, and maintain healthy blood sugar balance), you can target and control headaches.

THE RX TO BE HEADACHE-FREE

Numerous things can trigger a headache. I cannot possibly list all the potential offenders, but I can offer a few tips to end the suffering:

- *Keep a very strict sleep-wake cycle.* This is key to regulating your body's hormones and maintaining homeostasis — the body's preferred state of being, where its physiology is balanced.

- *Lose the fat.* The more you weigh, the more likely it is that you'll suffer from headaches.

- *Stay active.* Remaining sedentary breeds inflammation.

- *Watch caffeine and alcohol use.* Each of these in excess can stimulate a headache.

- *Don't keep erratic eating habits.* As with sleep, your eating patterns control many hormonal processes that can affect your risk for a headache.

- *Manage emotional stress, anxiety, worry, and even excitement.* These emotions are among the most common triggers of headaches. Migraine sufferers are generally sensitive to stressful events, which prompt the release of certain chemicals in the brain that can provoke vascular changes and cause a migraine. Adding insult to injury, emotions such as anxiety and worry can increase muscle tension and dilate blood vessels, intensifying the severity of the migraine.

- *Go gluten-, preservative-, additive-, and processed-free.* The low-glycemic, low-carb, high–healthy-fat diet outlined in chapter 11 will go a long way to reducing your risk for headaches. Be especially careful about aged cheese, cured meats, and sources of monosodium glutamate (MSG, commonly found in Chinese food), as these ingredients may be responsible for triggering up to 30 percent of migraines.

- *Track the patterns in your headache experience.* It helps to know when you're at a greater risk of getting a headache so you can pay extra attention during those times. Women, for example, can often trace patterns around their menstrual cycle. If you can define your patterns, you can better understand your unique situation and act accordingly.

The idea that we can treat—and in some cases, totally eliminate—common neurological ailments through diet alone is empowering. Most people immediately turn to drugs when seeking a solution, oblivious to the cure that awaits them in a few lifestyle shifts that are highly practical and absolutely free. Depending on my patients' unique circumstances, some of them need more short-term support for managing certain conditions, and this can come in the form of psychotherapy or even supplemental medication. But by and large, many of them respond positively to simply cleaning up their diet and expelling nerve-racking (literally) ingredients from their lives. And those who do require additional medical help often find that they can eventually wean themselves from pharmaceuticals and welcome the rewards that a drug-free life has to offer. Remember, if you do nothing else recommended in this book but eliminate gluten and refined carbohydrates, you will experience profound positive effects beyond those described in this chapter. In addition to watching your mood brighten up, you'll watch your weight go down and your energy soar in just a few weeks. Your body's innate healing capacities will be in high gear, as will your brain's functionality.

PART II

GRAIN BRAIN REHAB

Now that you've gotten a panoramic picture of "grain brain," which actually encompasses more than just grains and includes virtually all carbohydrates, it's time to turn to the ways in which you can support the ideal health and function of your brain. In this section of the book, we examine three key habits: diet, exercise, and sleep. Each of these plays a significant role in whether your brain thrives or begins to falter. And with the lessons gleaned in this part, you'll be fully prepared to execute the four-week protocol outlined in part III.

CHAPTER 7

Dietary Habits for an Optimal Brain

Hello, Fasting, Fats, and Essential Supplements

> *I fast for greater physical and mental efficiency.*
>
> — PLATO

THE SIZE OF OUR BRAIN IN COMPARISON to the rest of our body is one of the most important features distinguishing us from all other mammals. An elephant, for example, has a brain that weighs 7,500 grams, dwarfing our 1,400-gram brain. But its brain represents 1/550 of its total body weight, while our brain makes up 1/40 of our total body weight. So we can't make any comparisons about "brain power" or intelligence based on brain size alone. It's the ratio of brain size to body size that's key when considering the brain's functional capacity.[1]

But even more important than our impressive volume of brain matter is the fact that, gram for gram, our brain consumes a disproportionately huge amount of energy. It represents 2.5 percent of our total body weight but consumes an incredible 22 percent of our body's energy expenditure at rest. The human brain expends about 350 percent more energy than the brains of other anthropoids like gorillas, orangutans, and chimpanzees. So it takes a lot of dietary calories to keep our brains functioning. Fortunately for us, though, our large and powerful brains have allowed us to develop the skills and intelligence to survive extreme conditions like food scarcity. We can conceive of and plan for the future, a uniquely human trait. And having an understanding of our brain's amazing abilities can help inform the ways in which we can optimize our diet for a healthy, functioning brain.

THE POWER OF FASTING

One critical mechanism of the human body that I've already covered is its ability to convert fat into vital fuel during times of starvation. We can break down fat into specialized molecules called ketones, and one in particular that I've already mentioned—beta-hydroxybutyrate (beta-HBA)—is a superior fuel for the brain. This not only provides a compelling case for the benefits of intermittent fasting to nourish the brain, as contradictory as this may seem, but also serves as an explanation for one of the most hotly debated questions in anthropology: why our Neanderthal relatives disappeared between thirty and forty thousand years ago. While it's convenient and almost dogmatic to accept that Neanderthals were "wiped out" by clever *Homo sapiens*, many scientists now believe that food scarcity may have played a more prominent role in their disappearance. It may be that the Neanderthals didn't have the "mental endurance" to persevere because they lacked the biochemical pathway to utilize fat to feed the brain.

Unlike other mammals' brains, the human brain can use an alternative source of calories during times of starvation. Typically, our daily food consumption supplies our brain with glucose for fuel. In between meals, our brains are continually supplied with a steady stream of glucose that's made by breaking down glycogen, mostly from the liver and muscles. But glycogen stores can provide only so much glucose. Once our reserves are depleted, our metabolism shifts and we are able to create new molecules of glucose from amino acids taken from protein primarily found in muscle. This process is aptly named gluconeogenesis. On the plus side, this adds needed glucose to the system, but on the minus side, it sacrifices muscles. And muscle breakdown is not a good thing for a starving hunter-gatherer.

Luckily, human physiology offers one more pathway to power our brains.

When food is no longer available, after about three days, the liver begins to use body fat to create those ketones. This is when beta-HBA serves as a highly efficient fuel source for the brain, allowing us to function cognitively for extended periods during food scarcity. Such an alternative fuel source helps reduce our dependence on gluconeogenesis and, therefore, preserves our muscle mass.

But more than this, as the late Harvard Medical School professor George F. Cahill once stated, "Recent studies have shown that beta-hydroxybutyrate, the principal ketone, is not just a fuel, but a superfuel, more efficiently producing ATP energy than glucose. It has also protected neuronal cells in tissue cultures against exposure to toxins associated with Alzheimer's or Parkinson's."[2]

Indeed, Dr. Cahill and other researchers have determined that beta-HBA, which is easily obtainable just by adding coconut oil to your diet, improves antioxidant function, increases the number of mitochondria, and stimulates the growth of new brain cells.

In chapter 5 we explored the need to reduce caloric intake in order to increase BDNF as a means of stimulating the growth of new brain cells as well as enhancing the function of existing neurons. The idea of substantially reducing your daily calorie intake does not appeal to many people, even though it's a powerful approach to not only brain enhancement, but also overall health. But intermittent fasting—a complete restriction of food for twenty-four to seventy-two hours at regular intervals throughout the year—is more manageable, and I recommend and outline a fasting protocol in chapter 10. Research has demonstrated that many of the same health-providing and brain-enhancing genetic pathways activated by caloric restriction are similarly engaged by fasting, even for relatively short periods of time.[3] This is counter to conventional wisdom that says that fasting lowers the metabolism and forces the body to hold on to fat in a so-called starvation mode. Much to the contrary, fasting provides the body with benefits that can accelerate and enhance weight loss, not to mention boost brain health. In the early 1900s, doctors began recommending it to treat various disorders such as diabetes, obesity, and epilepsy. Today we have an impressive body of research to show that intermittent fasting can increase longevity and delay the onset of diseases that tend to cut life short, including dementia and cancer.[4]

Fasting not only turns on the genetic machinery for the production of BDNF, but also powers up the Nrf2 pathway, leading to enhanced detoxification, reduction of inflammation, and increased production of brain-protective antioxidants. Fasting causes the brain to shift away from using glucose as fuel to using ketones manufactured in the liver. When the brain is metabolizing ketones as fuel, even the process of cell suicide (apoptosis) is reduced, while mitochondrial genes are turned on, leading to mitochondrial replication. Simply put, fasting enhances energy production and paves the way for better brain function and clarity.

Fasting in spiritual quests is an integral part of religious history. All major religions promote fasting as far more than a ceremonial act. Fasting has always been a fundamental part of the spiritual practice, as in the Muslim fast of Ramadan and the Jewish fast of Yom Kippur. Yogis practice austerity with their diets, and shamans fast during their vision quests. Fasting is also a common practice among devout Christians, and the Bible has examples of one-day, three-day, seven-day, and forty-day fasts.

WHAT FASTING AND KETOGENIC DIETS HAVE IN COMMON

What happens when you substantially reduce your carbohydrate intake and derive more of your calories from fat? I just finished explaining the benefits of fasting, which stimulates the brain to turn to fat for fuel in the form of ketones. A similar reaction takes place when you follow a diet low in carbohydrates and rich in healthy fats and proteins. This is the foundation of the *Grain Brain* dietary protocol.

Throughout our history we sought fat as a calorie-dense food source. It kept us lean and served us well in our hunter-gatherer days. As you already know, eating carbohydrates stimulates insulin production, which leads to fat production, fat retention, and a reduced ability to burn fat. What's more, as we consume carbohydrates we stimulate an enzyme called lipoprotein lipase that tends to drive fat into the cells; the insulin secreted when we consume carbohydrates makes matters worse by triggering enzymes that lock fat tightly into our fat cells.

As I've also described, when we burn fat as opposed to carbohydrate, we enter ketosis. There's nothing inherently bad about it, and our bodies have been equipped for this activity for as long as we've roamed Earth. Being in a mild ketosis state is actually healthy. We are mildly ketotic when we first wake up in the morning, as our liver is mobilizing body fat to use as fuel. Both the heart and the brain run more efficiently on ketones than on blood sugar, by as much as 25 percent. Healthy, normal brain cells thrive when fueled by ketones. Certain brain tumor cells, however, can only use glucose as fuel. Standard treatment for glioblastoma, one of the most aggressive types of brain tumor, is surgery, radiation therapy, and chemotherapy. But quite honestly, results from these approaches are fairly dismal. Taking advantage of the fact that glioblastoma cells can only use glucose, and not ketones, Dr. Giulio Zuccoli, formerly of the University of Pittsburgh School of Medicine and now chief of neuroradiology at Children's Hospital of Philadelphia, reasoned that a ketogenic diet might actually prove effective in treating glioblastoma along with traditional treatments.[5] And, in fact, he published a case report of treating a glioblastoma patient using a ketogenic diet with impressive results. If a ketogenic diet can prolong the life of a cancer patient, what can it do in a healthy individual?

A purely ketogenic diet is one that derives 80 to 90 percent of calories from fat, and the rest from carbohydrate and protein. Certainly this is extreme, but again, recognize that ketones are a far more effective fuel for the brain. In 1921, when the Mayo Clinic's Russell Wilder developed the ketogenic diet, it was basically an all-fat proposition. In the 1950s, we learned about medium-chain triglycerides (MCTs), which act as precursors in the body for beta-HBA and can be consumed through coconut oil. Consuming MCT oil has in fact been shown to improve cognition and, essentially, brainpower. One such study out of Japan and published in 2016 concluded, "The ketogenic meal [with added MCTs] was suggested to have positive effects on working memory, visual attention, and task switching in non-demented elderly."[6] The researchers documented a direct correlation between heightened blood levels of beta-HBA and the improvement that people experienced on the MCT-rich ketogenic meals. The ketogenic diet has become popular in recent years, and even more popular in research circles. Today scientists are rigorously looking into how it can improve not only brain function overall, but help in treating difficult conditions like ALS, Parkinson's disease, and even type 1 diabetes.

Dr. Keith Runyan has written two books on conquering both types of diabetes with a ketogenic diet. Himself a type 1 diabetic, Dr. Runyan has challenged long-held approaches to his condition. He has practiced clinical medicine in the areas of emergency medicine, internal medicine, nephrology, and obesity medicine for nearly thirty years. Diagnosed in 1998, he achieved the "recommended" hemoglobin-A1C of 6.5 to 7 percent over the next fourteen years with conventional treatment. However, he was disturbed by frequent unpleasant and embarrassing hypoglycemic episodes, during which he'd become incredibly shaky, confused, sweaty, and irritated. After starting regular exercise to train for triathlons in 2007 and taking sports gels to prevent hypoglycemia, his glycemic control actually worsened. When he contemplated doing an Ironman Triathlon, he sought a better method to control his diabetes. He tried the ketogenic diet in 2012 and experienced not only an improvement in glycemic control, but also a reduction in hypoglycemia and its symptoms. He completed an Ironman Triathlon in 2012, without hypoglycemia or the need for sugar or food due to the fat adaptation afforded by the ketogenic diet. He is now an advocate for the use of the ketogenic diet for the management of diabetes (you can view my interview with him at DrPerlmutter.com or on my YouTube channel).

The powerful effects of a ketogenic diet in treating type 2 diabetes in particular were underscored in a 2018 paper by Dr. Sarah Hallberg (whom we met in chapter 3; she runs a medical weight loss program as part of Indiana University).[7] Dr. Hallberg and her colleagues conducted a study on a group of 349 type 2 diabetics. Part of the group received standard care under the direction of their physicians over a one-year period; the other group was placed on a ketogenic diet. They started out at 30 grams of carbohydrates each day, and the level of carbohydrates was adjusted to keep them in ketosis. What was unique about this study is the fact that the intervention group—the group put on the ketogenic diet—was in close touch with health coaches and physicians, with frequent measurements of their blood sugar and A1C, as well as their blood ketone levels to assure that they maintained ketosis. In addition, body weight and medication use were documented. The results of this study are breathtaking. After one year, the patients on the ketogenic diet had lost 12 percent of their body weight and their A1C levels went from 7.6 to 6.3. Incredibly, 94 percent of patients who had been prescribed insulin were able to reduce or stop their insulin altogether. And in those patients who were taking sulfonylureas, a common oral diabetic medication, all of them were able to discontinue the drug. The patients who did not go on the ketogenic diet had no changes in their A1C levels, their weight, or their use of diabetes medication. It's important to reiterate that the group on the ketogenic diet had continuous supervision by a health coach and a doctor, and this also may have factored into their dramatic improvement. This study demonstrates that a ketogenic diet in this setting represents the most effective intervention ever demonstrated for the treatment of type 2 diabetes. I had the opportunity to interview Dr. Hallberg a couple of weeks after this landmark study was published in the journal *Diabetes Therapy*. (You can watch the interview at DrPerlmutter.com or on my YouTube channel. I also encourage you to check out her 2015 TED Talk: "Reversing Type 2 Diabetes Starts with Ignoring the Guidelines"; it has been viewed more than 3 million times—and counting.)

The mechanisms for how the ketones that are produced on a ketogenic diet can be so helpful for the brain, apart from lowering risk of diabetes, include reduced inflammation, more efficient energy production, and increased production of antioxidants. Moreover, ketones increase BDNF by acting as cell-signaling molecules to turn on certain genetic pathways that increase the viability of cells. Put another way, getting into a state of ketosis changes your gene expression to help control your blood sugar, enhance energy availability for the brain, balance insulin levels, and reduce programmed cell death. A 2012 paper on the benefits of a ketogenic diet even called out how it increases sirtuin gene activation, a gene pathway associated with increased lifespan in animals.[8]

The diet protocol outlined in chapter 10 honors the main ketogenic principles of significantly reducing carbohydrates to the point that the body is pushed to burn fat while increasing dietary fat and adding nutrients to increase production of beta-HBA. You'll limit your consumption of net carbohydrates to just 20 to 25 grams a day during the first four weeks, after which you can increase that amount to 30 grams. Net carbs means total grams of carbs minus grams of fiber content, since fiber does not have any meaningful negative effect on blood sugar (and provided the food doesn't contain sugar alcohols). The degree of ketosis that you're able to achieve can easily be measured with a ketone meter. I have previously recommended ketone test strips (e.g., Ketostix) that detect ketones in urine, but this kind of testing is not nearly as precise as using a blood ketone meter that can measure glucose and ketones from a tiny finger prick. These devices, which are affordable and orderable online, usually measure beta-HBA; they are remarkably easy to use in monitoring your ketosis. To maintain mild ketosis, you'll want your beta-HBA levels to be in the range of 0.5 mmol/L to 4 mmol/L. This means that your body is effectively using ketones as energy.

If you follow my protocol, you can expect to become slightly ketotic after approximately the first week on the plan, and you may want to test yourself to see this effect. Many people feel better at higher levels of ketosis, though some do experience a temporary "breaking in" period during the first week or so during which they may feel sick (sometimes called "keto flu"). There is nothing wrong with this, as it is a natural reaction to the body entering ketosis and switching from a state of glucose-burning to fat-burning. Once you get used to eating in a way that sustains mild ketosis, you probably will not have to test yourself every day or even every week. During the four-week protocol, I will suggest that you stay in mild ketosis for the full course, but you do not have to remain in mild ketosis 365 days a year. I will advise that you break ketosis smartly once or twice a month by eating more healthy net carbs for two days. For many people, the weekends are ideal for upping your carb intake and cycling out of ketosis. Then come Monday morning, you get back into fat-burning mode.

BRAIN-BOOSTING SUPPLEMENTS

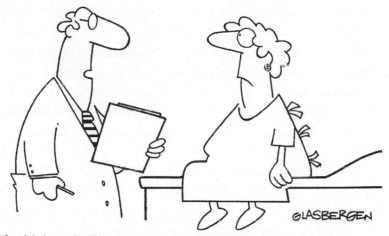

"The high-carb diet I put you on 20 years ago gave you diabetes, high blood pressure, and heart disease. Oops."

I love a cartoon that offers a nugget of wisdom in a matter of eyebrow-raising seconds, the time it takes to absorb the image and caption. The one above caught my eye years ago; I only wish more doctors were as smart as cartoonist Randy Glasbergen. Given all the science we've accumulated since this cartoon was first published in 2004, we can add "and set you up for brain disease" to the caption.

The painful reality in today's doctoring world is that you're not likely to get a lot of useful advice about staving off brain disorders during an office visit to your internist. Nowadays, you get fewer than fifteen minutes (if that) with a doctor who may or may not be aware of all the latest knowledge about how to preserve your mental faculties. What's more disturbing is that many of today's physicians, trained decades ago, don't have a firm grasp of nutrition and its effects on your health. I don't say this to pooh-pooh my industry; I'm merely pointing out a truth that's largely a consequence of economics. My hope is that our next generation of doctors will be better equipped to swing the pendulum to the side of prevention rather than focus so much on treatment. Which brings me to my recommended supplements. (Refer to pages 251–252 for exact dosages and instructions on when to take each of these daily.)

DHA: As I mentioned earlier, docosahexaenoic acid (DHA) is a star in the supplement kingdom. DHA is an omega-3 fatty acid that represents more than 90 percent of the omega-3 fats in the brain. Fifty percent of the weight of a neuron's plasma membrane is composed of DHA. And it's a key component in heart tissue. I could write an entire chapter on DHA alone, but I'll spare you that level of detail. Suffice it to say, DHA is one of the best-documented darlings in protecting the brain.

I often ask doctors in my lectures what they think the richest source of DHA is in nature. I hear all kinds of answers — cod liver oil, salmon oil, anchovy oil. Some guess flaxseed oil or avocado oil, but those don't contain adequate DHA. The richest source of DHA in nature is human breast milk, which explains why breast-feeding is continually touted as important for the neurologic health and long-term performance of a child.

Plenty of high-quality DHA supplements are available today, and there are more than five hundred food products that are enriched with DHA. It doesn't really matter whether you buy DHA that's derived from fish oil or from algae. Even though DHA beats its sibling, EPA, in its power and brain health effects, there is nothing wrong with buying DHA that comes in combination with EPA.

*   *   *

MCT or coconut oil: As previously mentioned, coconut oil is a great source of medium-chain triglycerides (MCT), an excellent form of saturated fatty acids that are easily digested and can increase HDL (good) cholesterol levels. The MCTs in coconut oil make it a superfuel for the brain—with the added benefit of reducing inflammation. It's known in the scientific literature as helping prevent and treat neurodegenerative disease as well as boost memory and cognition. Although the American Heart Association published a "Presidential Advisory" in 2017 that classifies coconut oil as an unhealthy saturated fat, let me be clear: Not only did the AHA get their science wrong, but they neglected to mention that the AHA received funding from Bayer Crop Science, the producer of Liberty Link soybeans, when they extolled the virtues of polyunsaturated oils such as soybean oil.[9] I recommend that you take 1 tablespoon daily of MCT oil derived from coconut oil or, if you prefer pure coconut oil, double the dose to 2 tablespoons. You can also cook with coconut oil and add MCT or coconut oil to coffee and tea. Coconut oil is heat stable, so you can cook with it at high temperatures—use it in place of extra virgin oil when cooking eggs or sautéing fish fillets, for example.

Turmeric: Turmeric *(Curcuma longa)*, a member of the ginger family, is the subject of intense scientific research, much of it evaluating the anti-inflammatory and antioxidant activities that stem from its active ingredient, curcumin. Turmeric is the seasoning that gives curry powder its yellow color, and as I mentioned earlier, it has been used for thousands of years in Chinese and Indian medicine as a natural remedy for a variety of ailments. In a report for the *American Journal of Epidemiology*, researchers investigated the association between curry consumption level and cognitive function in elderly Asians.[10] Those who ate curry "occasionally" and "often or very often" scored much better on specific tests designed to measure cognitive function than did people who "never or rarely" consumed curry.

One of curcumin's secret weapons is its ability to activate genes to produce a vast array of antioxidants that serve to protect our precious mitochondria. It also improves glucose metabolism. All these properties help reduce risk for brain disease. Unless you make lots of curry dishes at home, you probably don't get a lot of turmeric in your diet on a regular basis, so I suggest you take a supplement.

Probiotics: Stunning new research in just the last few years has shown that eating foods rich in probiotics—live microorganisms that support our intestine's resident bacteria—can influence brain behavior and help alleviate stress, anxiety, and depression.[11] These tribes of "good bacteria" that live in your intestines and help with digestion are enhanced and nourished by probiotics. They play a role in producing, absorbing, and transporting neurochemicals such as serotonin, dopamine, and nerve growth factor, which are essential for healthy brain and nerve function. (For all the details to this biology, see my book *Brain Maker*.)

Understanding how this is possible requires a quick lesson in the science of your microflora–gut–brain communication.[12] It's true that your gut is your "second brain."[13] This is an area of active, fascinating research, a large volume of which in recent years has demonstrated an intimate communication highway between the brain and the digestive system. Through this two-way connection, the brain receives information about what's going on in your intestines as the central nervous system sends information back to your gut to ensure optimal functioning.

All this transmission back and forth makes it possible for us to control our eating behavior and digestion, and even find restful sleep at night. The gut also sends out hormonal signals that relay to the brain feelings of fullness, hunger, and even pain from intestinal inflammation. In diseases and illnesses that affect the intestines, such as uncontrolled celiac, irritable bowel syndrome, or Crohn's disease, the gut can be a major influence on our well-being—how we feel, how well we sleep, what our energy level is, how much pain we experience, and even how we think. Researchers are currently looking at the possible role of some strains of intestinal bacteria in obesity, inflammatory and functional GI disorders, chronic pain, autism, and depression. They are also examining the role that these bacteria play in our emotions.[14]

So intricate and influential is this system that the health of our gut could be a much bigger player in our perception of overall health than we ever imagined. The information processed by the gut and sent up to the brain has everything to do with our sense of well-being. And if we can support this system just by consuming the gut's most important collaborators—healthy gut bacteria—then why not? Although lots of foods—such as yogurt and some beverages—are now fortified with probiotics, these products can often come with too much sugar. Ideally, you should get your probiotics either through natural, probiotic-rich foods like kefir, fermented foods, cultured condiments, and live-cultured yogurt, or through a non-GMO supplement that offers a variety of strains (at least ten), including *Lactobacillus acidophilus* and *Bifidobacterium lactis*, and contains at least thirty billion active bacteria per capsule. A few gems I recommend seeking based on their documented science:

Lactobacillus plantarum

Lactobacillus acidophilus

Lactobacillus brevis

Bifidobacterium lactis

If you're wanting to lose weight, I suggest looking for the following species in addition to those above:

Lactobacillus gasseri

Lactobacillus rhamnosus

For those with mood issues, including depression, look for:

Lactobacillus helveticus

Bifidobacterium longum

(Again, consult *Brain Maker* for more details about the science behind your microbiome and probiotics so you can choose the best formulas. You'll also want to consider *prebiotics,* the ingredients that gut bacteria love to eat to fuel their growth and activity; these can easily be ingested through certain foods such as dandelion greens, garlic, and sunchokes. Prebiotics can also come in combination with a probiotic supplement.)

Whole coffee fruit concentrate: This is one of the most exciting additions to my supplement regimen. You are likely familiar with coffee beans, from which we make coffee. But the coffee bean is actually a seed found inside a cherry-size, red fleshy berry that comes from the coffee plant. When the whole coffee fruit (coffee berries) are made into a supplement through a special process, we get an antioxidant-rich powerhouse for the brain. This extract, which contains chemicals called procyanidins that are known to protect brain cells, also has a unique profile of polyphenols that are credited for increasing blood levels of BDNF, which I introduced to you in chapter 5. I can't emphasize enough how important BDNF is, not only for keeping the brain healthy and maintaining its resistance to damage, but also for triggering the growth of new brain cells and increasing the connections between them. Study after study shows a relationship between levels of BDNF and risk for developing Alzheimer's disease. Recall the seminal 2014 study I mentioned in chapter 5 that was published in the *Journal of the American Medical Association* in which researchers at Boston University found that in a group of more than 2,100 elderly people followed for ten years, 140 of them developed dementia.[15] Those with the highest levels of BDNF in their blood had less than half the risk for dementia as compared to those who had the lowest levels of BDNF. Low levels of BDNF are documented in people with Alzheimer's as well as in people with obesity and depression. A single dosage of whole coffee fruit extract has been shown to double blood levels of BDNF during the first hour after consumption. And you don't have to worry about overdosing on caffeine, for this extract contains minimal levels of caffeine. It's not akin to a coffee concentrate, despite what its name suggests.

Alpha-lipoic acid: This fatty acid is found inside every cell in the body, where it's needed to produce the energy for the body's normal functions. It crosses the blood-brain barrier and acts as a powerful antioxidant in the brain in both watery and fatty tissues. Scientists are now investigating it as a potential treatment for strokes and other brain conditions involving free radical damage, such as dementia.[16] Although the body can produce adequate supplies of this fatty acid, our modern lifestyles and inadequate diets often require supplementation.

Vitamin B-complex: As I briefly mentioned earlier, high homocysteine levels increase risk for dementia, but you can lower your levels with B vitamins, notably vitamin B_6, folate, and vitamin B_{12}. (As an aside, plenty of studies in the literature now point to cases where a person suffering from depression is super low in B_{12} and relieves their depression through supplementation alone.) Many drugs can inhibit the B vitamins and therefore raise homocysteine (see the list at DrPerlmutter.com under Resources), which is why I recommend taking a B-complex, especially if your homocysteine levels come back on the high side (anything above 10 μmol/L in the blood).

Vitamin D: It's a misnomer to call vitamin D a "vitamin" because it's actually a fat-soluble steroid hormone. Although most people associate it strictly with bone health and calcium levels—hence its addition to fortified foods and beverages—vitamin D has far-reaching effects on the body and especially on the brain. We know that there are receptors for vitamin D throughout the entire central nervous system; we also know that vitamin D helps regulate enzymes in the brain and cerebrospinal fluid that are involved in manufacturing neurotransmitters and stimulating nerve growth. Both animal and laboratory studies have indicated that vitamin D protects neurons from the damaging effects of free radicals and reduces inflammation. Vitamin D also has a relationship with the microbiome. In 2010 we found out that gut bacteria interact with our vitamin D receptors, controlling them to either increase their activity or turn it down.[17] Let me state a few other key findings:[18]

- Reports have shown a 25 percent risk reduction in cognitive decline in individuals with higher levels of vitamin D (severely deficient individuals in one such study were 60 percent more likely to undergo cognitive decline over the six-year follow-up).[19]

- A paper published in 2014 in my favorite journal, *Neurology*, studied 1,658 elderly individuals who did not have dementia at the beginning of the study. Five and a half years later, those who had the lowest levels of vitamin D experienced more than double an increased risk of Alzheimer's.[20] Even those who were medically deficient at the start had about a 53 percent increased risk compared to those who had sufficient levels of vitamin D. The researchers concluded: "Our results confirm that vitamin D deficiency is associated with a substantially increased risk of all-cause dementia and Alzheimer disease."

- In another study, the mental states of 858 adults were evaluated between 1998 and 2006. The study found a substantial decline in mental function in those individuals with severe vitamin D deficiency.[21]

- Multiple studies link low levels of vitamin D with risk for Parkinson's and relapse in multiple sclerosis patients. In a 2017 editorial for *Neurology* that reflects on large-scale, well-designed studies linking low vitamin D and risk for multiple sclerosis (MS) in particular, two Canadian doctors write: "Vitamin D supplementation is a simple intervention that would be highly cost-effective even if it prevents only a proportion of MS cases. Harm from such a strategy is unlikely; doses of up to 4,000 IU/day are safe for adults even in pregnancy, so they could be used through late adolescence and adulthood as such doses would be adequate to achieve vitamin D sufficiency in most individuals. Vitamin D supplementation may also produce other benefits; supplementation during infancy is associated with greater bone mass among girls age 7–9 years. It is time to take an active approach to preventing MS, at a minimum targeting those individuals with an elevated risk of MS, including smokers, the obese, and those with a family history of MS."[22]

- Low vitamin D levels have long been shown in medical literature to contribute to depression and even chronic fatigue.[23] Adequate vitamin D is needed by the adrenal glands to help regulate an enzyme necessary for the production of dopamine, epinephrine, and norepinephrine — critical brain hormones that play a role in mood, stress management, and energy. People with mild to severe depression have been known to experience turnarounds and improvements through supplementation alone.

Correcting insufficient levels of vitamin D can take several months of supplementation, but doing so will significantly improve your entire body's chemistry—from bone health to brain health—and even its insulin sensitivity. My dietary protocol will also provide good sources of natural vitamin D found in nature, such as cold-water fish and mushrooms.

SPECIAL NOTE ABOUT MEDICATIONS

If you currently take any prescription medication, it's important that you talk with your physician before starting any supplement program. But I also want to remind you that popular drugs, some of which are over-the-counter, can be working against you and your brain health. Among the most problematic ones that new science is showing are those for acid reflux, the proton pump inhibitors (PPIs; e.g., Nexium, Prilosec, Protonix, and Prevacid). We've all seen the commercials: A man tries to eat a sausage sandwich, and the sausage turns away. The implication is that if he eats the sausage he'll get "indigestion," whatever that means. The call to action is to reach for an acid-blocking pill. Then, he can eat whatever he wants, and the world is supposedly a better place.

An estimated 15 million Americans use PPIs for gastroesophageal reflux disease, or GERD. These drugs block the production of stomach acid, something your body needs for normal digestion. Not only do they leave people vulnerable to nutritional and vitamin deficiencies and infections, some of which can be life threatening, but they also put people at greater risk of heart disease and chronic kidney failure. And they do a number on your beneficial gut bacteria. When researchers examined the diversity of microbes in stool samples of those taking two daily doses of proton pump inhibitors, they documented dramatic changes after just one week of treatment. These drugs can effectively ruin the integrity of your digestive system by dramatically changing your gut bacteria. Moreover, the studies of late have been so damning that they have moved the American Medical Association to print a bold statement in their journal in 2016: "The avoidance of PPI medication may prevent the development of dementia. This finding is supported by recent pharmacoepidemiological analyses on primary data and is in line with mouse models in which the use of PPIs increased the levels of β-amyloid in the brains of mice."[24] This incredible statement should be heeded by anyone wanting to preserve brain function.

Other drugs that I caution people on include acetaminophen (Tylenol), nonsteroidal anti-inflammatories such as ibuprofen (Advil, Motrin) and naproxen (Aleve), and antibiotics. Here's why:

Acetaminophen: New research shows that it compromises brain function, increasing the risk of making cognitive mistakes. A 2015 Ohio State University study revealed that acetaminophen blunts emotions, positive and negative.[25] Participants who took acetaminophen felt less strong emotions when they saw both pleasant and disturbing photos as compared to those who took placebos. Acetaminophen is also known to deplete one of the body's most vital antioxidants, glutathione, which helps control oxidative damage and inflammation in the body and especially in the brain. And in a 2014 study, Danish scientists collaborating with researchers at UCLA and the University of Arizona, among others, found that women who took acetaminophen during pregnancy were more likely to have children medicated for ADHD by age seven.[26]

Nonsteroidal anti-inflammatories (NSAIDs): These drugs work by reducing the amount of prostaglandins in the body, a family of chemicals produced by the cells that have several important functions. Prostaglandins promote the kind of short-term inflammation necessary for healing, they support the blood clotting function of platelets, and they protect the lining of the stomach from the damaging effects of acid. Because of these last two functions, NSAIDs that prevent prostaglandins from doing their thing can lead to unintended consequences on that intestinal lining; their number one side effect is stomach bleeding, ulcers, and stomach upset.[27] Research shows that they damage the small intestine and compromise the gut lining, thereby setting the stage for the very problem they are intended to address: inflammation.[28]

Antibiotics: They kill bacteria, both the good guys and the bad. Sometimes antibiotics are necessary in treating serious infections of bacterial origin, but often they are over-prescribed and misused. Antibiotics do not just change the microbial ecology in the body. They also drive adverse changes in insulin sensitivity, glucose tolerance, and fat accumulation due to how they alter the gut bacteria. The drugs tinker with our own physiology, changing how we metabolize carbohydrates and how the liver metabolizes fat and cholesterol.

No doubt there is a time and place for medications. But we live in a world where we are too quick to medicate, self-prescribe, and depend upon pills. I dream of the day when we can all minimize medications and maximize our body's innate ability to heal itself. If you rely on medications, I encourage you to work with your health-care provider to find alternative methods for treating and managing your conditions. I do believe that if you follow this program, you will experience a lessening of your symptoms, whether you need to continue treatment with drugs or not.

CHAPTER 8

Genetic Medicine

Jog Your Genes to Build a Better Brain

Old minds are like old horses; you must exercise them if you wish to keep them in working order.

— JOHN ADAMS

POP QUIZ! WHAT'S GOING TO MAKE YOU SMARTER and less prone to brain diseases? Is it (A) solving a complex brainteaser or (B) taking a walk? If you guessed (A), I won't come down hard on you, but I will encourage you to go for a walk first (as fast as you can) and then sit down to work on a brainy puzzle. The answer, it turns out, is (B). The simple act of moving your body will do more for your brain than any riddle, math equation, mystery book, or even thinking itself. In fact, nothing could be more positively powerful on brain health and function than plain old exercise. Studies going back decades and those coming out today (and tomorrow) have stated and will continue to irrefutably conclude: Exercise improves brain function. Period. It even acts as a "first aid kit" on damaged brain cells.

Exercise has numerous pro-health effects on the body—especially on the brain. It's a powerful player in the world of epigenetics. Put simply, when you exercise, you literally exercise your genetic makeup. Aerobic exercise not only turns on genes linked to longevity, but also targets the gene that codes for BDNF, the brain's "growth hormone." More exercise means more BDNF and less inflammation. Aerobic exercise has been shown to reverse memory decline in the elderly and increase growth of new brain cells in the brain's memory center. Follow-up studies to reports I originally talked about in this book, plus newer studies in the past few years, show time and time again that people who engage in physical activity regularly (forty-five to sixty minutes of moderate intensity most days of the week) significantly outpace sedentary counterparts in terms of cognitive performance and mental processing speed. There is an inverse relationship between "leisure time physical activity" and risk for cognitive decline, including how fast you can think and process information, as well as remember.[1] And regardless of cognitive status, those who move more enjoy bigger brains due to less atrophy with age. Here's a great quote to remember from one such collaborative study among many institutions and led by UCLA: "With the elderly population growing rapidly, a better understanding of preventive measures for maintaining cognitive function is crucial. Studies such as this one suggest that simply caloric expenditure, regardless of type or duration of exercise, may alone moderate neurodegeneration and even increase GM [gray matter] volume in structures of the brain central to cognitive functioning."[2]

For a long time now, we've known that exercise is good for the brain, but only in the past ten to fifteen years have we really been able to quantify and qualify the extraordinary relationship between physical fitness and mental fitness.[3] It has taken the collective force of many inquisitive researchers working from different camps, including neuroscientists, physiologists, bioengineers, psychologists, anthropologists, and doctors from various other fields of medicine. It has also taken the development of many advanced technologies for us to be able to analyze and understand the inner workings of brain matter itself, including its individual neurons. We can now image and view the brain like never before. The newest findings make it undeniably clear that the link between exercise and brain health isn't just a relationship. In the words of Gretchen Reynolds, science writer for the *New York Times*, "It is the relationship."[4] Exercise, according to the latest science, "appears to build a brain that resists physical shrinkage and enhances cognitive flexibility." And this, my friends, may mean that there is no greater tool at our fingertips than physical movement. Take a look at the following two graphics, one showing the percentage difference in one's risk for Alzheimer's

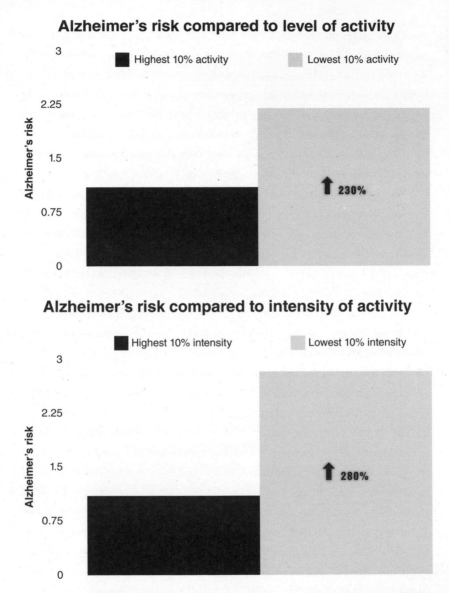

Alzheimer's risk compared to level of activity

■ Highest 10% activity   ▨ Lowest 10% activity

↑ 230%

Alzheimer's risk compared to intensity of activity

■ Highest 10% intensity   ▨ Lowest 10% intensity

↑ 280%

disease based on level of exercise, and another showing the difference based on intensity of exercise. I think these are quite telling.[5]

In early 2018, the American Academy of Neurology published a practice guideline for neurologists to indicate exactly what would represent the very best choices that we could pursue when dealing with a patient with mild cognitive impairment (MCI). As a reminder, MCI represents a situation in which not only does the patient recognize that there is some degree of problem with respect to brain function, but at this point the doctor is able to detect the deficit as well. The importance of diagnosing MCI cannot be understated as it typically represents the harbinger of full-blown Alzheimer's disease down the road. Neurologists have long debated what should be done in this situation to reduce the risk of developing Alzheimer's in these patients. To be sure, there's been a great effort to validate a medication that could possibly prove helpful in this circumstance. The subcommittee of the American Academy of Neurology that was tasked to come up with these recommendations reviewed no fewer than eight available medications that might possibly prove helpful in slowing the progression from MCI to full-blown Alzheimer's disease. And they determined that there was not a single drug on the list that proved effective in any way.

Now here's the key takeaway: The panel also had the opportunity to review exercise as a modality that might reduce the risks of cognitive decline and developing Alzheimer's. Their findings were stunning. They determined that exercise was in fact *the only meaningful recommendation* that clinicians could and should make for patients diagnosed with MCI. Can you imagine the most highly respected, peer-reviewed neurology journal advocating exercise — and not drugs? Yes, things are changing — for the better!

There are generally two ways that exercise benefits the brain (and body, really). Directly, exercise reduces insulin resistance and inflammation while stimulating the release of growth factors. These growth factors, BDNF among them, affect the health of neurons, the growth of new blood vessels in the brain, and even the abundance and survival of new neurons. Indirectly, exercise also boosts the brain by reducing stress and anxiety and improving sleep and mood. Is there any wonder how and why exercise can be such an antidote to risk for brain decline and dementia? It may as well be magic.

THE MAGIC OF MOVEMENT

As humans we have always been physically active — that is, until only quite recently. Modern technology has afforded us the privilege of a sedentary existence; virtually anything we need these days is available without having to exert much effort, much less get out of bed. But our genome, over millions of years, evolved in a state of constant challenge, from a physical perspective, in our quest to find food. In fact, our genome expects frequent exercise — indeed, it *requires* regular aerobic exercise to sustain life. But unfortunately, too few of us respect that requirement today. And we have the chronic illness and high mortality rates to show for it.

The idea that exercise can make us smarter has intrigued not just traditional researchers in biomedical labs, but also anthropologists searching for clues to the shaping of humankind through millennia. In 2004, the journal *Nature* published an article by evolutionary biologists Daniel E. Lieberman of Harvard and Dennis M. Bramble of the University of Utah, who argue that we survived this long in history by virtue of our athletic prowess.[6] It was our cavemen ancestors who were able to outpace predators and hunt down valuable prey for food that allowed for survival — producing meals and energy for mating. And those early endurance athletes passed on their genes. It's a beautiful hypothesis: We are designed to be athletes so that we can live long enough to procreate. Which is to say that natural selection drove early humans to evolve into supremely agile beings — developing longer legs, stubbier toes, and intricate inner ears to help us maintain better balance and coordination while standing and walking on just two feet as opposed to four.

For a long time, science couldn't explain why our brains had gotten so big — disproportionately so, when you consider our body's size in comparison to other animals'. Evolutionary scientists in the past liked to talk about our carnivore behaviors and need for social interaction, both of which demanded complicated thinking patterns (to hunt and kill, and to engage in relationships with others). But now science has another ingredient to add to the mix: physical activity. According to the latest research, we owe our tremendous brains to the need to think . . . and the need to run.

To arrive at this conclusion, anthropologists examined patterns between the brain size and endurance capacity of many animals, from guinea pigs and mice to wolves and sheep.[7] They noted that the species with the highest innate endurance capacity also had the highest brain volumes relative to their body size. Then the researchers took their experiment further by looking at mice and rats that were intentionally bred to be marathon runners. They created a line of lab animals that excelled at running by interbreeding those that ran the most in their cage's wheels. And then the truth began to emerge: Levels of BDNF and other substances that promote tissue growth and health began to increase in these newly bred animals. BDNF is also known to drive brain growth, which is why the new thinking is that physical activity may have helped us evolve into clever, quick-witted beings. David A. Raichlen, an anthropologist at the University of Arizona and leading scientist in the evolution of the human brain, summed up the concept brilliantly in his explanation to the *New York Times*, as reported and paraphrased by Gretchen Reynolds:[8]

> The more athletic and active survived and, as with the lab mice, passed along physiological characteristics that improved their endurance, including elevated levels of BDNF. Eventually, these early athletes had enough BDNF coursing through their bodies that some could migrate from the muscles to the brain, where it nudged the growth of brain tissue.
>
> With an enhanced ability to think, reason, and plan, early humans could then sharpen the skills that they needed to survive, such as hunting and killing prey. They benefited from a positive feedback loop: Being in motion made them smarter, and sharper minds further allowed them to stay in motion and move more effectively. Over time, humans would come to engage in complex thinking and invent things like math, microscopes, and MacBooks.
>
> The bottom line is that if physical activity helped us develop the brains we use today, then it's safe to say we need exercise to maintain those brains (not to mention to continue to evolve into a smarter, faster, more clever species).

BE NIMBLE AND QUICK

The biology of how exercise can be so beneficial to brain health goes far beyond the argument that it promotes blood flow to the brain and thus delivers nutrients for cell growth and maintenance. To be sure, cerebral blood flow is a good thing. But that's old news. The latest science behind the magic of movement in protecting and preserving brain function is stunning. It boils down to five benefits: controlling inflammation, increasing insulin sensitivity, influencing better blood sugar control, expanding the size of the memory center, and, as I've already mentioned, boosting levels of BDNF.

Some of the most compelling science has been performed in just the last decade.[9] In 2011, Dr. Justin S. Rhodes and his team at the Beckman Institute for Advanced Science and Technology at the University of Illinois made discoveries using four groups of mice in four different living arrangements.[10] One group lived in the lap of luxury in a setting that included lavish, mice-friendly meals (nuts, fruits and cheeses, and flavored waters) and lots of playful toys to explore, such as mirrors, balls, and tunnels. The second group of mice had access to the same treats and toys, but their living quarters included running wheels. A third group's cages resembled a cheap motel; they contained nothing extraordinary and the mice ate standard kibble. The fourth group of mice similarly lacked access to fancy amenities and food, but their home included running wheels.

At the start of the study, the mice underwent a series of cognitive tests and were injected with a substance that allowed the researchers to track changes in their brain structures. Over the next several months, the scientists let the mice do whatever they wanted in their respective homes, after which the researchers retested the mice's cognitive functions and examined their brain tissues.

The one variable that clearly stood out above all others was whether or not the mice had a running wheel. It didn't matter if they had things to play with in their cages. The animals that exercised were the ones that had healthier brains and outperformed on the cognitive tests. Those that didn't run, even if their world was otherwise stimulating, didn't improve cognitively. The researchers were specifically looking for cognitive improvements that implied a boost in complex thinking and problem solving. Only exercise proved key to that improvement.

We know that exercise spurs the generation of new brain cells. Scientists have actually measured this effect by comparing mice and rats that ran for a few weeks versus those that were sedentary. The running animals had about twice as many new neurons in their hippocampi as the couch potatoes. Other studies have looked at which types of exercise are the most effective. In 2011, when a group of 120 older men and women were split into two groups—one assigned to a walking program and the other to a stretching regimen—the walkers won over the stretchers.[11] They were the ones who showed larger hippocampi after a year and higher levels of BDNF in their bloodstreams. The stretchers, on the other hand, lost brain volume to normal atrophy and didn't perform as well on cognitive tests. Take a look at the results:

Change in size of the hippocampus over 1 year comparing aerobic exercisers to those doing stretching program

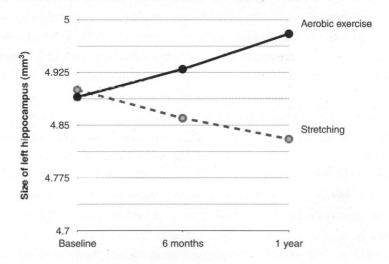

GROW NEW NETWORKS

Exercise has been proven to induce growth of new neurons in the brain, but the real miracle is that it has also been shown to help build novel networks in the brain. It's one thing to give birth to brain cells, but another to organize those cells into a network that functions in harmony. We don't get "smarter" just by making new brain cells. We have to be able to interconnect those cells into the existing neural network, otherwise they will roam around aimlessly and eventually die. One way to do this is to learn something new. In a

2007 study, newborn neurons in mice became integrated into the animals' brain networks if the mice learned to navigate a water maze.[12] This is a task that requires more cognitive power than physical ability. The researchers also noted that the newbie cells were limited in what they could do; they couldn't, for example, help the mice perform other cognitive tasks beyond the maze. To do that, the mice would need to exert themselves physically, which would encourage those new cells to become spry and cognitively limber.

And therein lies the secret benefit of exercise: It makes neurons nimble and able to multitask. We don't know how exercise facilitates mental make-overs on a molecular level, but we do know that BDNF plays a role by strength-ening cells and axons, fortifying the connections among neurons, and sparking neurogenesis. Neurogenesis increases the brain's ability to learn new things, which in turn strengthens those new brain cells and further fortifies the neural network. Remember, too, that higher levels of BDNF are associated with a decrease in appetite. So for those individuals who have trouble control-ling their appetite, this provides yet another impetus to exercise.

With an understanding of the relationship of BDNF to exercise, researchers have been examining the effect of physical exercise in people at risk for or already suffering from brain disorder and disease. In a recent report in the *Journal of the American Medical Association*, Professor Nicola Lautenschlager, then of the University of Western Australia and now at the University of Melbourne, found that elderly individuals who engaged in reg-ular physical exercise for a twenty-four-week period had an 1,800 percent improvement on measures of memory, language ability, attention, and other important cognitive functions compared to a control group.[13] The exercise group spent about 142 minutes in physical activity weekly, or about 20 min-utes a day. The researchers attributed these improvements to better blood flow, the growth of new blood vessels, growth of new brain cells, and improved brain "plasticity."

In a similar study, Harvard researchers identified a strong association between exercise and cognitive function in elderly women, concluding:

> In this large, prospective study of older women, higher levels of long-term regular physical activity were strongly associated with

higher levels of cognitive function and less cognitive decline. Specifically, the apparent cognitive benefits of greater physical activity were similar to being about three years younger in age and associated with a 20 percent lower risk of cognitive impairment.[14]

Multiple effects coalesce when the body is engaged in physical activity. Exercise is a potent anti-inflammatory. By activating the Nrf2 pathway I described earlier, physical exercise turns on the genes that suppress inflammation. And this can be measured in the laboratory. Scientists have documented time and time again that C-reactive protein — a commonly used laboratory marker of inflammation — is lower among people who follow an exercise routine. Exercise also improves insulin sensitivity. It helps manage blood sugar balance and reduce the glycation of proteins. We know this to be true from studies done on the effects of exercise on hemoglobin A1C. In one notable study, researchers told thirty participants to make no lifestyle changes while putting thirty-five others on an exercise program three days a week.[15] The control group did not participate in any form of exercise. After the sixteenth week, hemoglobin A1C decreased by 0.73 in the exercise group but increased by 0.28 in the nonexercise group. To put these numbers in context, if your hemoglobin A1C was 6.0, a reduction of 0.73 brought on by exercise represents a 12 percent reduction of hemoglobin A1C, and this rivals the effect of diabetes medications.

IT DOESN'T TAKE MUCH TO MAKE AN IMPACT

Okay, so exercise does a body and brain good. But how much? How rigorous? Do household chores and customary daily activities like gardening and taking out the trash count?

To answer this, let's turn to a study from Rush University's Memory and Aging Project — the study that led to the graphics I showcased on page 222. When Dr. Aron S. Buchman examined the effects of daily physical exercise on one's risk for Alzheimer's disease, he found dramatic differences between relatively sedentary people and those performing various types of activities, including simple acts like cooking, washing the dishes, playing cards, pushing a wheelchair, and cleaning. He managed to track people's activity levels using a device called an ActiGraph, which is worn on the wrist to detect and quantify movement. The average age of the individuals, who did not have dementia, was eighty-two years. Of the original 716 participants, 71 developed full-blown Alzheimer's disease over the course of approximately 3.5 years of follow-up.[16]

The results of the study revealed that those individuals in the lowest 10 percent of daily physical activity had a 230 percent increased risk of developing Alzheimer's disease compared to those in the highest 10 percent of physical activity. When the data was evaluated in terms of intensity of physical activity, the results were even more compelling. Comparing the people in the bottom 10 percent of intensity of physical activity to the individuals in the top 10 percent, Dr. Buchman and his team found that the risk of Alzheimer's was nearly tripled in those who exerted themselves the least. Dr. Buchman rightfully articulated in his conclusions that we cannot underestimate the power of low-cost, easily accessible, and side-effect-free activities that may not entail formal exercise. The mere actions of daily living can provide brain-protective benefits at any age. Whatever the activity, we have enough proof to confidently say that exercise needn't be exhausting to be effective for the brain.

You don't need to set your sights on climbing Mount Everest. Nor do you need to train for an endurance event. But regular exercise that gets your heart pumping is a must. Although a small number of studies have found cognitive benefits among older people who just lifted weights for a year, most studies to date, and all animal experiments, have involved running or other aerobic activities such as swimming, bicycling, hiking, and brisk walking at least five days a week for at least twenty minutes per session.

I realize that exercise is not on most people's list of top priorities, but I hope the evidence I've provided in this chapter will encourage you to rethink your to-dos if you don't already maintain an exercise routine. I'll ask that you devote one week during the program to focus on this important area of your life and commence a regular workout if you don't already have one. And if you do, then you can use that week to increase the duration and intensity of your workouts, or try something new.

CHAPTER 9

Good Night, Brain

*Leverage Your Leptin to Rule Your
Hormonal Kingdom*

*Finish each day before you begin the next,
and interpose a solid wall of sleep between the two.*

— RALPH WALDO EMERSON

WHEN SAMUEL, A FORTY-EIGHT-YEAR-OLD STOCKBROKER, came to see me on a late-November day, he asked me to "optimize his health." This wasn't the first time someone had made such a blanket, somewhat vague request, but I knew what he really wanted: He wanted me to get to the bottom of his misery and deliver him to a place of vibrant health like he'd never felt before. A tall order for any doctor to fill, but something in his bloated face instantly clued me in to what could have been the problem. I started by getting to know his medical history and chief complaints. He had a history of low thyroid function, for which he was taking medication. He said his life was quite stressful, but rated his overall health as "good." There wasn't much to report as far as past medical problems, but interestingly enough, he mentioned that his son had been "sensitive" to solid foods during his infancy and was diagnosed as having gluten sensitivity. We discussed his thyroid issue further, and it turned out that he had an autoimmune disease called Hashimoto's thyroiditis, which is caused by abnormal activation of the immune system that causes it to attack the thyroid gland.

As I used to do earlier in my practice, I ordered a gluten sensitivity test, which produced compelling results. He was indeed highly sensitive to gluten; only one of the twenty-four antibodies tested was in the normal range. He desperately needed to try a gluten-free diet.

His response to the diet was quite remarkable and, frankly, somewhat predictable in light of both his son's experience and his off-the-charts test. Four months after he started the diet, I received a letter from him that made me smile. He admitted in writing just how bad his life had gotten by the time he made his appointment to come see me. Evidently, he'd fibbed when he told me that his health was "good." It was far from that. He wrote:

> Prior to diagnosing me as gluten sensitive, my health was in a downward spiral. . . . Even though I was in my early forties and worked out daily, I was lethargic and struggled to make it through the day. . . . I was becoming more moody and would easily snap at the smallest things. . . . Depression set in, as I couldn't shake negative thoughts. I was convinced that I was dying. . . . [Today] I am a new person. I am once again happy-go-lucky, and I have energy throughout the day. I'm sleeping through the night regularly, and my joint pain is gone. I'm able to think clearly and not get sidetracked on my tasks. The best part is that the stubborn fat around my midsection virtually melted off in two weeks. I thank you for helping me get my life back.

Even though Samuel didn't mention his sleep problems when I first examined him, I had a hunch that restful sleep had evaded him for some time. He looked exhausted and had all the trademark signs of long-term, unfathomable sleep deprivation. For many of my patients prior to being treated, lack of sleep is so normal to them that they forget what it's like to have a good night's sleep until they experience it again. Samuel may have thought that sleeping through the night was just a side benefit to the relief he found from going gluten-free. But it was more than that. The moment Samuel began to have refreshing sleep night after night was the moment he began to deeply "re-plumb" his body—hormonally, emotionally, physically, and even spiritually. Casting aside all his issues with gluten and even his thyroid disorder, I can say without a doubt that achieving regular, restful sleep played a huge role in reversing his conditions and bringing him to exactly where he wanted to be: a place of optimal health.

Most of us undervalue the benefits of sleep, but it's one of the few assets in our lives that's totally free and absolutely essential to well-being. It's also, as you're about to find out, a fundamental tool in preventing brain decay.

THE SCIENCE OF SLUMBER

In the last fifteen years, the science of sleep has been a media darling. And for good reason: We understand the value of sleep from a scientific perspective as we never have before. Both laboratory and clinical studies have shown that virtually every system in the body is affected by the quality and amount of sleep we get, especially the brain.[1] Among the proven benefits: Sleep can dictate how much we eat, how fast our metabolism runs, how fat or thin we get, whether we can fight off infections, how creative and insightful we can be, how well we can cope with stress, how quickly we can process information and learn new things, and how well we can organize and store memories.[2] Adequate sleep, which for the vast majority of us means at least seven solid hours, also influences our genes. In early 2013, scientists in England found that a week of sleep deprivation altered the function of 711 genes, including some involved in stress, inflammation, immunity, and metabolism.[3] Anything that negatively affects these important functions in the body impacts the brain. We depend on those genes to produce a constant supply of proteins for replacing or repairing damaged tissue, and if they stop working after just a week of poor sleep, that says a lot about the power of sleep. Although we may not notice the side effects of poor sleep on a genetic level, we can certainly experience the other signs of chronic sleep deprivation: confusion, memory loss, brain fog, low immunity, obesity, cardiovascular disease, diabetes, and depression. All these conditions are uniquely tied to the brain.

While we know that many of us don't get enough sleep to support our bodies' true needs, I should point out that *too much sleep* is now considered a potential early marker for cognitive decline. In 2017, the journal *Neurology* reported that sleeping for more than nine hours a night could put one at a higher risk of progressing to clinical dementia within ten years.[4] That's quite a statement, and it's all the more powerful when you know that the same study measured smaller brain volume in the long sleepers. So clearly there has to be a sweet spot for leveraging sleep's benefits, and it appears that for most of us, seven to nine hours is it. But, also for most of us, we can't even get that.

About 10 percent of Americans suffer from chronic insomnia, while fully 25 percent of us report not getting enough sleep at least on occasion.[5] And beyond getting enough sleep, experts are now focused on the *quality* of sleep in terms of its ability to restore the brain. Is it better to sleep solidly for six hours or terribly for eight? One would think that questions like that are easy to answer, and that we'd know everything there is to know about something all of us do for a large portion of our lives. But science is still trying to unravel the mystery of sleep and even how it affects men and women differently. Apparently, the hormones influenced by sleep deprivation are different for men and women.[6] Although the outcome is the same for both sexes—an inclination to overeat—the underlying spark for that hunger is not the same for both sexes. In men, lack of sufficient sleep leads to elevated levels of ghrelin, a hormone that stimulates appetite. In women, on the other hand, ghrelin levels aren't influenced by lack of sleep, but levels of GLP-1, an appetite-suppressing hormone, are. Granted, such a subtle difference may seem insignificant since the overall result of eating more occurs either way, but it goes to show how little we know about the entire biochemistry of the human body in response to sleep.

If there's one thing we do know about sleep, it's that it increasingly becomes a challenge the older we get. This is true for a variety of reasons, many of them stemming from medical conditions that can put a dent in sound sleep. As many as 40 percent of older adults can't get a good night's sleep due to chronic problems like sleep apnea and insomnia. We even have evidence now for the relationship between disrupted sleep and cognitive decline. Kristine Yaffe is a psychiatrist at the University of California, San

Francisco, who studies people who have a higher risk of developing cognitive impairment and dementia. At her memory disorders clinic she sees a common thread in patients' complaints: difficulty falling asleep and staying asleep. They report being tired throughout the day and resorting to naps. When Yaffe led a series of studies analyzing more than thirteen hundred adults older than seventy-five over a five-year period, she noted that those with disrupted sleep, such as sleep-disordered breathing or sleep apnea, were more than twice as likely to develop dementia years later. Those who experienced breaks in their natural circadian rhythm or who awoke throughout the night were also at increased risk.[7] Newer research backs previous studies showing the relationship between sleep and risk for various health challenges. This research even reveals that our gut bugs — the intestinal microbiome — also share a relationship with not only our sleep habits but our circadian rhythm and whether it's healthy or hinging on a hiccup.[8]

Circadian rhythms are at the heart and soul of our well-being. By about six weeks old, all of us establish this pattern of repeated activity associated with the cycles of day and night that remains for the rest of our lives. As with sunrises and sunsets, these rhythms rerun roughly every twenty-four hours. We have many cycles that coincide with the twenty-four-hour solar day, from our sleep-wake cycle to the established patterns in our biological beats — the rise and fall of hormones, the fluctuations in body temperature, and the ebb and flow of certain molecules that feed into our health and wellness. When our rhythm is not in sync with the twenty-four-hour solar day, we can feel ill or tired, which is what happens, for instance, when we travel across time zones and force the body to adapt quickly to a new cycle.

I find that most people don't appreciate how much of their body's inherent rhythm is grounded in their sleep habits and controlled by their brain. Our body's natural day/night cycles pretty much command everything about us, when you consider that our hormonal secretion patterns are tethered to this cycle. A prime example is our body temperature, which, as a consequence of a dance of certain hormones in the body, rises during the day, takes a little dip in the afternoon (hence that late-day lull), peaks in the evening, then begins to decrease during the night. In the early morning hours, it reaches its nadir just as another pattern begins to peak, as cortisol levels reach their height in the morning and thereafter decrease throughout the day. Shift workers, who are notorious for keeping irregular sleep patterns due to their job responsibilities, live with a higher risk for a host of potentially serious illnesses as a result. Indeed, they don't call it the graveyard shift for nothing.

So the next time you're feeling uncharacteristically tired, moody, thirsty, hungry, mentally slow, forgetful, or even alert, aggressive, or horny, you can examine your recent sleep habits to glean insights. Suffice it to say we require a regular, reliable pattern of wakefulness and refreshing sleep to regulate our hormones. Volumes could be written on the body's hormones, but for purposes of this discussion and, in particular, the link between sleep and brain health, we're going to focus on one of the body's most underrated, unsung hormones: leptin. Because it essentially coordinates our body's inflammatory responses and helps determine whether or not we crave carbs, no conversation about brain health can exclude this important hormone. And it's powerfully impacted by sleep. If you can gain control of this biological master of ceremonies, you can rule your hormonal kingdom for the benefit of your brain and body.

GOT SLEEP?

You may not even be aware that you have poor sleep quality. Unless you truly know you're a good sleeper and wake up feeling refreshed each morning without the need for an alarm clock, I recommend you undergo a sleep study, known as a polysomnogram. This is a painless, noninvasive procedure that has you spending a night or two in a sleep facility. As you sleep, a sleep technologist records multiple biological functions to determine if you have any disorders like sleep apnea or restless leg syndrome. You'll want to find a certified sleep physician who is approved by the American Board of Sleep Medicine. Go to either absm.org and check "verification of diplomates" or abim .org and consult the "who is certified" section. Another good resource is the National Sleep Foundation, at sleepfoundation.org.

LEPTIN'S LORDSHIP

The year was 1994. It was a discovery that startled the medical community and forever changed how we view not only the human body and its complex hormonal system, but also sleep and its true value in orchestrating the empire. Just when we thought we had discovered all the hormones and their functions, we found a new hormone that we didn't previously know existed.[9] It's called leptin, and it turns out that this isn't just your average hormone; like insulin, leptin is a major one that ultimately influences all other hormones and controls virtually all the functions of the hypothalamus in the brain. Your hypothalamus is where your inner dinosaur lives; this ancient structure that pre-dates humans sits in the middle of your head and is responsible for your body's rhythmic activities and a vast array of physiological functions, from hunger to sex. But perhaps this finding came so late because leptin was identified in an unlikely place: fat cells.

Earlier I mentioned how we used to think that fat cells were just holding cells packed with unnecessary calories for a rainy day. But now we know that adipose tissue participates in our physiology as much as other "vital" organs, thanks to resident hormones like leptin that control whether or not we will end up with bulging bellies and small brains. First, a quick disclaimer: Leptin's function in the body, like most every hormone's, is extremely complex. The entire hormonal system, in fact, is extraordinarily intricate. There are untold numbers of interrelationships, and describing them all is beyond the scope of this book. I am going to keep it simple and reveal only what you need to know to take control of your hormones for the benefit of the brain.

Leptin is, at a most basic level, a primitive survival tool. It's uniquely tied to the coordination of our metabolic, hormonal, and behavioral response to starvation. As such, it has a powerful effect on our emotions and behavior. Leptin is a gatekeeper of sorts, and once you have an understanding of this hormone you'll know how to regulate the rest of your hormonal system and, in doing so, manage your health in unimaginable ways.

Although leptin is found in fat cells, that doesn't mean it's "bad." In excess it would indeed lead to problems, notably degenerative diseases and a shorter life. But healthy levels of leptin do the opposite—preventing most diseases of aging and supporting longevity. The more you can increase your sensitivity to this critical hormone, the healthier you will be. By "sensitivity," I'm referring to how your body's receptors to this hormone recognize and use leptin to carry out various operations. Nora T. Gedgaudas, an acclaimed nutritional therapist, defines leptin succinctly in her book *Primal Body, Primal Mind:*[10]

> Leptin essentially controls mammalian metabolism. Most people think that is the job of the thyroid, but leptin actually controls the thyroid, which regulates the rate of metabolism. Leptin oversees all energy stores. Leptin decides whether to make us hungry and store more fat or to burn fat. Leptin orchestrates our inflammatory response and can even control sympathetic versus parasympathetic arousal in the nervous system. If any part of your [hormonal] system is awry, including the adrenals or sex hormones, you will never have a prayer of truly resolving those issues until you have brought your leptin levels under control.

Gedgaudas calls leptin the "new kid on the block who runs the whole neighborhood," and I couldn't agree with her more. The next time you put down your fork and pull away from the dinner table, you can thank your leptin. When your stomach is full, fat cells release leptin to tell your brain to stop eating. It's your brake. And this explains why people with low levels of leptin are prone to overeating. A now-seminal study published in 2004 showed that people with a 20 percent drop in leptin experienced a 24 percent increase in hunger and appetite, driving them toward calorie-dense, high-carbohydrate foods, especially sweets, salty snacks, and starchy foods.[11] And what caused this leptin plunge? Sleep deprivation.[12] We've learned a lot about our hormones just from sleep studies alone. These, in turn, have informed us about the value of sleep in regulating our hormones.

Leptin and insulin have a lot in common, though they tend to antagonize each other. Both are pro-inflammatory molecules. Leptin is an inflammatory cytokine in addition to playing a big part in the body's inflammatory processes. It controls the creation of other inflammatory molecules in your fat tissue throughout your body. And it helps explain why overweight and obese people are susceptible to inflammatory problems, including those that substantially increase risk for brain disorders, mental health problems, and neurodegenerative disease. Both leptin and insulin are the higher-ups in the body's chain of command, so imbalances tend to spiral downward and wreak havoc on virtually every system of the body beyond those directly controlled by these hormones. What's more, leptin and insulin are negatively influenced by similar things, and their biggest transgressors are carbohydrates. The more refined and processed the carbohydrate, the more out of whack healthy levels of leptin and insulin become. Earlier I explained how continuous carbohydrate abuse on the body's insulin pumping and blood-sugar balancing will eventually lead to insulin resistance. The same happens with leptin. When the body is overloaded and overwhelmed by substances that cause continuous surges in leptin, the receptors for leptin stop hearing leptin's message; they start to turn off and you become leptin resistant. Put simply, they surrender the controls and you're left with a body vulnerable to illness and further dysfunction. So even though leptin is now elevated, it doesn't work — it won't signal to your brain that you're full so you can stop eating. And if you cannot control your appetite, then you're at a much greater risk for weight gain and obesity, which puts you at risk for brain disorders. Studies have also shown that elevated triglyceride levels, also a hallmark of too many carbs in the diet, cause leptin resistance.[13]

Not a single drug or supplement on the planet can balance leptin levels. But better sleep, as well as better dietary choices, will do the trick.

Are You Leptin Resistant?

It's a question we all have to ask ourselves. Unfortunately, millions of Americans qualify as bona fide members of the leptin-resistant club. It's practically a given if you've been eating a high-carb diet and don't sleep well. In Ron Rosedale and Carol Colman's book *The Rosedale Diet*, which takes a sweeping look at leptin in weight control, they enumerate the signs, many of which are common with insulin resistance, too:[14]

- being overweight
- being unable to change how your body looks, no matter how much you exercise
- being unable to lose weight or keep weight off
- constantly craving "comfort foods"
- feeling fatigue after meals
- feeling consistently anxious or stressed out
- feeling hungry all the time or at odd hours of the night
- having a tendency to snack after meals
- having high fasting triglycerides (over 100 mg/dL), particularly when equal to or exceeding cholesterol levels
- having osteoporosis
- having problems falling or staying asleep
- having high blood pressure
- regularly craving sugar or stimulants like caffeine
- having "love handles"

Don't panic if you have reason to believe you're leptin resistant. The program outlined in chapter 10 will get you back on track.

ON THE FLIP SIDE: GHRELIN

One more appetite-related hormone I should mention before moving on: ghrelin. It's the yin to leptin's yang. Ghrelin is secreted by the stomach when it's empty; it sends a message to your brain that you need to eat. As expected, a disruption in the tango between leptin and ghrelin will wage war on your cravings, sense of fullness, ability to resist temptations in the kitchen, and waistline. In sleep studies, ghrelin levels soared in response to inadequate pillow-time in men. This triggered a bigger appetite and a propensity to gravitate toward high-carb, low-nutrient foods that, once consumed, easily get turned into fat. When your appetite hormones are not behaving properly, your brain becomes essentially disconnected from your stomach. It deceives you into thinking you're hungry when you're not, and further stimulates hard-to-resist cravings for foods that will perpetuate that vicious cycle of fat formation. This cycle then feeds the larger feedback loops that play into blood sugar balance, inflammatory pathways, and, of course, risk for brain disorder and disease. Put simply, if you cannot control your hunger and appetite, good luck managing your blood chemistry, metabolism, waistline, and, in the bigger picture, the prospect of crippling your brain.

Dr. Matthew Walker, a professor of neuroscience and psychology at the University of California–Berkeley and the author of *Why We Sleep,* used to say that sleep is the third pillar of good health, alongside diet and exercise. But given his research into the impact of sleep on the brain and nervous system, he now teaches that sleep is the single most effective thing we can do to reset our brains and bodies, as well as increase a healthy life span.[15] In 2015, the National Sleep Foundation, along with a group of experts, issued its new general recommendations for sleep.[16] Babies, for instance, require more sleep than an elderly individual. But these recommendations are mostly generated by averaging how much we slept historically. There are very few studies that can say precisely how much sleep you or I need individually. Numbers will vary. I recommend to anyone unable to achieve restful sleep on a nightly basis to get a sleep study done, just as I have in the past. As noted in the box on page 236, I recommend a sleep study just to know if you sleep well in general because you might not know during which phase of sleep you falter.

During the third week of the program, I'll ask you to focus on achieving high-quality sleep so you can gain control of the hormones that have everything to do with the fate of your brain. And you won't have to reach for a sleep aid. The best sleep for the brain comes naturally.

PART III

SAY GOODBYE TO GRAIN BRAIN

Congratulations. You've learned more about the habits of a highly effective brain than most practicing doctors today. If you haven't already begun to change a few things in your life based on what you've read, now is your chance. In this section of the book, you'll follow a four-week program, during which you'll shift your diet from relying on carbs and rehabilitate your body back to optimal health. This will be the place where you feel vibrant, energetic, and mentally sharp. It's also where any doctor who examines your blood work will applaud you for having excellent control of your blood sugar, inflammatory markers, and even cholesterol level. It's the place we all dream of being—and it's much closer than you think.

Making lifestyle changes, even small ones, can seem overwhelming at first. You wonder how you can avoid your usual habits. Will you feel deprived and hungry? Will you find it impossible to keep this new way of life forever? Is this program doable given the time you have and the commitments you've already made? And can you reach a point where following these guidelines is second nature?

This program is the answer. It's a simple, straightforward strategy that has the right balance of structure and adaptability to honor your personal preferences and power of choice. You will finish my four-week program with the knowledge and inspiration to stay on a healthy path for the rest of your life. The closer you stick to my guidelines, the faster you will see results. Bear in mind that this program has many benefits beyond the obvious physical ones. Optimal brain health (and a smaller waistline) might be first and foremost on your mind, but the rewards don't end there. You will see change in every area of your life. You will feel more confident and have more self-esteem. You'll feel younger and more in control of your life and future. You'll be able to navigate through stressful times with ease, have the motivation to stay active and engage with others, and feel more accomplished at work and home. In short, you will be happier and more productive. And your success will breed more success. When your life becomes richer, fuller, and more energized as a result of your efforts, you won't want to revert to your old, unhealthy behaviors. I know you can do this. You must, for yourself and your loved ones. The payoffs—and the potentially calamitous consequences if you don't heed this advice—are huge.

A True GB Story

For as long as I can remember, I have always struggled with my body composition. I spent most of my youth overweight and battling depression. In 2005, I joined the U.S. Marines and spent most of the next four years overseas. Although I lost weight during my service time, the depression and anxiety I felt day to day never ceased. When I left the military, I moved back home and started attending college full-time. Everything changed: lifestyle, food, stress levels, and surely, over time, the weight started to come back on. I spent countless hours in the gym trying all sorts of things, to no avail. More than losing weight, I needed to find a way to resolve my depression. This depression had been a shroud covering me for years. It affected my work quality, learning was difficult, and my relationships with others suffered tremendously. I knew I had to make a change, so in

2011 I switched my major from computer science to start studying fitness and education with a minor in biology.

I started working as a personal trainer in 2012 and in 2014 I started working for a popular gym, where I had even more opportunities to learn about health and wellness. However, no matter how much information I got, no matter how much I played with my nutrition, it never seemed to "hit the nail on the head" when it came to dealing with my depression. And if I was having this problem myself, how could I ever give nutritional advice to anyone else?

That year I met a physician who referred me to a book that had helped her recover from a TBI [traumatic brain injury], and she thought it could help me, too. I bought the book, I read it, and as a fitness professional I was enlightened. Could the carbohydrates really be doing neurological damage?

There's no question about it at this point. After following the nutritional guidelines set out in *Grain Brain,* I have since been able to manage my body weight with ease, my depression has completely gone away, I am not bloated anymore, and my quality of life has tremendously improved.

I have given those recommendations to other clients who have also seen the results physically, emotionally, and psychologically. ~ Joseph M.

CHAPTER 10

A New Way of Life

The Four-Week Plan of Action

At home I serve the kind of food I know the story behind.

— Michael Pollan

Here's where the rubber meets the road. Some of you might be panicking at the thought of losing your beloved carbs. I realize that for some people, ditching bread, pasta, pastries, and most desserts (among other things) is going to be tough. Change is hard. And changing long-established habits is harder. I am often asked right off the bat, "What the heck am I going to eat?" Some worry about their withdrawal from sugar and wheat and their insatiable hunger for carbs. They anticipate colossal cravings that they won't be able to resist. They fear the body's reaction to a dietary U-turn. And they wonder if this is truly doable in the real world if willpower isn't in their vocabulary. Well, folks, let me be the first to say that yes, all of this is possible. You just need to take the initial plunge and experience the effects. Within a matter of days or just a couple of weeks I predict that you'll have clearer thoughts, better sleep, and improved energy. You'll suffer fewer headaches, manage stress effortlessly, and feel happier. Those of you who live with a chronic neurological condition, such as ADHD, anxiety disorder, or depression, may notice that your symptoms begin to wane or even vanish. Over time, you'll watch the weight fall off, and specific laboratory tests will show vast improvements in many areas of your biochemistry. If you could peer into your brain, you'd also see that it's functioning at its highest level.

It's a good idea to check with your doctor about beginning this new program, especially if you have any health issues such as diabetes. This is particularly important if you're going to opt for the one-day fast, outlined on pages 259–260. Over the course of the next month, you will achieve four important goals:

1. Shift your body away from relying on carbs for fuel and add brain-boosting supplements to your daily regimen.

2. Incorporate a fitness routine into your schedule if you don't already have one.

3. Work on getting restful, routine sleep seven days a week.

4. Establish a new rhythm and maintain healthy habits for life.

I've broken down the program into four weeks, with each week devoted to focusing on one of these specific goals. In the days leading up to the first week, you should see your doctor to have certain tests performed that will give you a baseline. You'll also use this time to get your kitchen organized, start your supplements, begin to wean yourself from carbs, and consider a one-day fast to kick-start the program.

During week 1, "Focus on Food," you'll start my menu plans and execute my dietary recommendations.

During week 2, "Focus on Exercise," I'll encourage you to start a regular workout program and give you ideas for moving more throughout the day.

During week 3, "Focus on Sleep," you'll turn your attention to your sleep habits and follow a few simple tips to ensure that you're achieving the best sleep possible every single night, weekends included.

During week 4, "Put It All Together," I'll help you put all the elements of this program together and equip you with strategies for permanently establishing these new behaviors in your life. Don't second-guess your ability to succeed at this; I've designed this program to be as practical and easy to follow as possible.

PRELUDE TO WEEK 1: PREPARE

Determine Your Baseline

Prior to beginning the dietary program, have the following laboratory studies performed, if possible. I've included target healthy levels where appropriate. Note that I've removed some tests that I don't think are as valuable as these below. You don't need to test for gluten sensitivity—assume that your body rejects this ingredient and eliminate it from your diet. The vitamin D test is optional; sometimes those test results are not as accurate as you'd think (and if you're in Canada, for example, the units by which they measure vitamin D are different). I'd prefer for you to assume you could boost your vitamin D levels, and as I've stated before, you cannot overdose on this brain-critical *hormone* using my supplement guidelines.

Test	Ideal level
fasting blood glucose	<95 mg/dL
fasting insulin	<8 µIU/ml (ideally, <3 µIU/ml)
hemoglobin A1C	4.8 to 5.4%
homocysteine	<8 µmol/L
C-reactive protein	0.00 to 3.0 mg/L
vitamin D (optional)	80 ng/mL

Upon completion of the four-week program, these laboratory studies should be repeated. Understand that it may take several months to see dramatic improvement in these parameters, especially the hemoglobin A1C, which is typically only measured every three to four months. But if you follow this program from day 1, you should nonetheless begin to see positive changes in your blood glucose and insulin levels within a month that will motivate you to keep going.

Homocysteine is an amino acid–like chemical, now generally regarded as being quite toxic to the brain; as noted above, you want to see a homocysteine level at around 8 μmol/L or less. If yours comes back above 8 (and especially over 10 μmol/L), be sure to add a B-complex supplement to your regimen. Note: Some people may have an elevated homocysteine despite taking B vitamins. If this is the case, you should consider genetic screening with the 23andMe company to determine if you (like me) have a genetic deficiency called MTHFR. If so, there are many health-care providers who can help you successfully lower your homocysteine with specific nutritional supplements.

An ideal level of C-reactive protein (CRP), a marker of inflammation in the body, is less than 1.0 mg/L. CRP may take several months to improve, but you may well see positive changes even after one month on the program.

Start Your Supplements

You will be starting a daily supplement regimen for life. All the supplements listed on pages 251–252 with their daily recommended dosage can be found at health food stores, most drugstores and supermarkets, and online. You'll find a list of some of my favorite brands at DrPerlmutter.com. Probiotics should be taken on an empty stomach right before a meal, but the other supplements can be taken with or without food. It's usually best to take the supplements at the same time every day so you don't forget, which for many people is in the morning, before leaving home. Only one of my suggested supplements, turmeric, should be taken twice daily; have one dose in the morning and another in the evening. For more details about each of these, refer back to chapter 7.

If you have any questions about dosage due to personal health challenges, ask your doctor for help in making proper adjustments. All of the dosages listed are generally ideal for both adults and children, but ask your pediatrician for specific recommendations based on your child's weight. At my clinic, for example, I prescribe 100 milligrams of DHA for children up to eighteen months and then 200 milligrams daily; for kids with ADHD, however, those dosages are usually higher—around 400 milligrams daily.

alpha-lipoic acid	300 to 500 mg daily
B-complex	Look for a whole-food vitamin B complex that contains all the essential water-soluble B vitamins and vitamin C. These include thiamine (vitamin B_1), riboflavin (vitamin B_2), niacin (vitamin B_3), pantothenic acid (vitamin B_5), pyridoxine (vitamin B_6), biotin, folate, and vitamin B_{12} in the form of methyl B_{12}. Take as directed on the packaging (usually 1 or 2 capsules daily). Remember: B vitamins are your best protection against elevated levels of homocysteine, an amino acid produced in the body that in excess can increase your risk of mood disorders, poor mental performance, and Alzheimer's disease.
DHA	1,000 mg daily (Reminder: It's okay to buy DHA that comes in combination with EPA; opt for a fish oil supplement or choose DHA derived from marine algae.)
MCT oil	1 tablespoon daily, taken straight or added to coffee or tea; or 2 tablespoons coconut oil daily, taken straight or used in cooking
turmeric	500 mg twice daily
vitamin D_3	5,000 IU daily (Once again, although you do not test your vitamin D levels, you can achieve the ideal dosage here by having your physician monitor your levels and adjust accordingly.)
whole coffee fruit concentrate	100 mg daily

| probiotics | 1 multi-strain capsule, taken daily at least 30 minutes before a meal. Look for a combination of species from *Lactobacillus* and *Bifidobacterium* (see page 213 for specific species to look for) |

Clear Out Your Kitchen

In the days leading up to your new way of eating, you'll want to take an inventory of your kitchen and eliminate items that you'll no longer be consuming. Start by removing the following:

• All sources of gluten (see pages 79–81 for the full list), including whole-grain and whole-wheat forms of bread, noodles, pastas, pastries, baked goods, crackers, and cereals. Don't forget to clear out alcoholic beverages that contain gluten, such as beer and wine coolers. (Gluten-free alcohols include rum, tequila, and wine. Unless gluten is added after distillation, all distilled alcohols are also gluten-free—but sometimes cereal grains are used in the production process, so check ingredients or contact the manufacturer to be sure.)

• All forms of processed carbs, sugar, and starch: chips, crackers, cookies, pastries, muffins, pizza dough, cakes, doughnuts, sugary snacks, candy, energy bars, ice cream/frozen yogurt/sherbet, jams/jellies/preserves, ketchup, processed cheese spreads, juices, dried fruit, sports drinks, soft drinks/soda, fried foods, honey, agave, sugar (white and brown), corn syrup, and maple syrup.

• All artificial sweeteners and products made with artificial sweeteners. Evict even the sugar substitutes that are marketed as "natural." These include the following: acesulfame potassium (Sunett, Sweet One); aspartame (NutraSweet, Equal); saccharin (Sweet'N Low, Sweet Twin, Sugar Twin); sucralose (Splenda); and neotame (Newtame). I would also be cautious about sugar alcohols that are marketed as healthy alternatives to regular and artificial sugars. These include ingredients like sorbitol, mannitol, xylitol, maltitol, erythritol, and isomalt. We don't know yet what these could be doing to your microbiome and, in turn, your brain.

• Packaged foods labeled "fat-free" or "low-fat" (unless they are authentically "fat-free" or "low-fat" and within the protocol, such as water, mustard, and balsamic vinegar).

• Margarine, vegetable shortening, and any commercial brand of cooking oil (soybean, corn, cottonseed, canola, peanut, safflower, grapeseed, sunflower, rice bran, and wheat germ oils)—even if they are organic. People often mistake vegetables oils as being derived from vegetables. They are not. The term is incredibly misleading, a relic from the days when food manufacturers needed to distinguish these fats from animal fats. These oils typically come from grains such as corn, seeds, or other plants such as soybeans. And they have been highly refined and chemically altered. The majority of Americans today get their fat from these oils, which are high in pro-inflammatory omega-6 fats as opposed to anti-inflammatory omega-3 fats. Do not consume them.

• Non-fermented soy (e.g., tofu and soy milk) and processed foods made with soy (look for "soy protein isolate" in list of ingredients; avoid soy cheese, soy burgers, soy hot dogs, soy nuggets, soy ice cream, soy yogurt). Note: Although some naturally brewed soy sauces are technically gluten-free, many commercial brands have trace amounts of gluten. If you need to use soy sauce in your cooking, use tamari soy sauce made with 100 percent soybeans and no wheat.

• Most starchy vegetables and those that grow below the ground: beets, corn, peas, potatoes, sweet potatoes, yams.

Watch out for foods marked (and marketed) "gluten-free." Some of these foods are fine because they never contained gluten to begin with. But many are labeled as such because they have been processed—their gluten has been replaced by another ingredient such as cornstarch, cornmeal, rice starch, potato starch, or tapioca starch, all of which can be equally as offensive, raising blood sugar enormously. Also, trace amounts of gluten can remain. The term "gluten-free" has no legal meaning at the moment; the FDA has proposed a definition but has not yet finalized it. Be extra cautious about gluten-free sauces, gravies, and cornmeal products (e.g., tacos, tortillas, cereals, and corn chips).

Restock

The following items can be consumed liberally (go organic, non-GMO, and local with your whole-food choices wherever possible; flash-frozen is fine, too):

- **Healthy fats:** extra virgin olive oil, sesame oil, coconut or MCT oil, avocado oil, grass-fed tallow and organic or pasture-fed butter, ghee, almond milk, avocados, coconuts, olives, nuts and nut butters, cheese (except for blue cheeses), and seeds (flaxseed, sunflower seeds, pumpkin seeds, sesame seeds, chia seeds)

- **Herbs, seasonings, and condiments:** You can go wild here as long as you watch labels. Kiss ketchup and chutney goodbye, but enjoy mustard, horse-radish, tapenade, and salsa if they are free of gluten, wheat, soy, and sugar. There are virtually no restrictions on herbs and seasonings; be mindful of packaged products, however, that are made at plants that process wheat and soy. Don't forget about cultured condiments (lacto-fermented mayonnaise, mustard, horseradish, hot sauce, relish, and salsa), which are rich in probiotics.

- **Low-sugar fruits:** avocado, bell pepper, cucumber, tomato, cour-gette, squash, pumpkin, aubergine, lemon, lime

- **Proteins:** whole eggs; wild fish (salmon, black cod, mahimahi, grouper, herring, trout, sardines); shellfish and mollusks (prawns, crab, lobster, mussels, clams, oysters); grass-fed meat, fowl, poultry, and pork (beef, lamb, liver, bison, chicken, turkey, duck, ostrich, veal); wild game

- **Vegetables:** leafy greens and lettuces, collards, spinach, broccoli, kale, chard, cabbage, onions, mushrooms, cauliflower, Brussels sprouts, sauerkraut, artichoke, alfalfa sprouts, green beans, celery, bok choy, radishes, watercress, turnips, asparagus, garlic, leeks, fennel, shallots, spring onions, ginger, jicama, water chestnuts

The following can be used in moderation ("moderation" means eating small amounts of these ingredients once a day or, ideally, just a couple of times weekly):

- Carrots and parsnips.

- Cottage cheese, yogurt, and kefir: Use sparingly in recipes or as a topping.

- Cow's milk and cream: Use sparingly in recipes or in coffee and tea.

- Legumes (beans, lentils, peas). Exception: You can have chickpeas and hummus. Watch out for commercially made hummus that's loaded with additives and inorganic ingredients. Classic hummus is simply chickpeas, tahini, olive oil, lemon juice, garlic, salt, and pepper.

- Non-gluten grains: amaranth, buckwheat, rice (brown, white, wild), millet, sorghum, teff. (Note: Although oats do not naturally contain gluten, they are frequently contaminated with gluten because they are processed at mills that also handle wheat; avoid them unless they come with a guarantee that they are gluten-free.) When non-gluten grains are processed for human consumption (e.g., milling whole oats and preparing rice for packaging), their physical structure changes, and this increases the risk of an inflammatory reaction. For this reason, we limit these foods.

- Quinoa: This is a seed, not a grain, but it's high in net carbs.

- Sweeteners: natural stevia and dark chocolate (at least 70 percent cacao).

- Whole sweet fruit. Berries are best; be extra cautious of sugary fruits such as apricots, mangos, melons, papaya, prunes, and pineapple.

- Wine: Have one glass a day if you so choose, preferably red.

Note about GMOs (Genetically Modified Organisms)

Since this book was first published, "GMO," which stands for genetically modified organism, has become a buzzword, along with "non-GMO" labeling on items in grocery stores. These terms were never mentioned in the first edition because they had not gone mainstream across the entire food and beverage industry. A lot has changed. Research is currently under way to study the effects of GMOs on our health and on the environment. GMOs are plants or animals that have been genetically engineered with DNA from other living things, including bacteria, viruses, plants, and animals. The genetic combinations that result cannot occur in nature or in traditional crossbreeding. GMO foods are commonly created to fight insects and viruses that can destroy crops, or to cultivate crops with certain desired characteristics. In the 1990s, for example, the ringspot virus decimated nearly half the crop of Hawaiian papaya in the state. In 1998, scientists developed a genetically engineered version of the papaya called the Rainbow papaya, which is resistant to the virus. Now 77 percent of the papayas grown in Hawaii are GMO.

Corn and soy are the top two GMO crops in the United States, and it's estimated that GMOs are in as much as 80 percent of conventional processed foods. Significant restrictions or outright bans have been placed on the production and sale of GMOs in more than sixty countries worldwide, including Australia, Japan, and all the countries in the European Union. But here in the United States, the government approves them. The problem: Many of the studies showing GMOs to be safe have been conducted by the same corporations that created and now profit from them. While it's true that not all genetically modified organisms are inherently bad, the methods used to create and farm GMOs can entail practices with far-reaching consequences, many of which we don't understand yet.

In addition to concerns about the effects of altered genetics in GMOs on human health, one of the most problematic—and contentious—aspects of GMOs has to do with current farming practices to grow GMO foods. No longer do farmers yank weeds from their fields by hand or machinery. They now spray a weed-killing chemical, glyphosate (the active ingredient in the common herbicide Roundup), on their crops. And they apply even more of this chemical just before the harvest to obtain a bigger yield and as a drying agent to prime the soil for a new crop. In order to protect crops from the herbicide, the seeds are genetically modified to be resistant to the herbicide's effects. In the world of agriculture, these seeds are known as "Roundup ready." The use of Roundup-ready GMO seeds has allowed farmers to use huge amounts of this herbicide. Which means that GMO foods—and foods conventionally farmed—are invariably contaminated with glyphosate, the "tobacco" of the twenty-first century that wreaks havoc on human health. Glyphosate is a poison like no other, toxic to the gut all the way up to the brain. Here's a list of my main concerns about this chemical (for more information, see *Brain Maker* and the focus area "GMO" on DrPerlmutter.com; also see my interview with Dr. Stephanie Seneff on *The Empowering Neurologist*). Glyphosate:[1]

- acts as a powerful antibiotic, slaughtering beneficial bacteria in your gut and thereby disrupting the healthy balance of your microbiome; in turn, this can trigger intestinal permeability and increased inflammation

- mimics hormones like estrogen, driving or stimulating the formation of hormone-sensitive cancers

- impairs the function of vitamin D, which as you know is an important player in human physiology

- depletes key compounds like iron, cobalt, molybdenum, and copper

- compromises your ability to detoxify toxins

- impairs the synthesis of tryptophan and tyrosine, important amino acids in protein and neurotransmitter production

It wouldn't surprise me in the least if it were soon revealed that the obesity epidemic could partly be blamed on the widespread use of glyphosate due to its effects on gut health and the microbiome. The importance of avoiding foods that have come into contact with glyphosate cannot be overemphasized. It can be found in unlikely places. In 2015, for instance, it was detected in PediaSure Enteral formula, which is widely used by hospitals in the United States for children in intensive care in need of nutrition. It is used in the wine industry. It has even been found in sanitary products because it is used by the cotton industry. Dr. Stephanie Seneff has devoted her time lately to studying the impact of this chemical on human health. When I interviewed her for my online vlog, she summarized the chief issue with glyphosate: "Wheat is now routinely sprayed with glyphosate right before harvest, and glyphosate in the wheat disrupts protein digestion and damages the gut microbes. Undigested proteins breach the leaky gut barrier and lead to inflammatory autoimmune diseases."

My hope is that stricter regulations are established to control the use of this harmful chemical. In 2017, California added new warning labels under Prop 65, calling glyphosate a potential carcinogen. That was the same year the *Journal of the American Medical Association* published data showing a stunning rise in glyphosate levels in a group of people evaluated first between 1993 and 1996 and then again between 2014 and 2016. The researchers found that glyphosate levels in their urine increased 500 percent over that time period of approximately twenty years! This is the reason we must choose non-GMO whenever we can. And again, even though wheat is not a GMO product, it is almost always sprayed with glyphosate.

Egg-Citing

I am compelled to say a few kind things in defense of eggs, since they are among the most wrongly accused foods in our modern era. I'll start by stating two important but seldom remembered facts: (1) Time and time again, science has failed to connect dietary fats of animal origin (i.e., saturated fats) and dietary cholesterol to either levels of serum cholesterol or risk for coronary heart disease; the belief that the cholesterol we eat converts directly into blood cholesterol is unequivocally false; and (2) when researchers compare serum cholesterol levels to egg intake, they note over and over that the levels of cholesterol in those who consume few or no eggs are virtually identical to those in people who consume bountiful numbers of eggs. Remember that contrary to popular wisdom, dietary cholesterol actually reduces the body's production of cholesterol, and more than 80 percent of the cholesterol in your blood that is measured on your cholesterol test is actually produced in your own liver.

To quote the authors of a cogent article by British researchers in the British Nutrition Foundation's newsletter: "The popular misconception that eggs are bad for your blood cholesterol and therefore bad for your heart persists among many people and still continues to influence the advice of some health professionals. The myth prevails despite strong evidence to show that the effects of cholesterol-rich foods on blood cholesterol are small and clinically insignificant."[2] The erroneous but strong messages about egg restriction that emanated primarily from the United States in the 1970s have unfortunately stuck around far too long. Scores of studies have confirmed the value of eggs, which are quite possibly the world's most perfect food; the yolk is the most nutritious part.[3] In fact, in a 2013 study, researchers at the University of Connecticut demonstrated that people on a low-carb diet, eating whole eggs—even on a daily basis—improved insulin sensitivity and other cardiovascular risk parameters.[4] Similar findings were published in 2016 following more than one thousand men in Finland and published in the *American Journal of Clinical Nutrition.*[5]

In addition to their healthy cholesterol, whole eggs contain all the essential amino acids we need to survive, vitamins and minerals, plus antioxidants known to protect our eyes. Moreover, they contain ample supplies of choline, which is particularly important for aiding healthy brain function as well as pregnancy. I cringe when I see an egg-white omelet on a menu. If only the people behind the old "incredible, edible egg" campaign would make some more noise!

You'll see that I recommend lots of eggs on this diet. Please don't be afraid of them. They could be the best way to start your day and set the tone for blood sugar balance. There are so many things you can do with eggs, too. Whether you scramble, fry, poach, boil, or use them in dishes, eggs are indeed among the most versatile ingredients. Hard-boil a carton of eggs on a Sunday night and you've got breakfast and/or snacks for the week.

Optional Fast

Ideally, start week 1 after you have fasted for one full day. Fasting is an excellent way to set the foundation and speed up your body's shift to burning fat for fuel and producing biochemicals that have astonishing pro-health effects on the body and brain. For many, it helps to do the fast on a Sunday (last meal is dinner Saturday night), and then begin the diet program on a Monday morning. Or have your last meal on Friday night and start the program on Sunday morning.

The fasting protocol is simple: No food but lots of water for a twenty-four-hour period. Avoid caffeine, too. If you take any medications, by all means continue to take them (if you take diabetes medications, please consult your physician first). If the idea of fasting is too painful for you, simply wean yourself from carbs for a few days as you prepare your kitchen. The more addicted your body is to carbs, the harder this will be. I prefer that my patients go cold turkey when it comes to nixing gluten, so do your best to at least eliminate sources of gluten entirely and cut back on other carbs. People whose bodies are not dependent on carbs can fast for longer periods, sometimes for days. When you've established this diet for life and want to fast for further benefits, you can try a seventy-two-hour fast (assuming you've checked with your doctor if you have any medical conditions to consider). I recommend that people fast at least four times a year; fasting during the seasonal changes (e.g., the last week of September, December, March, and June) is an excellent practice to keep.

GB CHALLENGE

As I described earlier, the body wakes up in mild ketosis. If you skip breakfast, you can keep this state going for a few hours before eating lunch at midday. Try skipping breakfast once or twice a week. That can help accelerate your transformation. For more resources on following a ketogenic diet, please go to my website at DrPerlmutter .com. Under the "Eat" pulldown tab, you'll find a wealth of information that will help you maintain ketosis. Remember: Aim to stay in mild ketosis throughout these four weeks, after which you can cycle in and out briefly once or twice a month. To break ketosis, simply increase your carb intake for two consecutive days, such as Saturday and Sunday. Increase carbs with healthy choices — choose whole fruit and rice, not processed sugars!

WEEK 1: FOCUS ON FOOD

Now that your kitchen is in order, it's time to get used to preparing meals using this new set of guidelines. In the next chapter, you'll find a day-by-day menu plan for the first week that will serve as a model for planning your meals the remaining three weeks. Unlike other diets, this one won't ask you to count calories, limit fat intake, or fret over portion sizes. I trust you can tell the difference between a supersize plate and a normal quantity. And I won't even ask you to worry about how much saturated versus unsaturated fat you're consuming.

The good news about this type of diet is that it's enormously "self-regulating"—you won't find yourself overeating and you'll enjoy feelings of fullness for several hours before needing another meal. When your body is running mostly on carbs, it's being driven by the glucose-insulin roller-coaster ride that triggers intense hunger when your blood sugar plunges, and then short-lived satiety. But eating a low-carb, higher-fat diet will have the opposite effect. It will eliminate cravings and prevent those mental shutdowns in the late afternoon that often occur on carb-based diets. It'll automatically allow you to control calories (without even thinking about it), burn more fat, put an end to mindless eating (i.e., the extra 500 calories or so many people unconsciously consume daily to bail out blood sugar chaos), and effortlessly boost your mental performance. Say goodbye to feeling moody, foggy, sluggish, and tired throughout the day. And say hello to a whole new you.

The only difference between this month and beyond is that you're going to aim for the fewest carbs now. It's imperative to lower net carb intake to just *20 to 25 grams a day for four weeks* (see the box on page 262). After that, you can increase your net carb intake to 30 grams a day. Adding more carbs into your diet after the first four weeks doesn't mean you can start eating pasta and bread again. What you'll do is simply add more of the items listed in the "moderate" category, such as whole fruit, non-gluten grains, and legumes. How to know how much you're getting? Use the food almanac on my website (DrPerlmutter.com), which lists grams of carbs per serving. If you follow the menu ideas and recipes in this book, you'll soon gain an understanding of what a low-carb meal looks like.

What about your fiber intake? Many people worry that reducing all those "fiber-rich" wheat products and breads will cause a dramatic loss of important fiber. Wrong. When you replace those wheat carbs with carbs from nuts and vegetables, your fiber intake will go up (and net carbs will go down). You will get your fill of essential vitamins and nutrients you were likely lacking previously, too.

Now that the low-carbohydrate dietary recommendations have taken hold in mainstream diet circles, we are beginning to see quite a bit more information about nutrition labeling that not only describes total carbohydrate content of a particular food, but also indicates "net carbs." Depending on the type of food, there may, in fact, actually be a significant difference between these two numbers. So let me remind you about this important difference.

The term *net carbs* simply describes the number of grams of total carbohydrates in a portion of food minus the grams of fiber. Fiber, you'll recall, is a form of carbohydrate, but is not a carbohydrate that has any effect on blood sugar or insulin response. Therefore, the idea of focusing on net carbs, meaning the carbs that are left over when the fiber is removed from the equation, does make a lot of sense because it is these residual carbohydrates that strongly influence blood sugar and, consequently, insulin response.

Let's look at an example. A ½-cup serving of baby carrots contains approximately 6 grams of total carbohydrate. But there is a fair amount of fiber in whole carrots, amounting to about 2 or 3 grams in this case. So the net carbs would be about 3 or 4 grams. An important place where this understanding comes into play is in looking at, for example, fruit juices. A 1-cup serving of regular orange juice provides 25.8 grams of total carbs and only 0.5 grams of fiber, so the net carbs are about 25.3 grams. That's enough to have a significant effect on blood sugar and insulin response.

Another way of looking at this calculation reveals that a larger difference between total carbs and net carbs is a good indication of the fiber content. The larger the difference, the better the food for your body and brain.

You might find it helpful to keep a food journal throughout the program. Make notes about recipes you like and foods that you think might still be giving you trouble (e.g., you experience symptoms such as stomach upset or headaches every time you eat sesame seeds). Some people are sensitive to foods that are included in this diet. For example, about 50 percent of those who are gluten intolerant are also sensitive to dairy. Surprisingly, researchers are also finding that coffee tends to cross-react with gluten. If, after embarking on this diet, you still sense a glitch somewhere, you may want to have a lab test done called the array 4, which can help pinpoint those foods that, for you, cross-react with gluten (see my website for details). It identifies reactions to the following:

amaranth	millet	spelt
buckwheat	oats	tapioca
chocolate	quinoa	teff
coffee	rice	whey
dairy	sesame	yeast
eggs	sorghum	
hemp	soy	

I recommend that you avoid eating out during the first three weeks on the program so you can focus on getting the dietary protocol down. This will prepare you for the day you do eat outside your home and have to make good decisions about what to order (see pages 271–272). The first three weeks will also eliminate your cravings so there's less temptation when you're looking at a menu filled with carbs.

During week 1, focus on mastering your new eating habits. You can use my recipes, including my sample seven-day meal plan, or venture out on your own as long as you stick to the guidelines. I've created an easy list of ideas categorized by type of meal (e.g., breakfast, lunch or dinner, salads), so you can pick and choose. Each meal should contain a source of healthy fat and protein. You can pretty much eat as many vegetables as you like with the exception of beets, peas, corn, potatoes, sweet potatoes, carrots, and parsnips. If you follow the first week's plan, configuring your own meals in the future will be a cinch.

WEEK 2: FOCUS ON EXERCISE

Aim to engage in aerobic physical activity if you're not already doing so for a minimum of twenty minutes a day. Use this week to establish a routine you enjoy that gets your heart rate up by at least 50 percent of your resting baseline. Remember, you are creating new habits for a lifetime, and you don't want to get burned out easily. But you also don't want to get too comfortable and shy away from challenging your body in ways that boost health and increase the brain's longevity.

To reap the benefits of exercise, make it a goal to break a sweat once a day and force your lungs and heart to work harder. Remember, in addition to all the cardiovascular and weight-management benefits you'll gain from exercise, studies show that people who exercise regularly, compete in sports, or just walk several times a week protect their brains from shrinkage. They also minimize the chance of becoming obese and diabetic—major risk factors in brain disease.

If you've been leading a sedentary lifestyle, then simply go for a twenty-minute walk daily and add more minutes as you get comfortable with your routine. You can also add intensity to your workouts by increasing your speed and tackling hills. Or carry a five-pound free weight in each hand and perform some bicep curls as you walk.

For those of you who already maintain a fitness regimen, see if you can increase your workouts to a minimum of thirty minutes a day, at least five days a week. This also might be the week you try something different, such as joining a group exercise class or dusting off that old bicycle in the garage. These days, opportunities to exercise are everywhere beyond traditional gyms, so there's really no excuse. You can even stream videos and exercise in the comfort of your own home. I really don't care which activity you choose. Just pick one!

Ideally, a comprehensive workout should entail a mix of cardio, strength training, and stretching. But if you're starting from scratch, begin with cardio and then add strength training and stretching over time. Strength training can be done with classic gym equipment, free weights, or the use of your own body weight in classes geared toward this activity such as yoga and

Pilates. These classes often entail lots of stretching, too, but you don't need a formal class to work on maintaining your flexibility. You can perform many stretching exercises on your own, even in front of the television.

Once you've gotten a regular workout down, you can schedule your daily routines around different types of exercise. For example, Mondays, Wednesdays, and Fridays could be the days you take a one-hour indoor cycling class; on Tuesdays and Thursdays you hit a yoga class. Then, on Saturday, you go for a hike with friends or swim laps in a pool and take Sunday off to rest. I recommend getting out your calendar and scheduling physical activity.

If you have a day during which there's absolutely no time to devote to a continuous segment of formal exercise, then think about the ways you can sneak in more minutes of physical activity during the day. All the research indicates that you can get similar health benefits from doing three ten-minute bouts of exercise as you would from doing a single thirty-minute workout. So if you are short on time on any given day, just break up your routine into bite-size chunks. And think of ways to combine exercise with other tasks; for example, conduct a meeting with a colleague at work while walking outside, or watch television at night while you complete a set of stretching exercises on the floor. If possible, limit the minutes you spend sitting down. Walk around if you can while you talk on the phone using a headset, take the stairs rather than the elevator, and park far away from the front door to your building. The more you move throughout the day, the more your brain stands to gain.

> Don't forget to use my online resources at DrPerlmutter.com. I have a library of useful information there, including videos where I demonstrate specific exercises to perform. In particular, pull down the "Focus" tab on the homepage.

WEEK 3: FOCUS ON SLEEP

In addition to continuing your new diet and exercise habits, use this week to focus on your sleep hygiene. Now that you've been on the protocol for a couple of weeks, your sleep should have improved. If you get fewer than six hours of sleep per night, you can start by increasing that period of time to at least seven hours. This is the bare minimum if you want to have normal, healthy levels of fluctuating hormones in your body.

To ensure that you're doing all that you can to maximize high-quality, restful sleep, below are some tips:

1. **Maintain regular sleep habits.** Experts in sleep medicine like to call this "sleep hygiene" — the ways in which we ensure refreshing sleep night after night. Go to bed and get up at roughly the same time seven days a week, 365 days a year. Keep your bedtime routine consistent; it might include reading, a warm bath, herbal tea, whatever you need to do to wind down and signal to your body that it's time for sleep. We do this with our young children but often forget about our own bedtime rituals. They work wonders in helping us to feel primed for slumber.

2. **Identify and manage ingredients hostile to sleep.** These can be any number of things, from prescription medicine to caffeine, alcohol, and nicotine. Both caffeine and nicotine are stimulants. Anyone who still smokes should adopt a plan to quit, for smoking alone will increase your risk of everything under the medical sun. As for caffeine, try to avoid it after two p.m. This will give your body time to process the caffeine so it doesn't impact sleep. Some people, however, are extra sensitive to caffeine, so you may want to back up this time to noon or move to less-caffeinated drinks. Ask your doctor or pharmacist about any potential sleep repercussions for medications you take on a routine basis. Be aware that lots of over-the-counter medications can contain sleep-disrupting ingredients, too. Popular headache drugs, for instance, can contain caffeine. Alcohol, while creating a sedative effect immediately upon consumption, can disrupt sleep while it's being processed by the body; one of the enzymes used to break down alcohol has stimulating effects. Alcohol also causes the release of adrenaline and disrupts the production of serotonin, an important brain chemical that initiates sleep.

3. **Time your dinner appropriately.** No one likes to go to bed on a full or empty stomach. Find your sweet spot, leaving approximately three hours between dinner and bedtime. Also be aware of ingredients in foods that can be problematic to digest easily before going to bed. Everyone's experience will be different in this department.

4. **Don't eat erratically.** Eat on a regular schedule. This will keep your appetite hormones in check. If you delay a meal too long, you will throw your hormones out of whack and trigger the nervous system, which can later impact your sleep.

5. **Try a bedtime snack.** Nocturnal hypoglycemia (low nighttime blood glucose levels) can cause insomnia. If your blood sugar drops too low, it causes the release of hormones that stimulate the brain and tell you to eat. Try a bedtime snack to avoid this midnight disaster. Go for foods high in the amino acid tryptophan, which is a natural promoter of sleep. Foods high in tryptophan include turkey, cottage cheese, chicken, eggs, and nuts (especially almonds). Just watch your portion, however. A handful of nuts might be perfect. You don't want to devour a three-egg omelet with turkey right before bedtime. Choose wisely.

6. **Beware of imposter stimulants.** You already know that regular coffee will keep you alert, but today caffeine-infused products are everywhere. If you follow my dietary protocol, you're not likely to encounter these. Also, certain food compounds such as colorings, flavorings, and refined carbs can *act as* stimulants, so avoid these, too.

7. **Set the setting.** It should come as no surprise that keeping brain- and eye-stimulating electronics in the bedroom is a bad idea. But people still break this most basic rule. Try to keep your bedroom a quiet, peaceful sanctuary free of rousing hardware (e.g., TVs, computers, phones, etc.), as well as bright lights and clutter. Invest in a comfortable bed and plush sheets. Maintain dim lighting. Cultivate a mood for sleep (and sex for that matter, which can also prepare one for sleep, but that's another story).

8. **Use sleep aids prudently.** The occasional sleep aid won't kill you. But chronic use of them can become a problem. The goal is to arrive at sound sleep on a routine basis without extra help. And I'm not referring to earplugs or eye masks here, both of which I approve of as sleep aids; I'm talking about over-the-counter and prescription drugs that induce sleep. Examples include "p.m." formulas that include sedating antihistamines such as diphenhydramine and doxylamine. Even if they claim to be nonaddictive, they can still create a psychological dependency. Better to regulate your sleep naturally. And consider a sleep study even if you think you're a good sleeper.

A Note About Bathroom Toiletries and Beauty Products

In addition to focusing on sleep, during week 3 you should overhaul your bathroom supplies. Gluten tends to find its way into many commercial products, and it can unintentionally end up in our bodies if we use these products on our skin—our largest organ. So pay attention to the beauty and makeup supplies you use regularly, including shampoos, conditioners, and other hair products. You may want to seek out brands that offer gluten-free products. Contact the manufacturer or a company representative if you're in doubt or cannot tell from a product's labeling whether it contains gluten.

WEEK 4: PUT IT ALL TOGETHER

By now you should be in the groove of this new way of life and feeling much better than you did three weeks ago. You can tell the difference between a grain-brain food and a healthier choice. Your sleep has improved and you've established a regular workout routine. Now what?

Don't panic if you don't feel like you've totally hit your stride yet. Most of us have at least one weak spot in our lives that requires extra attention. Perhaps you're the type who has a hard time getting to bed by ten p.m. every night, or maybe your Achilles' heel is finding time to work out most days of the week and avoiding the junk food that's always lying around your office's break room. Use this week to find a rhythm in your new routine. Identify areas in your life where you struggle to maintain this protocol and see what you can do to rectify that. A few tips that you might find helpful:

● **Plan each week in advance.** It helps to set aside a few minutes over the weekend to plan your upcoming week and take into consideration your agenda and appointments. Predict the hectic days when it will be harder to make time for a workout and see if you can build that into your schedule. Block out your sleeping zone every night and be sure to maintain the same bedtime; be religious about it. Map out the majority of your meals for the week, especially lunches and dinners. We tend to be pretty routine with breakfast, but can fall prey to last-minute decisions about lunch while at work, as well as dinner if we arrive home starving. Be on the lookout for those days when you know that you'll get home late and won't have energy to cook. Have a contingency plan in place. (I give you plenty of ideas in the next chapter for dealing with meals away from home and handling those moments when you need to have a little something to tide you over until you can eat a full meal.)

● **Prepare shopping lists.** Whether you shop for groceries every day or just once a week, you'll want to have a list in hand. This will help you be more efficient and avoid impulse buying. It will also take a lot of the guess-work out of trying to figure out what's a safe bet at the market to buy, cook, and eat. For the most part, stick to the perimeter of the grocery store, where the foods closest to nature are found. Avoid the middle aisles, which are overflowing with processed, packaged goods. And don't shop while hungry; if you do, you'll gravitate toward damaging foods of the sugary and salty variety. Keep in mind that fresh ingredients won't last more than three to five days unless you freeze them. A monthly trip to a store that sells foods in bulk might be helpful if you have a family to feed and extra room in your freezer for large quantities of meat, poultry, and frozen vegetables.

● **Create a few "non-negotiables."** If you have high hopes of getting to the farmers' market on Thursday afternoon in your neighborhood, then write that down in your calendar and make it a non-negotiable. If you dream of trying a new yoga studio that opened up in town, set aside a specific time and make it happen. Creating non-negotiable goals will help you dodge those excuses that surface when you get lazy or thwarted by other tasks. They are also excellent ways to fortify your weak spots. Be clear about your priorities when you set the course for your week and stick to them!

- **Use technology.** We use technology every day to make our lives easier. So why not capitalize on Internet resources and high-tech apps that can help us stick to our goals and stay tuned in to ourselves? The market for self-tracking apps, for instance, has exploded in the last few years. You can use nifty devices to track how many steps you take a day, how well you slept last night, and even how fast you eat. Some of these work on smartphones, while others require an actual device such as an accelerometer that tracks your bodily movements throughout the day. Granted, these tools are not for everyone, but you might just find a few programs that ultimately help you maintain a healthy lifestyle. For a few ideas, go to DrPerlmutter.com. There, you'll also find a list of apps that can help you maximize the information in this book, such as food almanacs that provide ingredient information about common foods and links to health-related services that can remind you to keep track of your habits. Google Calendar, for example, can be used as a comprehensive self-management application. If it works for you, use it.

- **Be flexible, but be consistent.** Don't beat yourself up when you momentarily fall off the program. We're all human. You might have a bad day and find yourself skipping the gym in favor of a night out with friends at a restaurant where pretty much everything served is off-limits. Or perhaps it's the holidays and a few indulgences are inevitable. As long as you get back on track once you catch yourself, you'll be fine. Just don't let a small slip derail you forever. To this end, remember to find consistency in your daily patterns. Consistency is not about rigidity. It's about eating and exercising in ways that serve you without making you feel like you're going to extremes or forcing yourself to do something you don't like. Finding your own unique version of consistency will be key to your success. You'll figure out what works best for you and what doesn't. Then you can adapt this program to your life based on the general guidelines and maintain it on a consistent basis.

- **Find motivators.** Sometimes it helps to have motivators. A motivator can be anything from the desire to run your town's 10K to planning a trip with your adult children to hike Mount Kilimanjaro. People who decide to focus on their health often do so for specific reasons, such as "I want more energy," "I want to live longer," "I want to lose weight," and "I don't want to die like my mother did." Keep the big picture in plain sight. This will help you not only maintain a healthy lifestyle, but also get back on track even if you do occasionally cheat. Progress is sometimes better than perfection.

Everyone's daily schedule will be different, but patterns should exist. Below is a sample of what a day might look like:

Wake up, walk the dog:	6:30 a.m.
Breakfast:	7:00 a.m.
Snack:	10:00 a.m.
Bagged lunch:	12:30 p.m.
20-minute walk:	1:00 p.m
Snack:	4:00 p.m.
Gym:	5:45 p.m.
Dinner:	7:00 p.m.
Walk the dog:	7:30 p.m.
Lights out:	10:30 p.m.

Eating Out

Toward the end of week 4, work on the goal of being able to eat anywhere. Many of us eat out several times a week, especially while we're at work. It's virtually impossible to plan and prepare every single meal and snack we eat, so make it a goal to navigate other menus. See if you can return to your favorite restaurants and order off the menu while still following this protocol. If you find it too challenging, then you may want to test new restaurants that cater to your needs. It's not that hard to make any menu work for you as long as you're savvy about your decisions. Baked fish with steamed vegetables is likely to be a safe bet (hold the potatoes, fries, and bread basket, and ask for a side salad with olive oil and vinegar). Watch out for elaborate dishes that contain multiple ingredients. And when in doubt, ask about the dishes.

In general, eating out should be minimized because eliminating all sources of bad ingredients is impossible. On most days of the week, commit to consuming foods that you prepare. Keep snacks on hand, too, so you don't get caught famished while at the gas station's convenience store. There are plenty of snack and "on-the-go" ideas in the next chapter, many of which are portable and nonperishable. Once you've gotten a handle on this way of eating, see if you can go back to your old recipes and modify them to fit my guidelines. You'd be surprised by what a little experimentation in the kitchen can do to turn a classic dish filled with gluten and inflammatory ingredients into an equally delicious but brain-friendly meal. Instead of regular flour or wheat, try coconut flour, nut meals like ground almonds, and ground flax-seed; in lieu of sugar, find ways to sweeten your recipe with a small pinch of stevia or whole fruits; and rather than cook with processed vegetable oils, stick with old-fashioned butter and extra virgin olive oil.

And when you're faced with temptation (the box of doughnuts at work or a friend's birthday cake), remind yourself that you'll pay for the indulgence somehow. Be willing to accept those consequences if you cannot say no. But keep in mind that a grain-brain-free way of life is, in my humble opinion, the most fulfilling and gratifying way of life there is. Enjoy it.

THE BALANCING ACT

As with so many things in life, discovering and establishing a new habit is a balancing act. Even once you've shifted your eating and exercise behaviors and changed the way you buy, cook, and order food, you'll still have moments when old habits emerge. I don't expect you to never eat a slice of crusty pizza or stack of steaming hot pancakes again, but I do hope that you stay mindful of your body's true needs now that you have the knowledge, and live out this newly found sensibility every day as best you can.

Many people have applied the famous 80/20 principle to diet—eat well 80 percent of the time and save that last 20 percent for splurges. But some of us find ourselves living the reverse! It's too easy to let an occasional splurge become a daily habit, like eating a bowl of ice cream several times a week. You should remember that there is always an excuse for not taking better care of yourself. We have parties and weddings to attend. We have work to address that leaves us high on stress and low on energy, time, and the mental bandwidth to make good food, exercise, and sleep choices. This is life, and accepting a certain give-and-take is okay. But see if you can stick to a 90/10 rule. For 90 percent of the time, eat within these guidelines and let the last 10 percent take care of itself, as it inevitably does in life. Then hit reboot whenever you feel like you've fallen too far off the wagon. You can do this by fasting for a day and committing again to the same four weeks of restricting carbs to 20 to 25 grams a day. This protocol can be your lifeline to a healthier way of living that supports the vision you have for yourself—and your brain.

Life is an endless series of choices. *This way or that way? Now or later? Red sweater or green one? Sandwich or salad?* The whole point of this book has been to help you learn to make better decisions that will ultimately allow you to participate in life at its fullest. My hope is that I've given you plenty of ideas to at least begin to make a difference in your life. I see the value that being healthy—and mentally sharp—brings to people every day in my practice. I also see what sudden illness and chronic disease can do, regardless of people's achievements and how much they are loved. For many, health may not seem to be the most important thing in life, but without it, nothing else matters. And when you have good health, pretty much anything is possible.

CHAPTER 11

Eating Your Way to a Healthy Brain

Meal Plans and Recipes

THE NUMBER OF MEAL IDEAS and recipes here goes to show how plentiful your choices are on this diet. You'll see an abundance of vegetables, fish, meat, poultry, nuts, eggs, and salads. But you could just as easily craft simpler dishes based on the themes presented here (e.g., pick a fish or meat to cook up with some side vegetables and a green salad for lunch or dinner and pack hard-boiled eggs for breakfast with a handful of nuts as a snack). You'll find a few ideas for dessert (yes, it's allowable!), as well as various salad dressings and dipping sauces.

Notice that you won't find nutritional content information in these recipes. As I mentioned earlier, one of my goals in this book has been to liberate you from ever having to count calories or grams of protein and fat (especially saturated fat) again. I want to teach you *what* to eat, not how to eat (i.e., how much of this or that). If you follow the guidelines and protocol, the fat, carbs, and protein intake will take care of itself. You won't overeat, you won't feel underfed, and you'll be maximally nourishing your body and brain.

At DrPerlmutter.com, you'll find my recommendations for specific brands of foods that follow the *Grain Brain* guidelines. Even though you're evicting gluten, wheat, and most sugar from your diet, you'd be surprised by the abundance of food options available to you. You'll also be astonished by the control you'll gain over your hunger levels, cravings, portion sizes, and caloric intake. Your taste buds will be rejoicing, too, as they experience a rebirth of sorts and bestow upon you a new appreciation for food.

In the past decade, there's been a huge shift in the variety of food available at our markets. If you live in an urban area, for instance, you're likely to be able to purchase any kind of ingredient within a matter of miles, whether that means visiting your usual grocery store that's now filled with organic foods or venturing to a local farmers' market. Get to know your grocers; they can tell you what just came in and where your foods are coming from. Aim for choosing produce that's in season, and be willing to try new foods you've never had before. Ten years ago, it was hard to buy bison or black cod, for instance, but today delicious and exotic meats and seafood are widely available. Remember, go organic or wild whenever possible. When in doubt, ask your grocer.

What to Drink: Ideally, stick with purified water. Drink half of your body weight in ounces of purified water daily. If you weigh 150 pounds, that means drinking at least 75 ounces, or about nine glasses, of water per day. You can also opt for tea or coffee (assuming you don't have any issues with coffee), but be careful about caffeine late in the day. For every caffeinated beverage you consume, include an extra 12 to 16 ounces of water. I highly recommend trying kombucha tea. This is a form of fermented black or green tea that contains naturally occurring probiotics. Fizzy and often served chilled, it's been used for centuries to help increase energy, and it may even help you lose weight in addition to contributing to the health of your gut microbes. Almond milk is also a healthy choice. At dinner, you have the option of having a glass of wine, preferably red. I have been asked a lot lately about alcohol in general. One day it's declared good for you, the next, bad. One 2017 study has emerged declaring *any* alcohol consumption—even if its moderate—as being bad for the brain, including hippocampal atrophy.[1] Other studies have shown that mild to moderate alcohol intake is associated with a lower risk of Alzheimer's disease, while heavy drinking increases the risk. My take? The balance of the research indicates that while no alcohol may be associated with a higher risk for the development of Alzheimer's disease, we know that there is also a higher risk of Alzheimer's disease in those who consume higher levels. Ultimately, my position is that there's a sweet spot and that red wine would be the best choice thanks to its brain-friendly ingredients, such as resveratrol and polyphenols. I recommend one glass for women and two for men per day.

Special Note about Coffee: Don't be deceived by cautionary warnings about coffee! The benefits of coffee consumption—three to five cups per day—far outweigh the risks. And it's not just about lowering one's risk for dementia to the tune of a 65 percent reduced risk. In 2017, the *Annals of Internal Medicine* reported on a massive, longitudinal study that involved ten European countries and more than half a million people. The results were quite powerful: Those who drank the most coffee had the lowest risk of dying—*of anything*—during the study, with a 12 percent reduction in risk for death in men and a 7 percent risk reduction in women.[2] And "higher consumption of coffee was associated with lower risk for death, particularly that due to digestive and circulatory diseases." What's important is that in women higher levels of coffee consumption correlated with lower A1C levels as well as lower C-reactive protein levels. More good news: If you don't like to drink coffee due to its caffeine content, decaf can be just as beneficial. Many of the components in coffee that make it brain- and body-friendly, notably those polyphenols, are not in the caffeine itself. Coffee is a potent antioxidant and BDNF stimulator, and is also involved in turning on the production of brain-loving ketones. So drink up!

Fruit: Choose whole fruit, and during the first four weeks, aim to save fruit for a snack or as a dessert. Try it with fresh, unsweetened cream or blended with coconut milk and a pinch of stevia or unsweetened cocoa powder.

Olive Oil Rule: You are free to liberally use olive oil (extra virgin and organic). It is in fact one of the easiest ways to add more good fat to your diet and automatically reduce your risk for stroke, dementia, and diabetes. Note that in many cases, you can substitute coconut oil for olive oil during the cooking process. For instance, pan-fry fish and sauté vegetables in coconut oil rather than olive oil or scramble eggs in coconut oil for breakfast. This will help you get your daily tablespoon of coconut oil as recommended in the supplement section.

On the Go: When you're strapped for time and don't have access to a kitchen, which is often the case during lunch at work, pack food. Having pre-cooked foods—such as roasted or broiled chicken, poached salmon, or strips of grilled sirloin steak or roast beef—in your refrigerator ready to go is helpful. Fill a container with salad greens and chopped raw veggies and add your protein and dressing of choice on top before eating. Many supermarkets now offer ready-to-go foods that list their ingredients so you know what you're getting.

And don't forget about leftovers. Many of the recipes in this chapter can be made over the weekend (and doubled for more) to cover multiple meals during the week while you're on the go. Just carry your food in an airtight container and eat cold or reheat in a microwave.

I always travel with avocados and cans of sockeye salmon. Canned foods can be excellent sources of good, portable nutrition, as long as you're careful about which canned products you're buying. Canned tomatoes, for instance, can be a great alternative to fresh. Just be watchful of added ingredients like sodium and sugar. When choosing canned fish, opt for sustainably caught, pole- or troll-caught fish. Also steer clear of any fish that is likely to be high in mercury. A great site to bookmark on your computer is the Monterey Bay Aquarium's Seafood Watch program at montereybayaquarium.org/cr /seafoodwatch.aspx. The site offers up-to-date information about where your fish is coming from and which fish to avoid due to contaminants and toxins.

What to Snack On: Due to the high satiety factor of the meals I suggest (not to mention the exquisite blood sugar control), you're not likely to find yourself hunting ravenously for food in between meals. But it's nice to know you can snack whenever you want to on this diet. Below are some ideas:

- A handful of raw nuts (with the exception of peanuts, which are a legume and not a nut). Or go for a mix of nuts and olives.
- A few squares of dark chocolate (anything above 70 percent cacao).
- Chopped raw vegetables (e.g., bell peppers, broccoli, cucumber, green beans, radishes) dipped in hummus, guacamole, goat cheese, tapenade, or nut butter. Or try a fermented condiment.
- Cheese and wheat-free, low-carb crackers.
- Slices of cold roasted turkey or chicken dipped in mustard or avocado mayonnaise.
- Half an avocado drizzled with olive oil, salt, and pepper.
- Two hard-boiled eggs, regular or fermented.
- Caprese salad: Tomato slices topped with fresh sliced mozzarella cheese, drizzled olive oil, basil, salt, and pepper.
- Cold peeled prawns with lemon and dill.
- One piece or serving of whole, low-sugar fruit (e.g., grapefruit, orange, apple, berries, melon, pear, cherries, grapes, kiwi, plum, peach, nectarine).
- Smoked salmon (wild, not farm-raised) or lox with a spread of ricotta.
- Grass-fed beef, turkey, or salmon jerky.

SAMPLE MENU FOR A WEEK

Here is what a weeklong, grain-brain-free diet approach could look like. All dishes accompanied by recipes are in boldface. The recipes, many of which are new, begin on page 283. I have kept all the original recipes from the first edition—now you get more! Note: You can use butter, organic extra virgin olive oil, or coconut oil when you pan-fry foods. Avoid processed oils and cooking sprays unless the spray is made from organic olive oil. Double or triple any recipe for which you want to yield more servings. Some of these recipes are more time-consuming to make than others, so plan ahead and feel free to swap one for another if you don't have the extra time. For even more ideas, go to my website for a gallery of additional recipes. I highly recommend checking out my "Brain Maker" foods under the "Eat" tab. There, you'll find a list of probiotic- and prebiotic-rich foods to incorporate into your diet to help nurture your microbiome. Finally, try skipping breakfast a couple of days a week, which will enhance your overnight ketosis. I've made that suggestion on two of the days here.

Monday

- Breakfast: 2 scrambled eggs with 25g/1oz Cheddar cheese and unlimited stir-fried veggies (e.g., onions, mushrooms, spinach, broccoli)
- Lunch: **Avocado Chicken Salad Stuffed Tomato** (page 309)
- Dinner: 75g/3oz grass-fed sirloin steak, roasted organic chicken, or wild fish with a side of greens and vegetables sautéed in butter and garlic
- Dessert: ½ cup berries topped with a drizzle of unsweetened cream

Tuesday

- Breakfast: Skip! Or have half an avocado drizzled with olive oil and 225g/8oz yogurt topped with crushed walnuts and fresh blueberries.
- Lunch: **Greek Village Salad with Prawns** (pages 309–310)
- Dinner: **Salmon & Vegetables in Parchment** (pages 303–304)
- Dessert: 2 **Chocolate Truffles** (page 324)

Wednesday

- Breakfast: **Two-Minute Microwave Frittata** (page 285)
- Lunch: **Chicken Fajita Salad** (pages 312–313)

- Dinner: **Chardonnay Baked Fish** (pages 293–294) with 75g/3oz wild rice and unlimited steamed vegetables
- Dessert: 1 apple, sliced and topped with a sprinkle of stevia and cinnamon

Thursday

- Breakfast: 3–4 slices of lox or smoked salmon with 25g/1oz goat cheese and 1 serving of **Quick Crunchy "Cereal"** (page 289)
- Lunch: **Curry Chickpea Salad** (page 313)
- Dinner: **Aubergine-Bun Burger** (page 291) with greens and vegetables sautéed in butter and garlic
- Dessert: 2–3 squares of dark chocolate

Friday

- Breakfast: Skip! Or try the **Coconut Oil Omelet** (pages 285–286).
- Lunch: **Fish Tacos with Avocado Slaw** (page 290)
- Dinner: **Greek Lemon Lamb** (pages 304–305) with unlimited green beans and broccoli
- Dessert: **Chocolate Coconut Mousse** (pages 324–325)

Saturday

- Breakfast: **Baked Grapefruit with Granola Crunch Topping** (pages 287–288)
- Lunch: **Rainbow Hummus Wraps** (pages 291–292)
- Dinner: **Sea Salt's Akaushi Beef Fillet with Brussels Sprouts** (page 297)
- Dessert: 115g/4oz whole strawberries dipped in 3 squares of melted dark chocolate

Sunday

- Breakfast: **Creamed Eggs over Asparagus** (pages 286–287)
- Lunch: **Goddess Gazpacho with Smoked Salmon** (pages 307–308)
- Dinner: **Sea Salt's Grilled Sardines with Tomato, Rocket, and Pecorino Cheese** (page 298)
- Dessert: 2 squares of dark chocolate dipped in 1 tablespoon almond butter

RECIPES

Abiding by the *Grain Brain* dietary principles is easier than you think. Even though this new way of eating significantly limits your intake of carbohydrates, especially wheat and sugar, there's really no shortage of foods and ingredients to play with in the kitchen. You'll have to get a little creative to adapt some of your beloved dishes, but once you learn how to effortlessly make certain substitutions, you'll be able to do the same with your own recipes and return to your classic cookbooks. These recipes will give you a general sense of how to apply the guidelines to virtually any meal, and help you master the art of grain-brain-free cuisine.

Knowing that most people maintain busy schedules and have limited time to cook, I've chosen simple dishes that are relatively easy to prepare and, above all, are filled with flavor and nutrition. Although I encourage you to follow my seven-day meal plan outlined on pages 279–281 so you don't even have to think about what to eat during the first week on the program, you could design your own protocol by choosing the recipes that appeal to you. Most of the ingredients used are widely available. Remember to go grass-fed, organic, and wild whenever possible. When choosing olive or coconut oil, reach for extra virgin varieties. Although all the ingredients listed in the recipes were chosen to be readily accessible as gluten-free, always check labels to be sure, particularly if you're buying a food processed by a manufacturer (e.g., mustard). You can never control what goes into products, but you can control what goes into your dishes.

BREAKFAST

Gruyère and Goat Cheese Frittatas

Eggs are one of the most versatile ingredients. They can serve as a meal on their own or be added to other dishes. Buy organic, free-range eggs whenever possible. Frittatas are quick and easy to make, and are great for serving large groups. You can make many different kinds of frittatas by changing the type of cheese, leafy greens, and vegetables you use. Here is one of my favorites.

Serves 4

1 tablespoon extra virgin olive oil

1 medium onion, chopped

½ teaspoon salt

½ teaspoon pepper

450g/1lb spinach leaves, chopped

1 tablespoon water

9 large eggs, beaten

75g/3oz goat cheese, crumbled

25g/1oz grated Gruyère cheese

Preheat the oven to 200°C/400°F/gas mark 6.

In an ovenproof frying pan, heat the oil over medium-high heat. Once hot, add the onion, salt, and pepper. Cook for 3 to 4 minutes, stirring occasionally, until the onion is translucent. Add the spinach and water and sauté until the spinach is wilted, 1 to 2 minutes. Pour in the eggs and sprinkle on the goat cheese and Gruyère. Cook for 1 to 2 minutes, until the mixture begins to set around the edges. Transfer the pan to the oven and bake until set, 10 to 12 minutes.

Remove from the oven and cut into wedges to serve.

Two-Minute Microwave Frittata

Here's an easy way to make a single-serving frittata for a quick breakfast when you are in a hurry. Feel free to swap in any other vegetables you have on hand.

Serves 1

2 large eggs

2 tablespoons diced red or orange bell pepper

2 tablespoons diced mushroom

2 teaspoons crumbled goat cheese

½ teaspoon dried oregano

Salt and pepper to taste

In a microwave-safe bowl (with at least a 500ml/18fl oz capacity to allow for "puffing" of the frittata as it cooks), beat the eggs, then stir in the remaining ingredients. Microwave on high power for 1½ minutes, then leave the frittata in the microwave for an additional 30 seconds before opening the door and removing.

Serve immediately from the bowl.

Coconut Oil Omelet

Omelets are a favorite in my house. Experiment with different vegetables and cook your omelet in coconut oil one day and olive oil the next.

Serves 1

2 large eggs

1 onion, chopped

1 ripe tomato, chopped

½ teaspoon salt

½ teaspoon pepper

1 tablespoon coconut oil

¼ avocado, sliced

2 tablespoons salsa

In a bowl, beat the eggs, then stir in the onion, tomato, salt, and pepper. In a small frying pan, heat the coconut oil over medium-high heat. Once hot, add the egg mixture and cook until the eggs begin to set, about 2 minutes. Flip the omelet with a spatula and cook until the eggs are no longer runny, about 1 more minute. Fold the omelet in half and continue to cook if the omelet is not yet slightly brown. Transfer to a plate and serve hot, topped with sliced avocado and salsa.

Huevos Rancheros

This classic Mexican dish has been modified so that instead of serving the eggs on tortillas, they are prepared over a bed of fresh greens.

Serves 2

> 1 tablespoon unsalted butter or extra virgin olive oil
> 4 large eggs
> 120g/4½oz coarsely torn curly endive
> 50g/2oz sharp Cheddar cheese, grated
> 4 tablespoons salsa
> 2 tablespoons chopped fresh coriander leaves
> Salt and pepper to taste

In a large frying pan, melt the butter over medium-high heat. When hot, crack the eggs into the pan and cook for 3 to 4 minutes for runny yolks, more for firmer yolks. Divide the endive between two plates and place two eggs on each. Top each with some cheese, salsa, and coriander and season with salt and pepper. Serve hot.

Creamed Eggs over Asparagus

Adding nutritional yeast to an egg dish is a great way to create a creamy, rich delight. Nutritional yeast is a deactivated yeast that happens to be a complete protein and has a nutty, cheesy flavor. Most grocery stores carry this ingredient; it's sold in the form of flakes or as a yellow powder and can be found in the health-food or baking aisle.

Serves 1

6 asparagus spears, tough ends snapped off

4 tablespoons canned coconut milk

1 tablespoon mashed avocado

1½ teaspoons nutritional yeast

Pinch salt

2 large eggs, hard-boiled, peeled, and chopped

Steam the asparagus spears in a shallow dish with 2 tablespoons water in the microwave on high power or in a steamer basket over boiling water on the hob for 4 to 5 minutes. Transfer the steamed asparagus to a serving plate. In a small saucepan, combine the milk, avocado, nutritional yeast, and salt. Heat over medium-high heat until warmed through and the mixture begins to thicken, about 4 minutes.

Turn off the heat and stir in the chopped eggs. Spoon the egg mixture over the asparagus and serve immediately.

Baked Grapefruit with Granola Crunch Topping

Something sweet and savory for breakfast will make you feel like you're eating dessert. This fruit- and nut-based dish is easy to put together and chock-full of nutrition that will fuel a bright morning.

Serves 1

½ grapefruit

⅛ teaspoon ground cinnamon

1 tablespoon unsalted nuts or seeds of choice

1 tablespoon hemp hearts (hulled hemp seeds)

1 tablespoon almond butter (no sugar added)

Preheat the oven to 190°C/375°F/gas mark 5 and line a small rimmed baking sheet with foil.

Score along the grapefruit segments with a paring knife to loosen the flesh, then place the grapefruit half on the baking sheet. Sprinkle the cinnamon over the grapefruit and set aside.

In a small bowl, combine the nuts or seeds, hemp hearts, and almond butter; stir until smooth. Spread the mixture on top of the grapefruit.

Bake until golden brown, 8 to 10 minutes, then transfer to a plate and serve.

Oatless "Oatmeal"

The following recipe, sometimes called "No Oat Oatmeal," was adapted from *The Paleo Diet Cookbook* by Loren Cordain and Nell Stephenson. If you enjoy a rich, thick, warm breakfast, try this instead of classic oatmeal.

Serves 2

25g/1oz raw, unsalted walnuts

40g/1½oz raw, unsalted almonds

2 tablespoons ground flaxseed

1 teaspoon ground allspice

3 large eggs

50ml/2fl oz unsweetened almond milk, plus more if needed

½ banana

1 tablespoon almond butter (no sugar added)

2 teaspoons pumpkin seeds (optional)

1 handful fresh berries (optional)

Combine the walnuts, almonds, flaxseed, and allspice in a food processor and pulse to a coarse grain but not a powder. Set aside.

In a bowl, whisk together the eggs and almond milk until thick like a custard. In another bowl, mash the banana together with the almond butter. Add the banana mixture to the custard and mix well. Stir in the coarse nut mixture.

Transfer the mixture to a small saucepan and heat over low heat, stirring frequently, until it reaches the desired consistency. Sprinkle the pumpkin seeds and berries on top and add more almond milk, if desired. Serve warm.

Quick Crunchy "Cereal"

Looking for a cereal that meets the *Grain Brain* guidelines? Try this one, and if walnuts are not your thing, you can substitute your favorite raw nut.

Serves 1

25g/1oz crushed raw, unsalted walnuts

25g/1oz coconut flakes

1 handful fresh berries

150ml/5fl oz whole milk or almond milk

Combine the ingredients in a bowl and enjoy.

LUNCH OR DINNER

Fish Tacos with Avocado Slaw

These fish tacos are fresh, delicious, simple, and clean. Instead of using traditional tortillas for the tacos, you'll use the leaves of romaine lettuce to wrap your fish and slaw.

Serves 1

- 1 (115g/4oz) boneless, skinless firm white fish fillet (such as halibut or cod)
- 1 lime, cut into 4 wedges
- ½ teaspoon ground cumin
- Salt and pepper to taste
- 100g/3 ½oz shredded cabbage
- 25g/1oz shredded carrot
- ¼ avocado
- 1 tablespoon salsa
- 3 large romaine lettuce leaves

Preheat the oven to 190°C/375°F/gas mark 5 and line a rimmed baking sheet with foil.

Place the fish on the lined baking sheet. Squeeze two of the lime wedges over, and sprinkle with the cumin, salt, and pepper. Bake until cooked through, 10 to 12 minutes.

While the fish bakes, prepare the slaw by tossing the cabbage and carrot together in a bowl. Add the avocado and mash it into the cabbage. Stir in the salsa and season with salt and pepper. Divide the slaw evenly among the romaine leaves.

When the fish is cooked, break it into bite-size pieces and divide it evenly on top of the slaw. Squeeze the remaining two lime wedges over the fish, roll up the tacos, and serve immediately.

Aubergine-Bun Burger

Who doesn't love a juicy burger once in a while? This classic skips the bun and uses sliced aubergine as a substitute. Another way to spin this is to grill large portobello mushroom caps and use those instead to bookend the beef.

Serves 1

- 2 (1cm/½-inch-thick) slices aubergine, about the same size and shape as a burger patty
- 2 teaspoons extra virgin olive oil
- 115g/4oz minced grass-fed beef, formed into a round patty
- Lettuce, tomato slice, mustard, and pickles, for serving (optional)

Brush the aubergine slices on both sides with the oil. Heat a large frying pan over medium heat, then add the aubergine slices and cook for 4 minutes per side. Transfer the aubergine slices to a serving plate and set aside.

Add the burger patty to the same pan and cook over medium heat until cooked through, about 5 minutes per side.

To serve, top one aubergine slice with the burger, add the lettuce, tomato slice, mustard, and pickles as desired, then top with the remaining aubergine slice. Serve immediately.

Rainbow Hummus Wraps

This dish can be put together quickly once you've got everything chopped. It can serve as a light lunch or a snack or even an appetizer when you host your next dinner party. If you don't make your hummus from scratch, be sure to buy organic hummus that contains no added sugars.

Serves 1 to 2

- 40g/1½oz diced red, yellow, or orange bell pepper
- 25g/1oz chopped dark leafy greens (such as kale, rocket, and/or spinach)
- 50g/2oz chopped water chestnuts
- 1½ teaspoons chopped fresh chives
- 1½ teaspoons fresh lemon juice
- 1½ teaspoons extra virgin olive oil
- Salt and pepper to taste
- 4 tablespoons hummus
- 2 large romaine lettuce leaves

In a small bowl, toss together the bell pepper, greens, water chestnuts, chives, lemon juice, oil, and salt and pepper. Divide the hummus evenly between the romaine leaves, spreading it down the center. Top with the vegetable mixture, roll up the wraps, and serve immediately.

Lemon Chicken

Here's an easy chicken recipe that you can have for dinner with a side salad and steamed veggies. Leftovers can be packed up for lunch the next day.

Serves 6

- 6 boneless, skinless chicken breasts
- 1 tablespoon chopped fresh rosemary leaves
- 2 garlic cloves, minced
- 1 shallot, minced
- Grated zest and juice of 1 lemon
- 120ml/4fl oz extra virgin olive oil

Place the chicken breasts in a single layer in a shallow baking dish. In a glass measuring jug, combine the rosemary, garlic, shallot, lemon zest, and lemon juice. Slowly whisk in the olive oil. Pour the marinade over the chicken, cover, and leave in the refrigerator for at least 2 hours or overnight.

Preheat the oven to 180°C/350°F/gas mark 4. Remove the chicken from the marinade and transfer to a roasting tin. Bake for 25 minutes, or until cooked through. Serve immediately.

Chicken with Mustard Vinaigrette

When you're strapped for time, this recipe takes just minutes to prepare as long as you have a roasted chicken on hand. You can double the dressing recipe and use it throughout the week on salads.

Serves 4

350g/12oz greens (such as mesclun, mixed greens, or baby spinach)
1 whole organic roasted chicken

For the mustard vinaigrette:

4 tablespoons extra virgin olive oil
2 tablespoons dry white wine
1 tablespoon red wine vinegar
1 tablespoon whole-grain mustard
1 teaspoon Dijon mustard
Salt and pepper to taste

Divide the greens evenly among four serving plates. Carve the chicken and divide it among the greens.

In a glass measuring jug, whisk together all the vinaigrette ingredients. Drizzle the vinaigrette over the chicken and greens and serve.

Chardonnay Baked Fish

Nothing could be simpler than baking your favorite fish and adding a rich, flavorful sauce. Although this sauce was originally prepared with salmon in mind, it goes well with any fish—buy the freshest wild-caught fish available at your market by asking what just came in. This fish goes great with Green Beans with Garlic Dressing (pages 316–317).

Serves 4

115g/4oz unsalted butter

250ml/8fl oz Chardonnay or other dry white wine

2 to 3 tablespoons Dijon mustard

3 tablespoons capers, drained and rinsed

Juice of 1 lemon

2 teaspoons chopped fresh dill

4 (115g/4oz) boneless, skin-on salmon fillets

Preheat the oven to 220°C/425°F/gas mark 7.

Melt the butter gently in a saucepan over medium heat, then stir in the Chardonnay, mustard, capers, and lemon juice. Heat for about 5 minutes to burn off the alcohol. Add the dill and remove from the heat.

Place the fish fillets in a baking tin, skin-side down. Pour the sauce over the fish and bake for 20 minutes, or until the fish is flaky. Serve immediately.

Balsamic-Glazed Steaks

Steak is a hassle-free meal because it takes just minutes to prepare. All you need is an excellent cut of grass-fed meat and a tasty marinade. Serve the steaks on a bed of greens with a side of your favorite veggies.

Serves 2

3 tablespoons balsamic vinegar

2 tablespoons extra virgin olive oil

½ teaspoon salt

½ teaspoon pepper

2 (2.5cm/1-inch-thick) steaks, such as fillet

225g/8oz greens (such as mesclun, mixed greens, or baby spinach)

Combine the vinegar, olive oil, salt, and pepper in a resealable plastic bag and add the steaks. Seal the bag and squish the steaks around to coat well. Marinate at room temperature for 30 minutes.

Heat the grill to high and oil the rack. Grill the steaks for 1 minute on each side, or to your liking. Brush the steaks with the marinade as they cook. Alternatively, you can sear the steaks in an oiled frying pan over high heat for about 30 seconds per side, then grill the steaks in the oven for about 2 minutes on each side (or longer if you like your steak well done). Let the steaks rest for 5 minutes.

To serve, divide the greens between two plates and top each with a steak.

Succulent Fore Ribs

The following recipe was adapted from one by winemaker-chef Steve Clifton. Steve loves to create dishes that go with his Palmina Italian wines, crafted in his California vineyards. I like to serve this dish with a side of Cauliflower "Couscous" (page 317).

Serves 6

100g/3½ oz almond flour

1 teaspoon salt

1 teaspoon pepper

1kg/2lb beef fore ribs

6 tablespoons extra virgin olive oil

4 medium yellow onions, coarsely chopped

3 garlic cloves, minced

3 carrots, peeled and coarsely chopped

6 celery stalks, coarsely chopped

3 tablespoons tomato purée

1 bottle Italian red wine

Grated zest and juice of 1 navel orange

4 tablespoons fresh thyme leaves

1 handful chopped fresh flat-leaf parsley leaves

In a large bowl, season the almond flour with the salt and pepper, then dredge the ribs in it.

Heat the olive oil in a 6-litre/10-pint saucepan or flameproof casserole over medium-high heat. Brown the ribs on all sides and transfer to a plate. Add the onions and garlic to the pan and sauté until translucent, about 5 minutes. Add the carrots and celery and cook until slightly softened, about 5 minutes. Return the ribs to the pan. Stir in the tomato purée to coat the ribs. Add the wine, orange zest, and orange juice. Cover and bring to a boil, then simmer, covered, for 2½ hours. Add the thyme leaves and simmer, uncovered, for another 30 minutes. Serve hot, with the parsley sprinkled on top.

Sea Salt's Tuna Carpaccio with Red Onion, Parsley, and Pink Peppercorns

The following seven recipes were created by my good friend, chef Fabrizio Aielli at Sea Salt (seasaltnaples.com), one of my favorite restaurants in Naples, Florida, which I frequently visit. Fabrizio was generous enough to give me a few of his recipes to share, and I recommend trying these when you have guests over for dinner and want to impress.

Serves 6

> 675g/1½lb sashimi grade tuna steaks, sliced 5mm/¼ inch thick
> ½ red onion, sliced
> 1 bunch fresh flat-leaf parsley, stems removed and leaves chopped
> 1 tablespoon ground pink peppercorns
> 4 tablespoons extra virgin olive oil
> Salt to taste
> 3 lemons, halved

Place three to five slices of tuna on each plate. Divide the red onion, parsley, pink pepper, and olive oil on top, and finish with a sprinkle of salt. Serve with a lemon half on the side.

Sea Salt's Akaushi Beef Fillet
with Brussels Sprouts

This dish is a crowd-pleaser for meat lovers. Beef from Akaushi cattle (Akaushi means "red cow") is famous for its healthy fats and mouthwatering flavor. If you have difficulty finding it, any richly marbled beef tenderloin will do.

Serves 6

> 1.4-litres/2½ pints water
> 6 tablespoons extra virgin olive oil
> Salt and pepper to taste
> 1kg/2lb Brussels sprouts, trimmed
> 250ml/8fl oz chicken stock
> 6 (175g/6oz) Akaushi beef fillet steaks
> 1 garlic clove, minced
> Leaves from 2 fresh rosemary sprigs, chopped

Combine the water, 2 tablespoons of the olive oil, and 2 teaspoons salt in a large saucepan. Bring to a boil over medium-high heat. Add the Brussels sprouts and cook for 9 minutes, or until tender. Drain. When the Brussels sprouts are cool enough to handle, cut them in half.

In a sauté pan, heat another 2 tablespoons of the olive oil over high heat. Add the Brussels sprouts, season with salt and pepper, and cook until the sprouts are lightly browned. Add the chicken stock and cook until it evaporates. Remove the pan from the heat.

Season the steaks with salt and pepper. Heat the remaining 2 tablespoons olive oil in another sauté pan over medium-high heat. Add the steaks and sear until golden brown on the first side, about 2 minutes. Turn them over and add the minced garlic and rosemary. Reduce the heat to medium and continue cooking and turning for a few more minutes until they are done to your liking, 3 to 6 minutes, depending on the steaks' thickness.

Place one steak on each serving plate. Pour the juices from the meat pan over the Brussels sprouts and serve on the side.

Sea Salt's Grilled Sardines with Tomato, Rocket, and Pecorino Cheese

Sardines are a fantastic way to boost your intake of protein, omega-3 fatty acids, vitamin B_{12}, and other nutrients. Although some like to eat these small, oily saltwater fish right out of the can, here's an easy, quick way to serve fresh sardines nicely on a plate with added flavor.

Serves 6

18 fresh Mediterranean sardines, cleaned
3 tablespoons extra virgin olive oil
Salt and pepper to taste
6 bunches baby rocket
4 ripe heirloom tomatoes, chopped
Juice of 3 lemons
1 bunch fresh flat-leaf parsley, stems removed and leaves chopped
150g/5oz Pecorino cheese, shaved

Heat the grill to medium-high (about 180°C/350°F) and oil the rack.

Brush the sardines with 1 teaspoon of the olive oil and season with salt and pepper. Grill for 4 minutes on each side. (Alternatively, you can pan-fry the sardines on the hob over medium-high heat.)

In a large bowl, toss together the rocket, tomatoes, remaining olive oil, lemon juice, and salt and pepper. Divide into six portions and top each portion with some sardines, chopped parsley, and shaved Pecorino cheese. Serve immediately.

Sea Salt's Red Snapper with Celery, Black Olives, Cucumber, Avocado, and Yellow Cherry Tomatoes

When red snapper arrives fresh at your market, pick some up and try this recipe. It takes less than 20 minutes to put together.

Serves 6

2 tablespoons extra virgin olive oil

6 (115g/4oz) boneless, skin-on red snapper fillets

Salt and pepper to taste

2 celery stalks, chopped

175g/6oz pitted black olives

1 cucumber, chopped

2 avocados, pitted, peeled, and chopped

450g/1lb yellow cherry tomatoes, halved

1 tablespoon red wine vinegar

Juice of 2 lemons

Heat 1 tablespoon of the olive oil in a large sauté pan over medium-high heat. Season the snapper fillets with salt and pepper and sear for 6 minutes on each side.

In a large bowl, toss together the celery, olives, cucumber, avocados, tomatoes, red wine vinegar, lemon juice, and remaining 1 tablespoon olive oil. Divide the salad among six plates and top with the seared snapper, skin-side up. Serve immediately.

Sea Salt's Courgette Yogurt Gazpacho with Saffron-Marinated Chicken Breast

It doesn't take much saffron, a spice derived from the flower of the crocus, to create an intensely delicious, flavorful dish. This one uses not just saffron but courgettes and coriander to elevate the dish to a whole new level.

Serves 6

250ml/8fl oz dry white wine

2 lemons

Pinch saffron

3 boneless, skinless chicken breasts

6 courgettes, roughly chopped

1-litre/1¾ pints vegetable stock

120ml/4fl oz extra virgin olive oil

Juice of 1 lime

2 tablespoons chopped fresh coriander, stems included

Salt and pepper to taste

1 cucumber, finely chopped

½ sweet onion, finely chopped

1 heirloom tomato, finely chopped

6 teaspoons plain full-fat Greek yogurt

Combine the wine, juice of 1 lemon, and saffron in a large bowl. Add the chicken breasts, cover, and marinate in the refrigerator overnight.

Heat the grill to medium-high (about 180°C/350°F) and oil the rack.

Remove the chicken breasts from the marinade and grill for 6 minutes on each side, or until cooked through. Cut into 5mm/¼-inch-thick slices. Transfer to a plate, cover, and chill in the refrigerator.

Combine the courgettes, vegetable stock, olive oil, juice of the remaining lemon, lime juice, and 1 tablespoon of the coriander in a blender and purée until smooth. Season with salt and pepper. Pour the soup into a large bowl and stir in the cucumber, onion, and tomato. Cover and chill for 1 to 2 hours. When ready to serve, divide the soup among six soup bowls and top each portion with 1 teaspoon yogurt. Divide the sliced chicken breast evenly on each serving. Season with salt and pepper, garnish with the remaining 1 tablespoon coriander, and serve.

Sea Salt's Liquid "Minestrone"

This version of minestrone soup swaps out the pasta and beans for more vegetables — and more flavor.

Serves 4 to 6

3 tablespoons extra virgin olive oil

3 celery stalks, chopped

1 onion, chopped

200g/7oz chopped broccoli

200g/7oz chopped cauliflower

135g/4¾oz chopped asparagus

3 medium-size courgettes, chopped

1 teaspoon dried thyme

450g/1lb celeriac, peeled and cut into 1cm/½-inch cubes

200g/7oz chopped kale leaves (stems removed)

150g/5oz chopped Swiss chard leaves (stems removed)

2 bay leaves

½ teaspoon dried sage

1½ teaspoons salt

¼ teaspoon pepper

2-litres/3½ pints chicken stock

150g/5oz chopped spinach leaves (stems removed)

6 tablespoons plain full-fat Greek yogurt

Heat the olive oil in a large stockpot over medium-high heat. Add the celery, onion, broccoli, cauliflower, asparagus, courgettes, and thyme. Sweat the vegetables until the onion is translucent, about 5 minutes. Add the celeriac, kale, Swiss chard, bay leaves, dried sage, salt, and pepper and cook for 4 minutes. Add the chicken stock. Bring the soup to a boil, then lower the heat to medium. Cook at a low boil until the vegetables are tender, 25 to 30 minutes. Let the soup stand for 10 minutes. Stir in the spinach. While stirring, locate the bay leaves and remove them. Working in batches, transfer the soup to a blender and purée until smooth. Rewarm gently over medium heat.

Garnish each serving with a dollop of Greek yogurt and serve.

Sea Salt's Tomato and Red Cabbage Soup

Whether it's the dead of winter or middle of summer, this refreshing, simple soup calls for ingredients that most people have on hand. This goes well with any main entrée in lieu of a side salad.

Serves 6

120ml/4fl oz extra virgin olive oil
1 sweet onion, chopped
2 celery stalks, chopped
2 tablespoons minced garlic
4 (400g/14oz) cans chopped tomatoes
1 head red cabbage, cored and chopped
10 basil leaves
1.5-litres/2½ pints chicken stock
1.5-litres/2½ pints vegetable stock
Salt and pepper to taste

In a large stockpot, heat half the olive oil over medium-high heat. Add the onion, celery, and garlic and sweat until translucent, about 5 minutes. Add the tomatoes, red cabbage, basil leaves, chicken stock, and vegetable stock and bring to a boil. Lower the heat to medium and continue to cook at a low boil for 25 to 30 minutes. Add the remaining olive oil, season with salt and pepper, and let the soup stand for 10 minutes. Working in batches, transfer the soup to a blender and purée. Rewarm gently over medium heat. Serve.

Quick Salmon with Mushrooms

It doesn't get any easier than pan-frying fresh fish fillets and adding flavor from mushrooms, herbs, spices, and a combination of olive and sesame oils. This recipe takes just minutes to prepare. Serve with a side of Roasted Seasonal Vegetables (see page 316).

Serves 4

    4 tablespoons extra virgin olive oil
    3 garlic cloves, crushed
    3 shallots, thinly sliced
    1 teaspoon dried or grated fresh ginger
    4 (115g/4oz) boneless, skinless salmon fillets
    1 tablespoon toasted sesame oil
    150g/5oz sliced button or cremini mushrooms
    25g/1oz chopped fresh coriander leaves

Heat 2 tablespoons of the olive oil in a sauté pan over medium heat, then add the garlic, shallots, and ginger. Cook until it sizzles, about 1 minute, then add the salmon fillets and cook until cooked through, about 3 minutes on each side. Remove the fillets and set aside.

Wipe out the pan carefully with a paper towel. Add the remaining 2 tablespoons olive oil and the sesame oil and heat over medium heat. Add the mushrooms and cook for 3 minutes, stirring constantly. Scatter the mushrooms over the salmon and garnish with the coriander. Serve immediately.

Salmon & Vegetables in Parchment

This dish has become a staple in my home. Nothing is cleaner and more nutritionally packed than fresh salmon and a mixture of vegetables all packed together in parchment paper. Experiment with different vegetables to vary this dish or simply add more to the mixture, such as bell peppers and broccoli or cauliflower florets.

Serves 1

  1 (115g/4oz) salmon fillet

  25g/1oz sliced button or cremini mushrooms

  75g/3oz sliced courgettes

  50g/2oz diced tomato

  1 or 2 fresh thyme sprigs

  Salt and pepper to taste

  1 teaspoon fresh lemon juice

  1 teaspoon extra virgin olive oil

Preheat the oven to 200°C/400°F/gas mark 6. Place a large piece of parchment paper on a rimmed baking sheet.

Place the salmon fillet on the parchment, skin-side down. Top with the mushrooms, courgettes, tomato, and thyme. Season with salt and pepper, then drizzle with the lemon juice and oil.

Wrap the salmon and veggies tightly in the parchment, crimping the edges to seal. Place the baking sheet with the fish packet in the oven and bake for 20 minutes. Remove from the oven and allow to sit for 5 minutes. Transfer the parchment packet to a serving plate, unwrap, and enjoy.

Greek Lemon Lamb

Whenever grass-fed lamb chops go on sale, pick some up. They make for a delicious, elegant entrée that takes little time to prepare and cook. All you need is a good marinade, like this one. Serve with a side of steamed veggies and Cauliflower "Couscous" (page 317).

Serves 4

  2 tablespoons extra virgin olive oil

  1½ lemons

  2 garlic cloves, minced

  Leaves from 2 fresh thyme sprigs

  1 teaspoon dried oregano

Salt and pepper to taste

12 lamb chops

In a bowl, whisk together the oil, juice of ½ lemon, garlic, thyme, oregano, and salt and pepper. Add the lamb chops and toss to coat well. Cover and refrigerate for 1 hour.

Heat the grill to high and oil the rack. Remove the lamb chops from the marinade and grill for 1 to 2 minutes on each side. (Alternatively, you can roast the lamb in a 200°C/400°F/gas mark 6 oven for about 10 minutes, or to the desired doneness.)

Serve the lamb with the remaining lemon, cut into wedges, for squeezing.

Quick Flat-Roasted Chicken

I like to keep small, whole chickens in the freezer and cook this recipe whenever I have friends coming over for dinner or want to have plenty of leftovers for the next day's lunch. If you start with a frozen chicken, thaw it in the refrigerator overnight. Serve with a side salad and Roasted Seasonal Vegetables (page 316).

Serves 6

1 (1.3–1.8kg/3–4lb) whole organic chicken

4 tablespoons extra virgin olive oil

Salt and pepper to taste

1 lemon, sliced

5 garlic cloves, peeled

7 fresh thyme, tarragon, or oregano sprigs

Preheat the oven to 200°C/400°F/gas mark 6.

Using kitchen scissors or a knife, cut along both sides of the backbone of the chicken. Open the chicken up and press down firmly on the breastbone to flatten it. Lay the chicken, skin-side up, in a large roasting tin. Brush the chicken with 2 tablespoons of the olive oil, then season with salt and pepper.

In a bowl, toss the lemon slices, garlic cloves, and herb sprigs with the remaining 2 tablespoons of the olive oil, then scatter them over the chicken. Bake until the chicken is cooked through, 45 to 55 minutes. Let rest for 5 minutes, then carve and serve.

Fish with Dill and Lemon

A little bit of dill, lemon, and Dijon will go a long way to bring out the best flavor of any fresh fish. You can use this recipe with any white fish. Serve with Cauliflower "Couscous" (page 317) and Sautéed Spinach and Garlic (page 318).

Serves 4

   Leaves from 1 bunch fresh dill or flat-leaf parsley, chopped

   2 tablespoons Dijon mustard

   Juice of 1 lemon

   2 tablespoons extra virgin olive oil

   Salt and pepper to taste

   4 (115g/4oz) boneless, skin-on firm white fish fillets (such as halibut or black cod)

   Preheat the oven to 200°C/400°F/gas mark 6.

   Process the dill, mustard, lemon juice, oil, and salt and pepper in a food processor until smooth.

   Place the fish fillets in a shallow baking dish, skin-side down, and coat with the dill sauce. Bake until cooked through, about 15 minutes.

Note: For an even quicker preparation, try topping the fish with Dill Spread (page 322) or Pecorino Pesto (page 322).

Broccoli Soup with Cashew Cream

When the day calls for a hot soup at lunch or dinner to go with your main entrée, here's one that you can prepare in advance and store in the refrigerator until you're ready to reheat. You can also use this as a snack to tide you over when your afternoon gets busy and dinner will be late.

Serves 4 to 6

- 100g/3½oz raw, unsalted cashews
- 175ml/6fl oz water
- Salt and pepper to taste
- 3 tablespoons extra virgin olive oil
- 1 large onion, chopped
- 3 shallots, chopped
- 1 garlic clove, chopped
- 1-litre/1¾ pints chicken stock
- 600g/1lb 5oz chopped broccoli florets
- 4 teaspoons fresh thyme leaves
- 250ml/8fl oz canned coconut milk
- 1 handful pumpkin seeds, for garnish (optional)

Purée the cashews, water, and a pinch of salt in a blender; set aside.

In a large stockpot, heat the olive oil over medium-high heat. Add the onion, shallots, and garlic and cook until translucent, about 4 minutes. Add the stock and broccoli and season with salt and pepper. Bring to a boil, then lower the heat and simmer until the broccoli is soft, about 10 minutes.

Working in batches, transfer the soup to the blender, add the thyme, and purée. Return the soup to the pot and stir in the coconut milk. Warm gently over medium heat.

Serve the soup with a drizzle of cashew cream on top and, if desired, a sprinkling of pumpkin seeds.

Goddess Gazpacho with Smoked Salmon

You might never have thought to pair a cold gazpacho-like soup with smoked salmon. This delectable dish will excite your taste buds and give you another terrific way to incorporate smoked salmon into a meal. To serve as a first course during a special dinner party, simply double or triple the recipe.

Serves 1

- 225g/8oz peeled, chopped cucumber, plus 1 cucumber slice, for garnish
- ¼ avocado
- 1 to 2 tablespoons water or canned coconut milk
- 1 teaspoon finely chopped fresh mint leaves, plus 1 mint sprig, for garnish
- Several drops hot sauce (optional)
- Pinch garlic powder
- Salt and pepper to taste
- 75g/3oz smoked wild salmon, chopped

Combine the chopped cucumber, avocado, 1 tablespoon water or coconut milk, chopped mint, hot sauce (if using), garlic powder, and salt and pepper in a blender and purée. Add the remaining 1 tablespoon water or coconut milk if needed to achieve the desired consistency.

Pour the soup into a serving bowl and add the salmon. Garnish with the cucumber slice and mint sprig. Serve immediately. (Alternatively, you can chill the soup before serving. If you do, wait until serving to add the salmon and the cucumber and mint garnishes.)

Note: Using coconut milk instead of water will make the soup creamier.

SALADS

Avocado Chicken Salad Stuffed Tomato

Throwing together a salad is often the easiest way to create a delicious, nutritious meal that can stand alone or serve as a side dish to any meal. I have one most every day. It helps if you keep any ingredients that need to be cooked, such as chicken in the case of this recipe, already done and ready to go in the fridge. That way, all you have to do is toss everything together and voilà! Feel free to double or triple this recipe to serve more people or keep extra in the fridge for the next day.

Serves 1

115g/4oz cooked boneless, skinless chicken breast, chopped
¼ avocado, mashed
1 tablespoon avocado oil mayonnaise (no sugar added)
1 teaspoon fresh lime juice
⅛ teaspoon garlic powder
Salt and pepper to taste
1 medium tomato, cored, insides scooped out

In a small bowl, combine the chicken, avocado, mayonnaise, lime juice, garlic powder, and salt and pepper. Stir to combine. Spoon the chicken salad into the hollowed-out tomato, packing it in. Plate and serve.

Greek Village Salad with Prawns

In this Greek-inspired dish, prawns take center stage, but if you don't like prawns, you can substitute chicken, steak, or fish. You can also be playful with the kind of vegetables you add to this super versatile salad. Don't be afraid to experiment.

Serves 1

> 3 teaspoons extra virgin olive oil
>
> 75–115g/3–4oz large raw prawns, peeled and deveined
>
> 150g/5oz cubed cucumber
>
> 1 small tomato, cubed
>
> 100g/3½oz diced yellow bell pepper
>
> ½ teaspoon dried oregano
>
> ½ teaspoon dried dill
>
> Salt and pepper to taste
>
> 2 romaine lettuce leaves

Warm 1 teaspoon of the olive oil in a frying pan over medium-high heat. Cook the prawns for about 2 minutes per side, until pink and cooked through. Transfer the prawns to a salad bowl and add the vegetables, remaining 2 teaspoons olive oil, and seasonings. Toss to combine. Spoon the prawn salad onto the romaine leaves to serve.

Herb Garden Salad with Balsamic Vinaigrette

This salad has become a staple for me. It can be used as a side to a main dish or stand alone as an entrée for lunch or dinner if you add your favorite protein (for example, slices of cooked chicken, fish, or steak). The vinaigrette recipe makes about 250ml/8fl oz, but because I rely on this salad throughout the week, I often double it so all I have to do is toss together the salad ingredients.

Serves 6

For the salad:

> 150g/5oz mixed salad leaves
>
> 25g/1oz fresh flat-leaf parsley leaves
>
> 25g/1oz chopped fresh chives
>
> 25g/1oz mixed fresh herb leaves (such as coriander, tarragon, sage, and/or mint)
>
> 50g/2oz chopped raw walnuts

For the balsamic vinaigrette:

4 tablespoons balsamic vinegar

Juice of 1 lemon

2 or 3 garlic cloves, minced

½ shallot, minced

1 tablespoon Dijon mustard

1 tablespoon chopped fresh rosemary leaves or dried, crumbled
    rosemary

1 teaspoon salt

1 teaspoon pepper

120ml/4fl oz extra virgin olive oil

Combine the salad ingredients in a salad bowl.

In a glass measuring jug, whisk together all the vinaigrette
ingredients except for the oil, then drizzle in the oil slowly so it emulsifies.

Add half of the balsamic vinaigrette to the salad, toss, and serve.
Store the remaining dressing in an airtight container in the refrigerator
for up to 1 week.

Niçoise Salad

This recipe is based on the classic niçoise salad that hails from Nice, France,
but without the potatoes, and you can use any type of cooked fish. Although
it takes a little extra time to prep the ingredients, the salad comes together
quickly and easily once you've gotten everything ready.

Serves 4

For the salad:

Salt

75g/3oz green beans, trimmed

150g/5oz rocket or mixed salad leaves

4 firm, ripe tomatoes, diced

1 green bell pepper, seeded and chopped

1 small cucumber, peeled and cubed

3 spring onions, thinly sliced

3 large eggs, hard-boiled and sliced

175g/6oz cooked fish (such as mahimahi, salmon, or black cod), cut into bite-size pieces

12 anchovy fillets, drained

75g/3oz black or Kalamata olives

10 fresh basil leaves, chopped

For the vinaigrette:

2 tablespoons extra virgin olive oil

2 teaspoons red wine vinegar

1 teaspoon Dijon mustard

Salt and pepper to taste

Bring a small saucepan of salted water to a boil over medium-high heat. Add the green beans and blanch until crisp-tender, about 4 minutes. Drain. Put the green beans in a salad bowl and add the remaining salad ingredients.

In a small bowl, whisk together the ingredients for the vinaigrette. Pour the dressing over the salad, toss, and serve.

Chicken Fajita Salad

I love a salad with Mexican flair — chilli powder and ground cumin light up any dish. This one comes together quickly.

Serves 1

1 (115g/4oz) boneless, skinless chicken breast

2 teaspoons extra virgin olive oil

½ teaspoon ground cumin

¼ teaspoon chilli powder

Salt and pepper to taste

50g/2oz sliced red, orange, and/or yellow bell pepper

200g/7oz torn dark, leafy greens

1 small tomato, cut into wedges

1 tablespoon salsa

Lime wedges, for serving

Heat a small frying pan over medium-high heat. Coat the chicken breast with the oil, cumin, chilli powder, and salt and pepper. Cook the chicken for 4 to 5 minutes per side, then add the bell pepper. Cook until the chicken is cooked through and the peppers are tender, about 5 minutes.

While the chicken cooks, arrange the greens in a serving bowl and top with the tomato wedges. Once the chicken is done, cut it into strips and add the chicken and peppers to the bowl. Top with the salsa and serve with lime wedges for squeezing over the top.

Curry Chickpea Salad

This curry-infused salad can stand alone or be served as a side dish. Curry powder is where we find turmeric, a veritable "brain food" that has been used for centuries in cooking and has now been shown to help boost the brain's ability to repair itself. Many people don't know how to incorporate turmeric into everyday dishes, so here's one recipe that takes just minutes to put together.

Serves 1

100g/3½oz shredded kale
1 teaspoon extra virgin olive oil
1 tablespoon diced onion
1 tablespoon shredded carrot
1 tablespoon diced green bell pepper
½ teaspoon curry powder
120g/4oz canned reduced-sodium chickpeas, rinsed and drained
1 tablespoon canned coconut milk

Put the kale in a salad bowl and set aside.

In a small saucepan, heat the oil over medium-high heat. Add the onion, carrot, and green pepper and sauté until tender, about 5 minutes. Add the curry powder and cook, stirring, for 1 minute. Add the chickpeas and coconut milk and stir until heated through. Spoon the chickpea mixture over the kale and serve immediately.

Roasted Walnut Oil Salad

You can turn any salad into Roasted Walnut Oil Salad just by using this dressing, which celebrates the robust flavor of walnuts. Although I've suggested goat cheese in this recipe, feel free to try another cheese such as crumbled feta or shaved Parmesan.

Serves 2

For the salad:

225g/8oz salad leaves (such as mesclun, mixed leaves, or baby spinach)

4 tablespoons crumbled goat cheese

50g/2oz chopped roasted, unsalted walnuts

3 tablespoons dried blueberries or cranberries

For the dressing:

2 tablespoons walnut oil

1 tablespoon balsamic or red wine vinegar

½ teaspoon whole-grain mustard

Salt and pepper to taste

Arrange the salad leaves in a salad bowl and top with the goat cheese, walnuts, and dried berries. In a glass measuring jug, whisk together the dressing ingredients until thoroughly combined. Pour the dressing over the salad, toss, and serve.

Lemon Rocket with Parmigiano-Reggiano

This salad is minimal in its ingredients but full of zesty flavor, thanks to peppery rocket mixed with tangy cheese and rich olive oil. I enjoy this as a complement to any Italian-inspired dish.

Serves 2

    200g/7oz baby rocket

    40g/1½oz raw, unsalted sunflower seeds

    8 to 10 shavings Parmigiano-Reggiano cheese

    Juice of 1 lemon

    6 tablespoons extra virgin olive oil

    Salt and pepper to taste

Combine the rocket, sunflower seeds, cheese, and lemon juice in a salad bowl. Drizzle with the olive oil, toss, season with salt and pepper, and serve.

Sea Salt's Kale Salad with Feta Cheese, Roasted Peppers, Black Olives, Artichokes, and Buttermilk Dressing

I'm known for ordering this salad pretty much every time I go to Sea Salt for lunch. It accompanies any main entrée beautifully.

Serves 6

    2 bunches kale, stems removed and leaves roughly torn

    300g/10oz feta cheese, crumbled

    3 roasted red bell peppers, sliced

    175g/6oz black olives, pitted and halved

    12 marinated baby artichokes, halved

    250ml/8fl oz buttermilk

    120ml/4fl oz extra virgin olive oil

    1 tablespoon red wine vinegar

    Salt and pepper to taste

In a salad bowl, toss together the kale, feta cheese, roasted peppers, olives, and artichokes. In a glass measuring jug, whisk together the buttermilk, olive oil, and red wine vinegar. Pour the dressing over the salad, toss, season with salt and pepper, and serve.

SIDES

Roasted Seasonal Vegetables

This recipe is good any time of the year. Just go with what's in season and be sure to use the best olive oil you can find alongside the freshest herbs. A drizzle of aged balsamic vinegar at the very end of the cooking process adds an extra treat.

Serves 4 to 6

> 1kg/2lb seasonal vegetables (such as asparagus, Brussels sprouts, bell peppers, courgettes, aubergines, and/or onion)
>
> 75ml/3fl oz extra virgin olive oil
>
> Salt and pepper to taste
>
> 4 tablespoons minced fresh herb leaves (such as rosemary, oregano, flat-leaf parsley, and/or thyme; optional)
>
> Aged balsamic vinegar (optional)

Preheat the oven to 220°C/425°F/gas mark 7. Line a roasting tin with foil.

Cut up any large vegetables into pieces. Spread out the vegetables in the lined tin. Drizzle the olive oil over the vegetables, then use clean hands to mix them so they are well coated with oil. Season with salt and pepper and add the herbs, if using. Roast the vegetables, stirring every 10 minutes, until they are cooked through and browned in spots, 35 to 40 minutes. Just prior to serving, drizzle lightly with aged balsamic vinegar, if desired.

Green Beans with Garlic Dressing

Just about any green vegetable can be dressed up with garlic and herbs.

Serves 4 to 6

> Salt and pepper to taste
>
> 1kg/2lb green beans, trimmed
>
> 2 tablespoons extra virgin olive oil

1 tablespoon fresh lemon juice

1 teaspoon Dijon mustard

2 garlic cloves, minced

½ teaspoon grated lemon zest

50g/2oz chopped raw, unsalted almonds

1 tablespoon fresh thyme leaves

Bring a large saucepan of salted water to a boil over medium-high heat. Add the green beans and blanch until al dente, about 4 minutes. Drain.

In a large bowl, whisk together the oil, lemon juice, mustard, garlic, lemon zest, and salt and pepper. Add the green beans, almonds, and thyme, toss, and serve.

Cauliflower "Couscous"

For a tasty stand-in for starchy vegetables like mashed potatoes, rice, or traditional couscous, try this dish made simply from cauliflower.

Serves 2

1 head cauliflower, cored and broken into florets

2 tablespoons extra virgin olive oil

2 garlic cloves, minced

25g/1oz toasted pine nuts

1 handful chopped fresh flat-leaf parsley leaves

In a food processor, process the cauliflower florets until they resemble small grains. (Alternatively, you can grate the entire cauliflower head on the large holes of a box grater until all the florets are grated and you're left with the stalk to discard.)

Heat the olive oil in a large frying pan over medium heat. Add the cauliflower, garlic, pine nuts, and parsley and sauté, stirring frequently, until the cauliflower begins to brown, about 5 minutes. Serve.

Note: For extra flavor, add 25g/1oz chopped olives or grated Parmesan cheese to the cauliflower while it's cooking.

Sautéed Spinach and Garlic

Just about any leafy green vegetable sautéed in garlic and olive oil is delightful. Here it's made with spinach, but feel free to experiment with other greens.

Serves 2

> 4 tablespoons extra virgin olive oil
>
> 225g/8oz baby spinach
>
> 6 garlic cloves, very thinly sliced
>
> 1 lemon
>
> 1 to 2 teaspoons chilli flakes
>
> Salt and pepper to taste

In a large sauté pan, heat the oil over high heat until almost smoking. Add the spinach and cook, stirring continuously, for 1 to 2 minutes. The spinach will begin to wilt slightly. Add the garlic and continue to cook, stirring rapidly, for about 1 more minute, then remove from the heat.

Squeeze the juice from the lemon over the top, add the chilli flakes, and season with salt and pepper. Toss well and serve.

DIPS & TOPPINGS

Guacamole Dip

You'll find many versions of guacamole that work with *Grain Brain*'s guidelines, so feel free to experiment. The following was adapted from Alton Brown's recipe on FoodNetwork.com. I love his use of spices for an added kick. Use it for snacking with cut-up raw veggies like bell peppers, celery, and radishes, or add a dollop to dishes for a boost of flavor where you feel it works.

Serves 4

> 2 large, ripe avocados, pitted and peeled
> Juice of 1 lime
> 1 teaspoon salt
> ¼ teaspoon ground cumin
> ¼ teaspoon cayenne
> ½ small red onion, diced
> 1 garlic clove, minced
> ½ jalapeño pepper, seeded and minced
> 2 medium ripe tomatoes, diced
> 1 tablespoon chopped fresh coriander leaves

In a large bowl, mash the avocado flesh with the lime juice. Add the salt, cumin, and cayenne. Fold in the onion, garlic, jalapeño, tomatoes, and coriander. Serve immediately or store in an airtight container in the refrigerator for up to 2 days.

Avocado-Tahini Dip

Here's a dip that's in between guacamole and hummus. Try it with cut-up raw veggies or cooked cubed chicken.

Makes about 375ml/13fl oz

> 1 tablespoon extra virgin olive oil
> 115g/4oz rocket
> 1 large, ripe avocado, pitted and peeled
> 50g/2oz tahini
> 4 tablespoons water
> Juice of 1 lemon
> ½ teaspoon ground cumin
> 2 tablespoons minced fresh flat-leaf parsley or coriander leaves

Heat the olive oil in a large frying pan or saucepan over medium-high heat. Add the rocket and cook until it is wilted. Transfer the rocket to a food processor, add the remaining ingredients, and process until smooth. Add more water if necessary to achieve a medium-thick consistency. Serve immediately or store in an airtight container in the refrigerator for up to 2 days.

Creamy Cashew Dip

Cashew nuts are rich in flavor and brain-healthy fats. In addition to serving as a dip for raw vegetables, this recipe also works well as a topping on many soups and chicken dishes.

Makes 250 ml/8fl oz

> 60g/2½oz raw, unsalted cashews
> 250ml/8fl oz water
> 4 tablespoons fresh lemon juice
> 2 teaspoons light miso
> ¼ teaspoon ground nutmeg
> Salt to taste

In a blender, purée the cashews, 120ml/4fl oz of the water, lemon juice, miso, and nutmeg until smooth. With the machine running, slowly add the remaining water until the mixture is the consistency of whipped cream. If you prefer a thinner consistency, add more water. Season with salt and serve immediately, or store in an airtight container in the refrigerator for up to 4 days.

Hummus Dip

Hummus is one of the most versatile dips and can be used in a variety of ways. It's delicious with veggies as a snack and can be used to add depth to meat dishes.

Serves 4

1 (400g/14oz) can reduced-sodium chickpeas
4 tablespoons fresh lemon juice
2 tablespoons extra virgin olive oil, plus more for serving
1½ tablespoons tahini
2 garlic cloves, peeled
½ teaspoon salt
1 handful chopped fresh flat-leaf parsley leaves

Drain the chickpeas but reserve 4 tablespoons of the liquid from the can. In a food processor, combine the chickpeas and reserved liquid, lemon juice, olive oil, tahini, garlic, and salt. Process for 3 minutes on low speed until smooth. Scoop the hummus into a serving bowl and drizzle olive oil on top. Garnish with the parsley and serve immediately, or store in an airtight container in the refrigerator for up to 4 days.

Dill Spread

When you've run out of ideas for cooking fish, try this spread on any fresh fish you want to bake or grill.

Makes about 120ml/4fl oz

3 bunches fresh dill fronds

Leaves from 1 bunch fresh flat-leaf parsley

2 garlic cloves, peeled

3 tablespoons extra virgin olive oil

2 tablespoons Dijon mustard

1 tablespoon fresh lemon juice

Salt and pepper to taste

Process all the ingredients in a food processor or blender until smooth. Serve immediately or store in an airtight container in the refrigerator for up to 1 week.

Pecorino Pesto

Here's a tasty spread to use with baked or grilled fish.

Makes about 120ml/4fl oz

50g/2oz raw, unsalted almonds, walnuts, or pine nuts

2 garlic cloves, peeled

60g/2½oz fresh basil leaves

40g/1½oz grated Pecorino cheese

Salt and pepper to taste

75ml/3fl oz extra virgin olive oil

Process the nuts, garlic, basil, cheese, and salt and pepper in a food processor while slowly pouring in the oil through the feed tube; the pesto should be rich, creamy, and spreadable. Serve immediately or store in an airtight container in the refrigerator for up to 1 week.

Sofrito

Sofrito is a seasoned tomato-based sauce used frequently in Latin cooking. Incredibly versatile, it can be added to roasted chicken, stews, and scrambled eggs, as well as grilled or baked fish.

Makes about 850ml/1½ pints

2 tablespoons extra virgin olive oil
1 medium onion, finely chopped
1 green bell pepper, seeded and finely chopped
2 garlic cloves, minced
2 (400g/14oz) cans chopped tomatoes
Leaves from 1 bunch fresh coriander, chopped
1 teaspoon paprika
Salt and pepper to taste

In a large frying pan, heat the olive oil over medium heat. Add the onion and sauté until translucent, about 5 minutes. Add the green pepper and cook for 5 minutes, stirring often. Add the garlic and sauté for 1 minute more. Add the tomatoes, coriander, and paprika and stir well. Continue to cook for 10 to 15 minutes. Season with salt and pepper and serve immediately, or store in an airtight container in the refrigerator for up to 1 week.

DESSERT

Chocolate Truffles

These are a fantastic treat for dessert or to serve at your next dinner party. The higher the quality of the chocolate, the better. Experiment with different flavorings depending on your mood.

Makes 30–40 truffles

225g/8oz dark chocolate (at least 70% cacao), chopped into small
  pieces
120ml/4fl oz double cream
1 teaspoon almond, orange, vanilla, or hazelnut extract
Unsweetened cocoa powder or finely chopped nuts, for coating

Put the chocolate in a small heat-safe bowl; set aside.

In a small saucepan, bring the cream to a simmer over medium-low heat. Stir in your choice of flavoring, then pour the mixture over the chocolate in the bowl. Let stand for a few minutes before stirring until smooth. Allow to cool, then cover and refrigerate for 2 hours.

Line a rimmed baking sheet with parchment paper. Using a teaspoon, form the chocolate mixture into 2.5cm/1-inch balls and roll them quickly between your palms. Place the balls on the lined baking sheet. Cover and refrigerate overnight.

Roll the truffles in cocoa powder or chopped nuts. Store in an airtight container in the refrigerator for up to 1 week.

Chocolate Coconut Mousse

Looking for a quick dessert? Keep a can of coconut milk in the refrigerator so it's ready to go when you feel like indulging in a decadent treat.

Serves 2

1 (400ml/14fl oz) can full-fat coconut milk
3 tablespoons unsweetened cocoa powder

1 to 2 teaspoons stevia

Shredded unsweetened coconut, almond butter, or ground
   cinnamon, for topping (optional)

Chill the unopened can of coconut milk in the refrigerator for several hours or overnight.

Open the can and scoop the solidified coconut cream into a mixing bowl (use the remaining coconut milk for smoothies or soups). Beat the cream vigorously with a whisk or electric mixer until softened; it shouldn't liquefy. Add the cocoa powder and stevia and continue to beat until the mousse is light and fluffy. Top with shredded coconut, a dollop of almond butter, or a sprinkling of cinnamon, if desired, and serve.

Epilogue

The Mesmerizing Truth

IN THE EIGHTEENTH CENTURY, a German physician who studied in Vienna set up a clinic following an interest in so-called animal magnetism, which he developed into a system of treatment through hypnotism. It was called mesmerism, after his name: Franz Anton Mesmer. Dr. Mesmer claimed he could cure nervous system problems using magnetism. According to Mesmer, a proper balance of a "subtle fluid" maintained the body's health. This subtle fluid was the same one responsible for heat, light, and gravity, and it floated throughout the universe. Dr. Mesmer created animal magnetism by focusing on the magnetic poles of the body, which he thought helped direct this fluid. Under his theory, the poles had to be aligned properly to work and to maintain a correct, smooth, and harmonious flow of fluid. If the fluid balance was off, a person could develop "nervous afflictions," and he or she would need to be "mesmerized" to get the poles realigned and the fluid rebalanced.

It didn't take long for Dr. Mesmer to generate publicity as well as notoriety. He received a lot of attention and got a lot of people—educated and not—curious. The medical and scientific community feared Mesmer; the government worried about secrecy and subversion of his growing group. In 1777 he was expelled from Vienna, so he went to Paris and established himself all over again.

By the 1780s he had accumulated new disciples and set up shops with them in Paris. These believers "mesmerized" people by claiming to locate their poles and control their fluid. One can picture a dramatic scene of the mad scientist waving his arms in the air, gathering his powers, and then administering the power of his touch to hapless people with "nervous afflictions," in a futile attempt at drawing demons from them. His popularity became part mystery, part fashion. Getting treated by Mesmer and his "mesmerists" became a trendy thing to do. They would use a very elaborate apparatus, complete with mesmeric tubes, bottles of mesmerized water, and iron bars that carried the subtle fluid. These mesmeric treatments happened in secluded areas, hence the mystery and notoriety.

Dr. Mesmer didn't last very long in Paris, either. Investigations commenced. A royal government commission that included Antoine-Laurent Lavoisier and Benjamin Franklin looked into his independent practice. In 1785, Mesmer left Paris for London, then went back to Austria, and then on to Italy, Switzerland, and eventually to his native Germany, where he returned to a village near his birthplace and died in 1815. No matter where he went, he tried to win the universal acclaim he believed he deserved for his therapies.

It's now generally accepted that Mesmer was actually treating psychosomatic illness, and he profited mightily from people's gullibility. In retrospect, his theories and practices sound ridiculous, but in truth, the story of Mesmer parallels many stories of today. It's not so ridiculous to imagine people falling prey to products, procedures, and health claims that are brilliantly marketed. Every day we hear of some news item related to health. We are bombarded by messages about our health—good, bad, and confusingly contradictory. And we are literally mesmerized by these messages. Even the smart, educated, cautious, and skeptical consumer is mesmerized. It's hard to separate truth from fiction, and to know the difference between what's healthful and harmful when the information and endorsements come from "experts."

If you consider some of the advice doled out in the past century from these so-called experts, you'll quickly realize that things do not always appear as they seem. It's quite common to witness a complete about-face when it comes to the validity of a certain fact, claim, or practice. Bloodletting was still common in the late nineteenth century. We used to think that eggs were evil and margarine was magical, but now we know that eggs are among the world's most nutrient-dense foods and that margarine contains deadly trans fats. Doctors in the mid-twentieth century used to pose for cigarette advertisements, and later on, they began to say that baby formula was much better than breast milk for children. And while it's hard to conceive of today, not too long ago we thought that diet had absolutely no effect on disease. We now know otherwise.

When I imagine the world fifty years from now, I wonder what kind of bogus claims that many of us accept today will have been evicted from society. I also wonder whether I'll have had any influence, given the work I've been doing to change people's misguided perspectives on carbs, fat, and cholesterol. Indeed, there are powerful forces behind our viewpoints today. Walk into any supermarket and you'll be met with dozens of reasons why you should eat this or that—many of those assertions perpetuating false facts and promises. This is especially true for foods labeled healthy, wholegrain, low-fat, and cholesterol-free. In addition to telling you that these goods are your ticket to a longer, more vibrant life, food manufacturers somehow tie them to a lower risk of cancer, heart disease, diabetes, and obesity. But now you know the truth.

We live in an exciting time in medicine; we finally have the technology at our fingertips to help us diagnose, treat, and cure many illnesses that shortened life just a few decades ago. But we also live in a time when deaths from chronic disease outpace people dying from infectious disease by a long shot. It's common knowledge that our country's health-care system is in need of repair. Despite numerous attempts in the past decade to remedy the problems, the system remains on life support itself. Health-care costs are exorbitant. We devote far more of our economy to health-care—nearly 20 percent of our gross domestic product—than any other country. Health insurance premiums for the average family continue to rise sharply, costing some families more than twenty thousand dollars a year. And although we are presently ranked first in the world in health-care spending, we are ranked thirty-seventh in overall health-system performance, according to the World Health Organization's most recent estimations,[1] and twenty-second in life expectancy among the thirty developed countries. In 2016 and 2017, the average life expectancy *dropped* in the United States for the first time in more than two decades.[2] A surge in drug overdoses seems to be part of the picture here, but incidence of Alzheimer's disease climbed as well.

What will save our system and our future generations? We cannot wait for the massively complicated health-care system to fix itself, just as we cannot expect change to happen as fast as we need it. We also cannot rely on drugs to keep us alive and well. In many cases, as I've described in this book, drugs push us further away from where we really want to be. We must start individually with small shifts in our daily habits that amount to huge gains in our health quotient today and in the future.

Though some consider the beating heart to be the center of life, it's really the brain that takes center stage. Our heart wouldn't beat without our brain, and it is our brain that allows us to experience the world on every level—to feel pleasure and pain, to love and to learn, to make decisions, and to participate in life in ways that make it worth living!

Until we face a health challenge that affects our brain's functionality, we tend to take our mental faculties for granted. We assume that our mind will travel with us wherever we go. But what if that doesn't happen? And what if we can in fact guarantee our mental prowess and brainpower just by actively nurturing the brain in the ways I've described? We all cherish the right to free speech, the right to privacy, and the right to vote, among others. These are fundamental to our way of life. But what about the right to a long life, free of cognitive decline and mental disease? You can claim this right today. I hope you do.

Acknowledgments

As anyone who has ever written a book knows, it takes an army of creative, bright, and tireless people to put it all together. And just when you think you're done, another troop of equally brilliant people emerges on the scene to help see things through until a reader like you can absorb the very first page.

If I had my way, I'd list everyone who has ever contributed to my thinking and supported me throughout my life and career. But that would entail hundreds of people and many pages here, so I will keep this short and sweet. I am indebted to all the scientists and my fellow colleagues who have worked to understand the mysteries of the human brain and body. I am also forever grateful to my patients, who teach me every day and provide insights that cannot be found elsewhere. This book is as much yours as it is mine.

Thanks to my friend and literary agent, Bonnie Solow. It was your recognition of the importance of this message that catalyzed all that has followed. But more than anything else, I am appreciative that this project has brought us our friendship. Thanks for your gracious leadership and attention to details. I know that you've gone beyond the call of duty—protecting, guiding, and helping this book reach the masses.

To Kristin Loberg: While the content of this work represents my research and professional experience, it is wholly through your artistic mastery that our message is now conveyed.

Thanks to the indefatigable team at Little, Brown Spark that has championed this book and the others that followed since our first meeting. A special thanks goes to Tracy Behar, my editor with an unparalleled gift for making sure the message remains clear, succinct, and practical. Your talented editorial genius made this a much better book through all its iterations. And another special shout-out to Marisa Vigilante, who oversaw this new edition's revisions with her own editorial brilliance. Thanks also to Michael Pietsch, Reagan Arthur, Ian Straus, Jessica Chun, Juliana Horbachevsky, Craig Young, Pamela Brown, Sabrina Callahan, Jayne Yaffe Kemp, Karen Wise, Kathryn Blatt, Pat Jalbert-Levine, Charlee Trantino, Giraud Lorber, and Stacy Schuck. It's been a pleasure to work with such a dedicated, professional group.

The management team at Proton Enterprises has done and continues to do an incredible job managing and directing the many moving parts involved in our projects. Thanks to James Murphy, Sharon Green, Lou Cowell, and Blake Brown.

Thanks to Digital Natives, the savvy tech team responsible for making my website come alive as a companion to the book.

Thanks to Gigi Stewart, who helped with some of the recipes from her own tasty kitchen that abide by my rules and make cooking fun.

To my wife, Leize: Thank you for all the time and commitment in lovingly preparing the recipes. I am grateful beyond measure to have you in my life.

And finally, I wish to acknowledge my children, Austin and Reisha, who have never ceased to encourage and support me on this journey.

Illustration Credits

Page 7   Adapted from: Maureen M. Leonard, et al., "Celiac Disease and Nonceliac Gluten Sensitivity," *JAMA* 318, no. 7 (2017): 647–56.

Page 8   Alzheimer's Association, "2017 Alzheimer's Disease Facts and Figures." *Alzheimer's & Dementia* 13 (2017): 325–73, https://www.alz.org/documents_custom/2017-facts-and-figures.pdf.

Page 10   Alzheimer's Disease International, "World Alzheimer Report 2015," https://www.alz.co.uk/research/WorldAlzheimerReport2015.pdf.

Page 35   Adapted from: K. A. Walker, et al., "Midlife Systemic Inflammatory Markers Are Associated with Late-Life Brain Volume: The ARIC Study," *Neurology* 89, no. 22 (2017): 2262–70.

Page 70   Reprinted from *The Lancet Neurology*, Volume 9, Issue 3, M. Hadjivassiliou, MD, et al., Gluten sensitivity: from gut to brain, pages 318–30, March 2010, with permission from Elsevier.

Page 99   Centers for Disease Control and Prevention, "Long-Term Trends in Diabetes," April 2017, https://www.cdc.gov/diabetes/statistics/slides/long_term_trends.pdf.

Page 102   Adapted from: S. Yoon, et al., "Brain Changes in Overweight/Obese and Normal-Weight Adults with Type 2 Diabetes Mellitus," *Diabetologia* 60, no. 7 (2017): 1207–17.

Page 102   Ibid.

Page 103   Ibid.

Page 103   Ibid.

Page 111   Adapted from: A. L. Culver, et al., "Statin Use and Risk of Diabetes Mellitus in Postmenopausal Women in the Women's Health Initiative," *Archives of Internal Medicine* 172, no. 2 (2012): 144–52.

Page 134   Adapted from: C. Enzinger, et al., "Risk Factors for Progression of Brain Atrophy in Aging: Six-Year Follow-Up of Normal Subjects," *Neurology* 64, no. 10 (2005): 1704–11.

Page 144   Adapted from: Matthew P. Pase, et al., "Sugar- and Artificially Sweetened Beverages and the Risks of Incident Stroke and Dementia," *Stroke* 48, no. 5 (2017): 1139–46.

Page 144   Ibid.

Page 145   Ibid.

Page 209   © Randy Glasbergen. glasbergen.com. Reprinted with permission.

Page 222   Adapted from: A. S. Buchman, et al., "Total Daily Physical Activity and the Risk of AD and Cognitive Decline in Older Adults," *Neurology* 78, no. 17 (2012): 1323–29.

Page 222   Ibid.

Page 227   Adapted from: K. I. Erikson, et al., "Exercise Training Increases Size of Hippocampus and Improves Memory," *Proceedings of the National Academy of Sciences U.S.A.* 108, no. 7 (2011): 3017–22.

Notes

The following is a list of books and scientific papers that you might find helpful in learning more about some of the ideas and concepts expressed in this book. These materials can also open doors for further research and inquiry. For access to these and more studies, and for an ongoing updated list of references, please visit DrPerlmutter.com. Our database is robust and fully searchable by topic; also check out the "Focus" tab on the main menu. Bonus: Subscribe to my free newsletter to become part of my email community.

Introduction

1. David Perlmutter, "Why We Can and Must Focus on Preventing Alzheimer's," *The Daily Beast*, August 22, 2013, https://www.thedailybeast.com/why-we-can-and-must -focus-on-preventing-alzheimers.
2. Alessio Fasano, et al., "Effect of Gliadin on Permeability of Intestinal Biopsy Explants from Celiac Disease Patients and Patients with Non-Celiac Gluten Sensitivity," *Nutrients* 7, no. 3 (2015): 1565–76.
3. Maureen M. Leonard, et al., "Celiac Disease and Nonceliac Gluten Sensitivity," *JAMA* 318, no. 7 (2017): 647–56.
4. Michal Schnaider-Beeri and Joshua Sonnen, "Brain BDNF Expression as a Biomarker for Cognitive Reserve Against Alzheimer's Disease Progression," *Neurology* 86, no. 8 (2016): 702–3.
5. Alzheimer's Association, "2017 Alzheimer's Disease Facts and Figures." *Alzheimer's & Dementia* 13 (2017): 325–73, https://www.alz.org/documents_custom/2017-facts -and-figures.pdf.
6. Alzheimer's Disease International, https://www.alz.co.uk/.
7. Alzheimer's Disease International, "World Alzheimer Report 2015," https://www .alz.co.uk/research/WorldAlzheimerReport2015.pdf.

8. N. Scarmeas, et al., "Physical Activity, Diet, and Risk of Alzheimer's Disease," *JAMA* 302, no. 6 (2009): 627–37.

9. Jonathan Graff-Radford, "Alzheimer's: Can a Mediterranean Diet Lower My Risk?" *The Mayo Clinic's FAQ*, February 2, 2018, https://www.mayoclinic.org/diseases -conditions/alzheimers-disease/expert-answers/alzheimers-disease/faq-20058062.

10. Allison Aubrey, "The Average American Ate (Literally) a Ton This Year," *The Salt* (blog), NPR, December 31, 2011, https://www.npr.org/sections/thesalt/2011/12/31/ 144478009/the-average-american-ate-literally-a-ton-this-year.

11. Annie L. Culver, et al., "Statin Use and Risk of Diabetes Mellitus in Postmenopausal Women in the Women's Health Initiative," *Archives of Internal Medicine* 172, no. 2 (2012): 144–52.

12. H. Cederberg, et al., "Increased Risk of Diabetes with Statin Treatment Is Associated with Impaired Insulin Sensitivity and Insulin Secretion: A 6-Year Follow-Up Study of the METSIM Cohort," *Diabetologia* 58, no. 5 (2015): 1109–17.

13. Åsa Blomström, et al., "Maternal Antibodies to Dietary Antigens and Risk for Nonaffective Psychosis in Offspring," *American Journal of Psychiatry* 169 (2012): 625–32.

14. Q. Hu, et al., "Homocysteine and Alzheimers' Disease: Evidence for a Causal Link from Mendelian Randomization," *Journal of Alzheimer's Disease* 52, no. 2 (2016): 747–56; L. Shen and H. F. Ji, "Associations Between Homocysteine, Folic Acid, Vitamin B_{12} and Alzheimer's Disease: Insights from Meta-Analyses," *Journal of Alzheimer's Disease* 46, no. 3 (2015): 777–90.

15. Fei Ma, et al., "Plasma Homocysteine and Serum Folate and Vitamin B_{12} Levels in Mild Cognitive Impairment and Alzheimer's Disease: A Case-Control Study," *Nutrients* 9, no. 7 (2017): 725.

Chapter 1

1. Eric Steen, et al., "Impaired Insulin and Insulin-like Growth Factor Expression and Signaling Mechanisms in Alzheimer's Disease — Is This Type 3 Diabetes?" *Journal of Alzheimer's Disease* 7, no. 1 (2005): 63–80.

2. R. O. Roberts, et al., "Relative Intake of Macronutrients Impacts Risk of Mild Cognitive Impairment or Dementia," *Journal of Alzheimer's Disease* 32, no. 2 (2012): 329–39; R. Kandimalla, et al., "Is Alzheimer's Disease a Type 3 Diabetes? A Critical Appraisal," *Biochimica et Biophysica Acta* 1863, no. 5 (2017): 1078–89.

3. Mark Bittman, "Is Alzheimer's Type 3 Diabetes?" *Opinionator* (blog), *New York Times*, September 25, 2012, http://opinionator.blogs.nytimes.com/2012/09/25/bitt man-is-alzheimers-type-3-diabetes/. Bittman's piece provides a great explanation of type 3 diabetes. A more recent article that also offers a layman's review of the studies is Olga Khazan, "The Startling Link Between Sugar and Alzheimer's," *The Atlantic*, January 26, 2018, https://www.theatlantic.com/health/archive/2018/01/ the-startling-link-between-sugar-and-alzheimers/551528/.

4. American Diabetes Association, "Statistics About Diabetes," http://www.diabetes .org/diabetes-basics/statistics/. Updated March 22, 2018.

5. Centers for Disease Control and Prevention, National Center for Health Statistics, "Leading Causes of Death," https://www.cdc.gov/nchs/fastats/leading-causes-of-death .htm. Last modified March 17, 2017.

6. F. Zheng, et al., "HbA1C, Diabetes and Cognitive Decline: The English Longitudinal Study of Ageing," *Diabetologia* 61, no. 4 (2018): 839–48.

7. Alzheimer's Association, "2018 Alzheimer's Association Facts and Figures," https:// www.alz.org/facts/.

8. Ibid.

9. Centers for Disease Control and Prevention, National Center for Chronic Disease Prevention and Health Promotion, "National Diabetes Statistics Report 2017," https://www.cdc.gov/diabetes/pdfs/data/statistics/national-diabetes-statistics -report.pdf. Also see: Andy Menke, et al., "Prevalence of and Trends in Diabetes Among Adults in the United States, 1988–2012," *JAMA* 314, no. 10 (2015): 1021–29.

10. J. M. Silverman and J. Schmeidler, "Outcome Age-Based Prediction of Successful Cognitive Aging by Total Cholesterol," *Alzheimer's & Dementia* (published online March 1, 2018).

11. Framingham Heart Study, http://www.framinghamheartstudy.org.

12. Penelope K. Elias, et al., "Serum Cholesterol and Cognitive Performance in the Framingham Heart Study," *Psychosomatic Medicine* 67, no. 1 (2005): 24–30.

13. Nicolas Cherbuin, et al., "Higher Normal Fasting Plasma Glucose Is Associated with Hippocampal Atrophy: The PATH Study," *Neurology* 79, no. 10 (January/ February 2012): 1019–26. doi: 10.1212/WNL.0b013e31826846de. Also see the follow-up study: Nicolas Cherbuin, et al., "Higher Fasting Plasma Glucose Is Associated with Striatal and Hippocampal Shape Differences: The 2sweet Project," *BMJ Open Diabetes Research & Care* 4, no. 1 (2016): e000175.

14. American Academy of Neurology (AAN), "Even in Normal Range, High Blood Sugar Linked to Brain Shrinkage," *Science Daily*, September 4, 2012, http://www .sciencedaily.com/releases/2012/09/120904095856.htm.

15. Walter F. Stewart, et al., "Risk of Alzheimer's Disease and Duration of NSAID Use," *Neurology* 48, no. 3 (March 1997): 626–32; Angelika D. Wahner, et al., "Nonsteroidal Anti-inflammatory Drugs May Protect Against Parkinson's Disease," *Neurology* 69, no. 19 (November 6, 2007): 1836–42.

16. Jose Miguel Rubio-Perez, et al., "A Review: Inflammatory Process in Alzheimer's Disease, Role of Cytokines," *Scientific World Journal* (April 1, 2012). doi: 10.1100/2012/756357.

17. K. A. Walker, et al., "Midlife Systemic Inflammatory Markers Are Associated with Late-Life Brain Volume: The ARIC Study," *Neurology* 89, no. 22 (2017): 2262–70.

18. M. Berk, et al., "So Depression Is an Inflammatory Disease, but Where Does the Inflammation Come From?" *BMC Medicine* 11 (2013): 200.
19. William Davis, *Wheat Belly* (New York: Rodale Books, 2011).

Chapter 2

1. Heather Wood, "Motor Neuron Disease: Can Gluten Sensitivity Mimic Amyotrophic Lateral Sclerosis?" *Nature Reviews Neurology* 11, no. 6 (2015): 308.
2. Statista, "Global Gluten-Free Food Market Size from 2013 to 2020 (in Million U.S. Dollars)," https://www.statista.com/statistics/248467/global-gluten-free-food-market-size/.
3. Katie Forster, "Gluten-Free Diet Can Do More Harm than Good for People without Coeliac Disease, Scientists Say," *The Independent*, May 2, 2017, https://www.independent.co.uk/news/health/gluten-free-diet-harmful-people-without-coeliac-disease-health-benefits-a7713711.html.
4. Catherine M. Bulka, et al., "The Unintended Consequences of a Gluten-free Diet," *Epidemiology* 28, no. 3 (2017): e24–e25.
5. Benjamin Lebwohl, et al., "Long Term Gluten Consumption in Adults without Celiac Disease and Risk of Coronary Heart Disease: Prospective Cohort Study," *BMJ* 357 (2017): j1892.
6. "Gluten-Free Diet May Increase Risk of Arsenic, Mercury Exposure," University of Illinois Press Release for UCI Today, February 13, 2017, https://today.uic.edu/gluten-free-diet-may-increase-risk-of-arsenic-mercury-exposure.
7. The Celiac Disease Foundation, "What Is Celiac Disease?," https://celiac.org/celiac-disease/understanding-celiac-disease-2/what-is-celiac-disease/.
8. Q. Mu, et al., "Leaky Gut As a Danger Signal for Autoimmune Diseases," *Frontiers in Immunology* 8 (2017): 598.
9. David Perlmutter, "Gluten Sensitivity and the Impact on the Brain," http://www.huffingtonpost.com/dr-david-perlmutter-md/gluten-impacts-the-brain_b_785901.html, November 21, 2010. Updated May 25, 2011. Also go to my website at DrPerlmutter.com for more on this discussion.
10. David Perlmutter and Alberto Villoldo, *Power Up Your Brain: The Neuroscience of Enlightenment* (New York: Hay House, 2011).
11. Dr. Alessio Fasano of Boston's Center for Celiac Research and Treatments, which is part of Massachusetts General Hospital, has written extensively on gluten sensitivity and the many ways it can manifest in people—sometimes mimicking other disorders. You can visit his website and access his publications at http://www.celiaccenter.org/.
12. Marios Hadjivassiliou, et al., "Does Cryptic Gluten Sensitivity Play a Part in Neurological Illness?" *Lancet* 347, no. 8998 (February 10, 1996): 369–71.

13. Marios Hadjivassiliou, et al., "Gluten Sensitivity As a Neurological Illness," *Journal of Neurology, Neurosurgery, and Psychiatry* 72, no. 5 (May 2002): 560–63.

14. Justin Hollon, et al., "Effect of Gliadin on Permeability of Intestinal Biopsy Explants from Celiac Disease Patients and Patients with Non-Celiac Gluten Sensitivity," *Nutrients* 7, no. 3 (2015): 1565–76.

15. The Celiac Disease Foundation, "Non-Celiac Wheat Sensitivity Is Official," Press Release, August 4, 2016; https://celiac.org/blog/2016/08/non-celiac-wheat-sensi tivity-is-official/; M. Uhde, et al., "Intestinal Cell Damage and Systemic Immune Activation in Individuals Reporting Sensitivity to Wheat in the Absence of Coeliac Disease," *Gut* 65, no. 12 (2016): 1930–37.

16. Beyond Celiac, http://www.beyondceliac.org.

17. Uhde, et al., "Intestinal Cell Damage and Systemic Immune Activation in Individuals Reporting Sensitivity to Wheat in the Absence of Coeliac Disease" (see n. 15).

18. Bernadette Kalman and Thomas H. Brannagan III, "Neurological Manifestations of Gluten Sensitivity," in *Neuroimmunology in Clinical Practice* (Wiley-Blackwell, 2007). This book provides an excellent review of the history of celiac disease.

19. Henry W. Woltman and Frank J. Heck, "Funicular Degeneration of the Spinal Cord without Pernicious Anemianeurologic Aspects of Sprue, Nontropical Sprue and Idiopathic Steatorrhea," *Archives of Internal Medicine* (Chicago) 60, no. 2 (1937): 272–300.

20. Marios Hadjivassiliou, et al., "Gluten Sensitivity: From Gut to Brain," *Lancet Neurology* 9, no. 3 (March 2010): 318–30. This article provides another wonderful overview of celiac through the ages.

21. T. William, et al., "Cognitive Impairment and Celiac Disease," *Archives of Neurology* 63, no. 10 (October 2006): 1440–46; Mayo Clinic, "Mayo Clinic Discovers Potential Link Between Celiac Disease and Cognitive Decline," *Science Daily,* October 12, 2006, http://www.sciencedaily.com/releases/2006/10/061010022602.htm.

22. Hadjivassiliou, et al., "Gluten Sensitivity: From Gut to Brain" (see no. 20).

23. The following website is a gateway to Dr. Aristo Vojdani's work and publications: http://www.yourmedicaldetective.com/public/148.cfm.

24. Rodney P. Ford, "The Gluten Syndrome: A Neurological Disease," *Medical Hypotheses* 73, no. 3 (September 2009): 438–40.

25. E. Lionetti, et al., "Gluten Psychosis: Confirmation of a New Clinical Entity," *Nutrients* 8, no. 7 (2015): 5532–39.

26. Gianna Ferretti, et al., "Celiac Disease, Inflammation and Oxidative Damage: A Nutrigenetic Approach," *Nutrients* 4, no. 4 (April 2012): 243–57.

27. Ibid.

28. Davis, *Wheat Belly* (see chap. 1, n. 19).

29. Christine Zioudrou, et al., "Opioid Peptides Derived from Food Proteins (the Exorphins)," *Journal of Biological Chemistry* 254, no. 7 (April 10, 1979): 2446–49.

30. Davis, *Wheat Belly* (see chap. 1, n. 19).

31. Lucy Goodchild van Hilten, "How Digesting Bread and Pasta Could Be Affecting Our Brains," posted to Elsevier Connect on July 2, 2015, https://www.elsevier.com/connect/how-digesting-bread-and-pasta-could-be-affecting-our-brains.
32. Grażyna Czaja-Bulsa, "Non Coeliac Gluten Sensitivity: A New Disease with Gluten Intolerance," *Clinical Nutrition* 24, no. 2 (2015): 189–94.

Chapter 3

1. Statista, "U.S. Population: Do You Eat Breakfast Cereals (Cold)?," https://www.statista.com/statistics/279999/us-households-consumption-of-breakfast-cereals-cold/.
2. Office of Disease Prevention and Health Promotion, "2015–2020 Dietary Guidelines for Americans," https://health.gov/dietaryguidelines/2015/.
3. R. F. Gottesman, et al., "Midlife Hypertension and 20-Year Cognitive Change: The Atherosclerosis Risk in Communities Neurocognitive Study," *JAMA Neurology* 71, no. 10 (2014): 1218–27.
4. R. F. Gottesman, et al., "Association Between Midlife Vascular Risk Factors and Estimated Brain Amyloid Deposition," *JAMA* 317, no. 14 (2017): 1443–50.
5. Roberts, et al., "Relative Intake of Macronutrients Impacts Risk of Mild Cognitive Impairment or Dementia" (see chap. 1, n. 2).
6. M. Mulder, et al., "Reduced Levels of Cholesterol, Phospholipids, and Fatty Acids in Cerebrospinal Fluid of Alzheimer Disease Patients Are Not Related to Apolipoprotein E4," *Alzheimer Disease and Associated Disorders* 12, no. 3 (September 1998): 198–203.
7. P. Barberger-Gateau, et al., "Dietary Patterns and Risk of Dementia: The Three-City Cohort Study," *Neurology* 69, no. 20 (November 13, 2007): 1921–30.
8. Y. Zhang, et al., "Intakes of Fish and Polyunsaturated Fatty Acids and Mild-to-Severe Cognitive Impairment Risks: A Dose-Response Meta-Analysis of 21 Cohort Studies," *American Journal of Clinical Nutrition* 103, no. 2 (2016): 330–40.
9. P. M. Kris-Etherton, et al., "Polyunsaturated Fatty Acids in the Food Chain in the United States," *American Journal of Clinical Nutrition* 71, no. 1 (January 2000): S179–88.
10. Rebecca West, et al., "Better Memory Functioning Associated with Higher Total and Low-Density Lipoprotein Cholesterol Levels in Very Elderly Subjects Without the Apolipoprotein e4 Allele," *American Journal of Geriatric Psychiatry* 16, no. 9 (September 2008): 781–85.
11. L. M. de Lau, et al., "Serum Cholesterol Levels and the Risk of Parkinson's Disease," *American Journal of Epidemiology* 164, no. 10 (August 11, 2006): 998–1002.
12. X. Huang, et al., "Low LDL Cholesterol and Increased Risk of Parkinson's Disease: Prospective Results from Honolulu-Asia Aging Study," *Movement Disorders* 23, no. 7 (May 15, 2008): 1013–18.

13. H. M. Krumholz, et al., "Lack of Association Between Cholesterol and Coronary Heart Disease Mortality and Morbidity and All-Cause Mortality in Persons Older Than 70 Years," *JAMA* 272, no. 17 (November 2, 1994): 1335–40.

14. H. Petousis-Harris, "Saturated Fat Has Been Unfairly Demonised: Yes," *Primary Health Care* 3, no. 4 (December 1, 2011): 317–19.

15. George V. Mann, "Diet-Heart: End of An Era," *New England Journal of Medicine* (September 22, 1977): 644–50.

16. George V. Mann, *Coronary Heart Disease: The Dietary Sense and Nonsense* (Harry Ransom Humanities Research Center: Austin, 1993); see also http://www.survive diabetes.com/lowfat.html.

17. A. W. Weverling-Rijnsburger, et al., "Total Cholesterol and Risk of Mortality in the Oldest Old," *Lancet* 350, no. 9085 (October 18, 1997): 1119–23.

18. L. Dupuis, et al., "Dyslipidemia Is a Protective Factor in Amyotrophic Lateral Sclerosis," *Neurology* 70, no. 13 (March 25, 2008): 1004–9.

19. P. W. Siri-Tarino, et al., "Meta-Analysis of Prospective Cohort Studies Evaluating the Association of Saturated Fat with Cardiovascular Disease," *American Journal of Clinical Nutrition* 91, no. 3 (March 2010): 535–46.

20. Michael I. Gurr, et al., *Lipid Biochemistry: An Introduction*, 5th ed. (New York: Wiley-Blackwell, 2010).

21. A. Astrup, et al., "The Role of Reducing Intakes of Saturated Fat in the Prevention of Cardiovascular Disease: Where Does the Evidence Stand in 2010?" *American Journal of Clinical Nutrition* 93, no. 4 (April 2011): 684–88.

22. For an engrossing, sweeping view of our dietary habits over the past century, see Dr. Donald W. Miller Jr., "Health Benefits of a Low-Carbohydrate, High-Saturated-Fat Diet," https://www.lewrockwell.com/1970/01/donald-w-miller-jr-md/low-carbo hydrate-high-saturated-fat/.

23. United States Department of Agriculture, "Choose My Plate," http://www.choose myplate.gov/.

24. Miller, "Health Benefits of a Low-Carbohydrate, High-Saturated-Fat Diet" (see n. 22).

25. International Atherosclerosis Project, "General Findings of the International Atherosclerosis Project," *Laboratory Investigation* 18, no. 5 (May 1968): 498–502.

26. Centers for Disease Control and Prevention, "Long-Term Trends in Diabetes," April 2017, https://www.cdc.gov/diabetes/statistics/slides/long_term_trends.pdf.

27. R. Stocker and J. F. Keaney Jr., "Role of Oxidative Modifications in Atherosclerosis," *Physiology Review* 84, no. 4 (October 2004): 1381–478.

28. Y. Kiyohara, "The Cohort Study of Dementia: The Hisayama Study," *Rinsho Shinkeigaku* 51, no. 11 (November 2011): 906–9. Note that the article is in Japanese. Also see Ann Harding's coverage of this study for CNN Health at http://www.cnn.com/2011/09/19/health/diabetes-doubles-alzheimers.

29. Melissa A. Schilling, "Unraveling Alzheimer's: Making Sense of the Relationship between Diabetes and Alzheimer's Disease," *Journal of Alzheimer's Disease* 51, no. 4 (2016): 961–77.

30. S. Yoon, et al., "Brain Changes in Overweight/Obese and Normal-Weight Adults with Type 2 Diabetes Mellitus," *Diabetologia* 60, no. 7 (2017): 1207–17.

31. M. Dehghan, et al., "Associations of Fats and Carbohydrate Intake with Cardiovascular Disease and Mortality in 18 Countries from Five Continents (PURE): A Prospective Cohort Stud," *Lancet* 390, no. 10107 (2017): 2050–62.

32. R. H. Swerdlow, et al., "Feasibility and Efficacy Data from a Ketogenic Diet Intervention in Alzheimer's Disease," *Alzheimer's & Dementia: Translational Research & Clinical Interventions* 4 (2018): 28–36.

33. C. Valls-Pedret, et al., "Mediterranean Diet and Age-Related Cognitive Decline: A Randomized Clinical Trial," *JAMA Internal Medicine* 175, no. 7 (2015): 1094–103.

34. Michele G. Sullivan, "Fueling the Alzheimer's Brain with Fat," *Clinical Neurology News,* August 23, 2017, https://www.mdedge.com/clinicalneurologynews/article/145220/alzheimers-cognition/fueling-alzheimers-brain-fat; Ling Wu, et al., "Olive Component Oleuropein Promotes β-cell Insulin Secretion and Protects β-cells from Amylin Amyloid Induced Cytotoxicity," *Biochemistry* 56, no. 38 (2017): 5035–39.

35. D. Jacobs, et al., "Report of the Conference on Low Blood Cholesterol: Mortality Associations," *Circulation* 86, no. 3 (September 1992): 1046–60.

36. Duane Graveline, *Lipitor, Thief of Memory: Statin Drugs and the Misguided War on Cholesterol* (Duane Graveline, MD, 2006).

37. Culver, et al., "Statin Use and Risk of Diabetes Mellitus in Postmenopausal Women in the Women's Health Initiative" (see introduction, n. 11).

38. David Perlmutter, Beatrice Golomb, and Stephen Sinatra, "Appropriate Clinical Use of Statins: A Discussion of the Evidence, Scope, Benefits, and Risk," *Alternative Therapies, Heart Health* vol. 19, suppl. 1 (2013).

39. Stephanie Seneff, "APOE-4: The Clue to Why Low Fat Diet and Statins May Cause Alzheimer's," December 15, 2009, http://people.csail.mit.edu/seneff/alzheimers_statins.html.

40. Iowa State University, "Cholesterol-Reducing Drugs May Lessen Brain Function, Says Researcher," *Science Daily,* February 26, 2009, http://www.sciencedaily.com/releases/2009/02/090223221430.htm.

41. Center for Advancing Health, "Statins Do Not Help Prevent Alzheimer's Disease, Review Finds," *Science Daily,* April 16, 2009, http://www.sciencedaily.com/releases/2009/04/090415171324.htm. See also B. McGuinness, et al., "Statins for the Prevention of Dementia," *Cochrane Database of Systematic Reviews* 2 (2009).

42. Ibid.

43. Seneff, "APOE-4: The Clue to Why Low Fat Diet and Statins May Cause Alzheimer's" (see n. 39).

44. Ibid.

45. Ibid.

46. K. Rizvi, et al., "Do Lipid-Lowering Drugs Cause Erectile Dysfunction? A Systematic Review," *Journal of Family Practice* 19, no. 1 (February 2002): 95–98.

47. G. Corona, et al., "The Effect of Statin Therapy on Testosterone Levels in Subjects Consulting for Erectile Dysfunction: Part 1," *Journal of Sexual Medicine* 7, no. 4 (April 2010): 1547–56.

48. C. J. Malkin, et al., "Low Serum Testosterone and Increased Mortality in Men with Coronary Heart Disease," *Heart* 96, no. 22 (November 2010): 1821–25.

49. David Perlmutter, *Brain Maker: The Power of Gut Microbes to Heal and Protect Your Brain—for Life* (New York: Little, Brown, 2015).

Chapter 4

1. R. H. Lustig, et al., "Public Health: The Toxic Truth About Sugar," *Nature* 482, no. 7383 (February 1, 2012): 27–29.

2. Gary Taubes, *Good Calories, Bad Calories: Challenging the Conventional Wisdom on Diet, Weight Control, and Disease* (New York: Knopf, 2007); Gary Taubes, *Why We Get Fat: And What to Do About It* (New York: Knopf, 2010).

3. Gary Taubes, "Is Sugar Toxic?" *New York Times*, April 13, 2011, http://www.nytimes.com/2011/04/17/magazine/mag-17Sugar-t.html.

4. Gary Taubes, *The Case Against Sugar* (New York: Knopf, 2016).

5. Robert Lustig, *Fat Chance: Beating the Odds Against Sugar, Processed Food, Obesity, and Disease* (New York: Hudson Street Press, 2012).

6. U.S. Department of Agriculture Economic Research Service, "Food Availability and Consumption," https://www.ers.usda.gov/data-products/ag-and-food-statistics-charting-the-essentials/food-availability-and-consumption. Updated October 18, 2016.

7. E. E. Ventura, J. N. Davis, and M. I. Goran, "Sugar Content of Popular Sweetened Beverages Based on Objective Laboratory Analysis: Focus on Fructose Content," *Obesity* (Silver Spring) 19, no. 4 (2011): 868–74.

8. R. H. Lustig, "Sugar: The Bitter Truth," http://youtu.be/dBnniua6-oM (2009). This video gives a captivating overview of sugar metabolism.

9. Taubes, *Why We Get Fat*, 138 (see n. 2).

10. Ibid., 134.

11. National Institute of Diabetes and Digestive and Kidney Diseases, "Diabetes Statistics," September 2017, https://www.niddk.nih.gov/health-information/health-statistics/diabetes-statistics.

12. K. Yaffe, et al., "Diabetes, Glucose Control, and 9-Year Cognitive Decline Among Older Adults Without Dementia," *Archives of Neurology* 69, no. 9 (September 2012): 1170–75.

13. R. O. Roberts, et al., "Association of Duration and Severity of Diabetes Mellitus with Mild Cognitive Impairment," *Archives of Neurology* 65, no. 8 (August 2008): 1066–73.

14. Amy Dockser Marcus, "Mad-Cow Disease May Hold Clues to Other Neurological Disorders," *Wall Street Journal*, December 3, 2012, http://online.wsj.com/article/SB10001424127887324020804578151291509136144.html.

15. J. Stöhr, et al., "Purified and Synthetic Alzheimer's Amyloid Beta (Aβ) Prions," *Proceedings of the National Academy of Sciences* 109, no. 27 (July 3, 2012): 11025–30.

16. L. C. Maillard, "Action of Amino Acids on Sugars: Formation of Melanoidins in a Methodical Way," *Comptes Rendus Chimie* 154 (1912): 66–68.

17. P. Gkogkolou and M. Böhm, "Advanced Glycation End Products: Key Players in Skin Aging?" *Dermato-Endocrinology* 4, no. 3 (July 1, 2012): 259–70.

18. Q. Zhang, et al., "A Perspective on the Maillard Reaction and the Analysis of Protein Glycation by Mass Spectrometry: Probing the Pathogenesis of Chronic Disease," *Journal of Proteome Research* 8, no. 2 (February 2009): 754–69.

19. Sonia Gandhi and Audrey Abramov, "Mechanism of Oxidative Stress in Neuro-degeneration," *Oxidative Medicine and Cellular Longevity* (2012).

20. Yoon, et al., "Brain Changes in Overweight/Obese and Normal-Weight Adults with Type 2 Diabetes Mellitus" (see chap. 3, n. 30).

21. C. Enzinger, et al., "Risk Factors for Progression of Brain Atrophy in Aging: Six-Year Follow-Up of Normal Subjects," *Neurology* 64, no. 10 (May 24, 2005): 1704–11.

22. M. Hamer, et al., "Haemoglobin A1c, Fasting Glucose and Future Risk of Elevated Depressive Symptoms over 2 Years of Follow-Up in the English Longitudinal Study of Ageing," *Psychological Medicine* 41, no. 9 (September 2011): 1889–96.

23. C. Geroldi, et al., "Insulin Resistance in Cognitive Impairment: The InCHIANTI Study," *Archives of Neurology* 62, no. 7 (2005): 1067–72.

24. E. I. Walsh, et al., "Brain Atrophy in Ageing: Estimating Effects of Blood Glucose Levels vs. Other Type 2 Diabetes Effects," *Diabetes & Metabolism* 44, no. 1 (2018): 80–83.

25. H. Haimoto, et al., "Effects of a Low-Carbohydrate Diet on Glycemic Control in Outpatients with Severe Type 2 Diabetes," *Nutrition & Metabolism* (London) 6 (2009): 6.

26. M. Adamczak and A. Wiecek, "The Adipose Tissue as an Endocrine Organ," *Seminars in Nephrology* 33, no. 1 (January 2013): 2–13.

27. E. L. de Hollander, et al., "The Association Between Waist Circumference and Risk of Mortality Considering Body Mass Index in 65- to 74-Year-Olds: A Meta-Analysis of 29 Cohorts Involving More Than 58,000 Elderly Persons," *International Journal of Epidemiology* 41, no. 3 (June 2012): 805–17.

28. F. Item and D. Konrad, "Visceral Fat and Metabolic Inflammation: The Portal Theory Revisited," pt. 2, *Obesity Reviews* 13 (December 2012): S30–S39.

29. C. Geroldi, et al., "Insulin Resistance in Cognitive Impairment" (see n. 23).

30. C. A. Raji, et al., "Brain Structure and Obesity," *Human Brain Mapping* 31, no. 3 (March 2010): 353–64.

31. R. A. Whitmer, et al., "Central Obesity and Increased Risk of Dementia More Than Three Decades Later," *Neurology* 71, no. 14 (September 30, 2008): 1057–64.

32. A. Singh-Manoux, et al., "Obesity Trajectories and Risk of Dementia: 28 Years of Follow-Up in the Whitehall II Study," *Alzheimer's & Dementia* 14, no. 2 (2018): 178–86.

33. C. Mason, et al., "Dietary Weight Loss and Exercise Effects on Insulin Resistance in Postmenopausal Women," *American Journal of Preventive Medicine* 41, no. 4 (2011): 366–75.

34. C. B. Ebbeling, et al., "Effects of Dietary Composition on Energy Expenditure During Weight-Loss Maintenance," *JAMA* 307, no. 24 (June 27, 2012): 2627–34.

35. R. Estruch, et al., "Primary Prevention of Cardiovascular Disease with a Mediterranean Diet," *New England Journal of Medicine* (February 25, 2013), http://www.nejm.org/doi/full/10.1056/NEJMoa1200303#t=article.

36. R. Estruch, et al., "Primary Prevention of Cardiovascular Disease with a Mediterranean Diet," *New England Journal of Medicine* (June 21, 2018), https://www.nejm.org/doi/10.1056/NEJMoa1800389.

37. Michelle Luciano, et al., "Mediterranean-Type Diet and Brain Structural Change from 73 to 76 Years in a Scottish Cohort," *Neurology* 88, no. 5 (2017): 449–55.

38. Segal, et al., "Artificial Sweeteners Induce Glucose Intolerance by Altering the Gut Microbiota," *Nature* 514, no. 7521 (2014). 181–86, Sofia Carlsson, et al., "Sweetened Beverage Intake and Risk of Latent Autoimmune Diabetes in Adults (LADA) and Type 2 Diabetes," *European Journal of Endocrinology* 175 (2016): 605–14; G. Fagherazzi, et al., "Consumption of Artificially and Sugar-Sweetened Beverages and Incident Type 2 Diabetes in the Etude Epidemiologique aupres des femmes de la Mutuelle Generale de l'Education Nationale-European Prospective Investigation into Cancer and Nutrition Cohort," *American Journal of Clinical Nutrition* 97, no. 3 (2013): 517–23.

39. Matthew P. Pase, et al., "Sugar- and Artificially Sweetened Beverages and the Risks of Incident Stroke and Dementia," *Stroke* 48, no. 5 (2017): 1139–46.

Chapter 5

1. Nicholas Wade, "Heart Muscle Renewed over Lifetime, Study Finds," *New York Times*, April 2, 2009, http://www.nytimes.com/2009/04/03/science/03heart.html.

2. Santiago Ramón y Cajal, *Cajal's Degeneration and Regeneration of the Nervous System* (History of Neuroscience) (New York: Oxford University Press, 1991).

3. Charles C. Gross, "Neurogenesis in the Adult Brain: Death of a Dogma," *Nature Reviews Neuroscience* 1, no. 1 (October 2000): 67–73. See this op-ed piece for a summation of how we've come to understand neurogenesis in mammals.

4. P. S. Eriksson, et al., "Neurogenesis in the Adult Human Hippocampus," *Nature Medicine* 4, no. 11 (November 1998): 1313–17.

5. Perlmutter and Villoldo, *Power Up Your Brain* (see chap. 2, n. 10).

6. Norman Doidge, *The Brain That Changes Itself: Stories of Personal Triumph from the Frontiers of Brain Science* (New York: Viking, 2007); Norman Doidge, *The Brain's Way of Healing: Remarkable Discoveries and Recoveries from the Frontiers of Neuroplasticity* (New York: Viking, 2015).

7. J. Lee, et al., "Decreased Levels of BDNF Protein in Alzheimer Temporal Cortex Are Independent of BDNF Polymorphisms," *Experimental Neurology* 194, no. 1 (July 2005): 91–96.

8. G. Weinstein, et al., "Serum Brain-Derived Neurotrophic Factor and the Risk for Dementia: The Framingham Heart Study," *JAMA Neurology* 71, no. 1 (2014): 55–61.

9. Schnaider-Beeri and Sonnen, "Brain BDNF Expression as a Biomarker for Cognitive Reserve Against Alzheimer's Disease Progression" (see introduction, n. 4).

10. A. Y. Kudinova, et al., "Circulating Levels of Brain-Derived Neurotrophic Factor and History of Suicide Attempts in Women," *Suicide & Life-Threatening Behavior* (September 28, 2017).

11. A. E. Autry and L. M. Monteggia, "Brain-Derived Neurotrophic Factor and Neuropsychiatric Disorders," *Pharmacological Reviews* 64, no. 2 (2012): 238–58.

12. Weinstein, et al., "Serum Brain-Derived Neurotrophic Factor and the Risk for Dementia" (see n. 8).

13. Perlmutter and Villoldo, *Power Up Your Brain* (see chap. 2, n. 10); T. Kishi, et al., "Calorie Restriction Improves Cognitive Decline via Up-Regulation of Brain-Derived Neurotrophic Factor: Tropomyosin-Related Kinase B in Hippocampus of Obesity-Induced Hypertensive Rats," *International Heart Journal* 56, no. 1 (2015): 110–15.

14. A. V. Witte, et al., "Caloric Restriction Improves Memory in Elderly Humans," *Proceedings of the National Academy of Sciences* 106, no. 4 (January 27, 2009): 1255–60.

15. M. P. Mattson, et al., "Prophylactic Activation of Neuroprotective Stress Response Pathways by Dietary and Behavioral Manipulations," *NeuroRx* 1, no. 1 (January 2004): 111–16.

16. H. C. Hendrie, et al., "Incidence of Dementia and Alzheimer Disease in 2 Communities: Yoruba Residing in Ibadan, Nigeria, and African Americans Residing in Indianapolis, Indiana," *JAMA* 285, no. 6 (February 14, 2001): 739–47.

17. Joe Sugarman, "Are There Any Proven Benefits to Fasting?" *Johns Hopkins Health Review* 3, no. 1 (Spring/Summer 2016), http://www.johnshopkinshealthreview .com/issues/spring-summer-2016/articles/are-there-any-proven-benefits-to-fasting.

18. Drew Desilver, "What's on Your Table? How America's Diet Has Changed Over Decades," Pew Research Center, December 13, 2016, http://www.pewresearch.org/ fact-tank/2016/12/13/whats-on-your-table-how-americas-diet-has-changed-over -the-decades/. Data from the USDA's Food Availability (Per Capita) Data System.

19. Skye Gould, "6 Charts That Show How Much More Americans Eat Than They Used To," *Business Insider*, May 10, 2017, http://www.businessinsider.com/daily-calories -americans-eat-increase-2016-07.

20. US Department of Agriculture Economic Research Service, "Food Availability and Consumption," https://www.ers.usda.gov/data-products/ag-and-food-statistics -charting-the-essentials/food-availability-and-consumption/n. Updated September 14, 2017.

21. A. V. Araya, et al., "Evaluation of the Effect of Caloric Restriction on Serum BDNF in Overweight and Obese Subjects: Preliminary Evidences," *Endocrine* 33, no. 3 (June 2008): 300–304.

22. R. Molteni, et al., "A High-Fat, Refined Sugar Diet Reduces Hippocampal Brain-Derived Neurotrophic Factor, Neuronal Plasticity, and Learning," *Neuroscience* 112, no. 4 (2002): 803–14.

23. S. Srivastava and M. C. Haigis, "Role of Sirtuins and Calorie Restriction in Neuroprotection: Implications in Alzheimer's and Parkinson's Diseases," *Current Pharmaceutical Design* 17, no. 31 (2011): 3418–33.

24. Y. Nakajo, et al., "Genetic Increase in Brain-Derived Neurotrophic Factor Levels Enhances Learning and Memory," *Brain Research* 1241 (November 19, 2008): 103–9.

25. C. E. Stafstrom and J. M. Rho, "The Ketogenic Diet As a Treatment Paradigm for Diverse Neurological Disorders," *Frontiers in Pharmacology* 3 (2012): 59; M. Gasior, et al., "Neuroprotective and Disease-Modifying Effects of the Ketogenic Diet," *Behavioral Pharmacology* 17, nos. 5–6 (September 2006): 431–39; Z. Zhao, et al., "A Ketogenic Diet As a Potential Novel Therapeutic Intervention in Amyotrophic Lateral Sclerosis," *BMC Neuroscience* 7 (April 3, 2006): 29. For a history of the ketogenic diet, see http://www.news-medical.net/health/History-of-the-Ketogenic-Diet.aspx. For more about ketogenic diets and to stay abreast of this ongoing research, see my website: http://www.DrPerlmutter.com/ketogenic-diet-benefits.

26. T. B. Vanitallie, et al., "Treatment of Parkinson Disease with Diet-Induced Hyperketonemia: A Feasibility Study," *Neurology* 64, no. 4 (February 22, 2005): 728–30.

27. M. A. Reger, et al., "Effects of Beta-Hydroxybutyrate on Cognition in Memory-Impaired Adults," *Neurobiology of Aging* 25, no. 3 (March 2004): 311–14.

28. Mary Newport, "What If There Was a Cure for Alzheimer's Disease and No One Knew?," July 22, 2008, http://www.coconutketones.com/whatifcure.pdf.

29. I. Van der Auwera, et al., "A Ketogenic Diet Reduces Amyloid Beta 40 and 42 in a Mouse Model of Alzheimer's Disease," *Nutrition & Metabolism* 2 (October 17, 2005): 28.

30. D. R. Ziegler, et al., "Ketogenic Diet Increases Glutathione Peroxidase Activity in Rat Hippocampus," *Neurochemical Research* 28, no. 12 (December 2003): 1793–97.

31. K. W. Barañano and A. L. Hartman, "The Ketogenic Diet: Uses in Epilepsy and Other Neurologic Illnesses," *Current Treatment Options in Neurology* 10, no. 6 (November 2008): 410–19.

32. Taubes, *Why We Get Fat: And What to Do About It*, 178 (see chap. 4, n. 2).

33. R. Krikorian, et al., "Dietary Ketosis Enhances Memory in Mild Cognitive Impairment," *Neurobiology of Aging* 33, no. 2 (2012): 425.

34. A. V. Witte, et al., "Caloric Restriction Improves Memory in Elderly Humans," *Proceedings of the National Academy of Sciences of the United States of America* 106, no. 4 (2009): 1255–60.

35. Gary Small, et al., "Memory and Brain Amyloid and Tau Effects of a Bioavailable Form of Curcumin in Non-Demented Adults: A Double-Blind, Placebo-Controlled 18-Month Trial," *American Journal of Geriatric Psychiatry* 26, no. 3 (2018): 266–77.

36. J. V. Pottala, et al., "Higher RBC EPA + DHA Corresponds with Larger Total Brain and Hippocampal Volumes: WHIMS-MRI Study," *Neurology* 82, no. 5 (2014): 435–42.

37. Z. S. Tan, et al., "Red Blood Cell ω-3 Fatty Acid Levels and Markers of Accelerated Brain Aging," *Neurology* 78, no. 9 (2012): 658–64.

38. K. Allaire, et al., "Randomized, Crossover, Head-to-Head Comparison of EPA and DHA Supplementation to Reduce Inflammation Markers in Men and Women: The Comparing EPA to DHA Study," *American Journal of Clinical Nutrition* 104, no. 2 (2016): 280–87.

39. K. Yurko-Mauro, et al., "Beneficial Effects of Docosahexaenoic Acid on Cognition in Age-Related Cognitive Decline," *Alzheimer's and Dementia* 6, no. 6 (November 2010): 456–64.

40. M. C. Morris, et al., "Consumption of Fish and n-3 Fatty Acids and Risk of Incident Alzheimer Disease," *Archives of Neurology* 60, no. 7 (July 2003): 940–46.

41. E. J. Schaefer, et al., "Plasma Phosphatidylcholine Docosahexaenoic Acid Content and Risk of Dementia and Alzheimer Disease: The Framingham Heart Study," *Archives of Neurology* 63, no. 11 (November 2006): 1545–50.

42. Mattson, et al., "Prophylactic Activation of Neuroprotective Stress Response Pathways by Dietary and Behavioral Manipulations" (see n. 15). See also: M. P. Mattson, et al., "Modification of Brain Aging and Neurodegenerative Disorders by Genes, Diet, and Behavior," *Physiological Reviews* 82, no. 3 (July 2002): 637–72.

43. G. L. Xiong and P. M. Doraiswamy, "Does Meditation Enhance Cognition and Brain Plasticity?" *Annals of the New York Academy of Sciences* 1172 (August 2009): 63–69. See also: E. Dakwar and F. R. Levin, "The Emerging Role of Meditation in Addressing Psychiatric Illness, with a Focus on Substance Use Disorders," *Harvard Review of Psychiatry* 17, no. 4 (2009): 254–67.

44. Some of the material here was adapted from Perlmutter and Villoldo, *Power Up Your Brain* (see chap. 2, n. 10) and from David Perlmutter, "Free Radicals: How They Speed the Aging Process," *Huffington Post*, January 25, 2011, http://www.huffingtonpost.com.

45. D. Harman, "Aging: A Theory Based on Free Radical and Radiation Chemistry," *Journal of Gerontology* 11, no. 3 (July 1956): 298–300.

46. D. Harman, "Free Radical Theory of Aging: Dietary Implications," *American Journal of Clinical Nutrition* 25, no. 8 (August 1972): 839–43.

47. W. R. Markesbery and M. A. Lovell, "Damage to Lipids, Proteins, DNA, and RNA in Mild Cognitive Impairment," *Archives of Neurology* 64, no. 7 (July 2007): 954–56.

48. L. Gao, et al., "Novel n-3 Fatty Acid Oxidation Products Activate Nrf2 by Destabilizing the Association Between Keap1 and Cullin3," *Journal of Biological Chemistry* 282, no. 4 (January 26, 2007): 2529–37.

49. U. Boettler, et al., "Coffee Constituents as Modulators of Nrf2 Nuclear Transloca-tion and ARE (EpRE)-Dependent Gene Expression," *Journal of Nutritional Bio-chemistry* 22, no. 5 (May 2011): 426–40.

50. National Institute on Aging, http://www.nia.nih.gov.

Chapter 6

1. Centers for Disease Control and Prevention, "Attention-Deficit/Hyperactivity Disorder (ADHD)," https://www.cdc.gov/ncbddd/adhd/data.html. Updated March 20, 2018.

2. Ibid.

3. Alan Schwarz and Sarah Cohen, "A.D.H.D. Seen in 11% of U.S. Children as Diagnoses Rise," *New York Times*, March 31, 2013, https://www.nytimes.com/2013/04/01/health/more-diagnoses-of-hyperactivity-causing-concern.html.

4. Ibid.

5. Sara G. Miller, "1 in 6 Americans Takes a Psychiatric Drug," *Scientific American* December 13, 2016, https://www.scientificamerican.com/article/1-in-6-americans-takes-a-psychiatric-drug/.

6. Thomas Insel, "Post by Former NIMH Director Thomas Insel: Are Children Overmedicated?" National Institutes of Mental Health, June 6, 2014, https://www.nimh.nih.gov/about/directors/thomas-insel/blog/2014/are-children-overmedi cated.shtml.

7. N. Zelnik, et al., "Range of Neurologic Disorders in Patients with Celiac Disease," *Pediatrics* 113, no. 6 (June 2004): 1672–76. See also: M. Percy and E. Propst, "Celiac Disease: Its Many Faces and Relevance to Developmental Disabilities," *Journal on Developmental Disabilities* 14, no. 2 (2008).

8. L. Corvaglia, et al., "Depression in Adult Untreated Celiac Subjects: Diagnosis by the Pediatrician," *American Journal of Gastroenterology* 94, no. 3 (March 1999): 839–43; James M. Greenblatt, MD, "Is Gluten Making You Depressed? The Link between Celiac Disease and Depression," *The Breakthrough Depression Solution* (blog), *Psychology Today*, May 24, 2011, https://www.psychologytoday.com/us/blog/the-breakthrough-depression-solution/201105/is-gluten-making-you-depressed.

9. American Academy of Pediatrics, "Gastrointestinal Problems Common in Chil-dren with Autism," *Science Daily*, May 3, 2010, http://www.sciencedaily.com/releases/2010/05/100502080234.htm. See also: L. W. Wang, et al., "The Prevalence of Gastrointestinal Problems in Children Across the United States with Autism Spectrum Disorders from Families with Multiple Affected Members," *Journal of Developmental and Behavioral Pediatrics* 32, no. 5 (June 2011): 351–60.

10. T. L. Lowe, et al., "Stimulant Medications Precipitate Tourette's Syndrome," *JAMA* 247, no. 12 (March 26, 1982): 1729–31.

11. M. A. Verkasalo, et al., "Undiagnosed Silent Coeliac Disease: A Risk for Underachievement?" *Scandinavian Journal of Gastroenterology* 40, no. 12 (December 2005): 1407–12.

12. S. Amiri, et al., "Pregnancy-Related Maternal Risk Factors of Attention-Deficit Hyperactivity Disorder: A Case-Control Study," *ISRN Pediatrics* (2012). doi: 10.5402/2012/458064.

13. A. K. Akobeng, et al., "Effect of Breast Feeding on Risk of Coeliac Disease: A Systematic Review and Meta-Analysis of Observational Studies," *Archives of Disease in Childhood* 91, no. 1 (January 2006): 39–43. For an update to this kind of research, see: H. Szajewska, et al., Systematic Review: Early Infant Feeding and the Prevention of Coeliac Disease," *Alimentary Pharmacology & Therapeutics* 36, no. 7 (2012): 607–18.

14. Centers for Disease Control and Prevention, National Center for Health Statistics, "National Health Interview Survey," https://www.cdc.gov/nchs/nhis/index.htm. Updated June 7, 2018.

15. Centers for Disease Control and Prevention, "Autism Spectrum Disorder," https://www.cdc.gov/ncbddd/autism/data.html. Updated April 26, 2018.

16. S. J. Genuis, et al., "Celiac Disease Presenting as Autism," *Journal of Child Neurology* 25, no. 1 (January 2013): 114–19.

17. P. Whiteley, et al., "A Gluten-Free Diet as an Intervention for Autism and Associated Spectrum Disorders: Preliminary Findings," *Autism* 3, no. 1 (March 1999): 45–65.

18. K. L. Reichelt and A. M. Knivsberg, "Can the Pathophysiology of Autism Be Explained by the Nature of the Discovered Urine Peptides?" *Nutritional Neuroscience* 6, no. 1 (February 2003): 19–28. See also: A. E. Kalaydjian, et al., "The Gluten Connection: The Association Between Schizophrenia and Celiac Disease," *Acta Psychiatrica Scandinavia* 113, no. 2 (February 2006): 82–90.

19. C. M. Pennesi and L. C. Klein, "Effectiveness of the Gluten-Free, Casein-Free Diet for Children Diagnosed with Autism Spectrum Disorder: Based on Parental Report," *Nutritional Neuroscience* 15, no. 2 (March 2012): 85–91. See also: Penn State, "Gluten-Free, Casein-Free Diet May Help Some Children with Autism, Research Suggests," *Science Daily*, February 29 2012, http://www.sciencedaily.com/releases/2012/02/120229105128.htm.

20. C. J. L. Murray and A. D. Lopez, "The Global Burden of Disease: A Comprehensive Assessment of Mortality and Disability from Diseases, Injuries and Risk Factors in 1990 and Projected to 2020," World Health Organization, Geneva, Switzerland (1996).

21. J. W. Smoller, et al., "Antidepressant Use and Risk of Incident Cardiovascular Morbidity and Mortality Among Postmenopausal Women in the Women's Health Initiative Study," *Archives of Internal Medicine* 169, no. 22 (December 14, 2009): 2128–39.

22. J. C. Fournier, et al., "Antidepressant Drug Effects and Depression Severity: A Patient-Level Meta-Analysis," *JAMA* 303, no. 1 (January 6, 2010): 47–53.

23. J. Y. Shin, et al., "Are Cholesterol and Depression Inversely Related? A Meta-Analysis of the Association Between Two Cardiac Risk Factors," *Annals of Behavioral Medicine* 36, no. 1 (August 2008): 33–43.

24. S. Shrivastava, et al., "Chronic Cholesterol Depletion Using Statin Impairs the Function and Dynamics of Human Serotonin1A Receptors," *Biochemistry* 49 (2010): 5426–5435.

25. James Greenblatt, "Low Cholesterol and Its Psychological Effects: Low Cholesterol Is Linked to Depression, Suicide, and Violence," *The Breakthrough Depression Solution* (blog), *Psychology Today*, June 10, 2011, http://www.psychologytoday.com/blog/the-breakthrough-depression-solution/201106/low-cholesterol-and-its-psychological-effects.

26. R. E. Morgan, et al., "Plasma Cholesterol and Depressive Symptoms in Older Men," *Lancet* 341, no. 8837 (January 9, 1993): 75–79.

27. M. Horsten, et al., "Depressive Symptoms, Social Support, and Lipid Profile in Healthy Middle-aged Women," *Psychosomatic Medicine* 59, no. 5 (September October 1997): 521–28.

28. P. H. Steegmans, et al., "Higher Prevalence of Depressive Symptoms in Middle-Aged Men with Low Serum Cholesterol Levels," *Psychosomatic Medicine* 62, no. 2 (March–April 2000): 205–11.

29. M. M. Perez-Rodriguez, et al., "Low Serum Cholesterol May Be Associated with Suicide Attempt History," *Journal of Clinical Psychiatry* 69, no. 12 (December 2008): 1920–27.

30. J. A. Boscarino, et al., "Low Serum Cholesterol and External-Cause Mortality: Potential Implications for Research and Surveillance," *Journal of Psychiatric Research* 43, no. 9 (June 2009): 848–54.

31. Sarah T. Melton, "Are Cholesterol Levels Linked to Bipolar Disorder?" Medscape Today News, Ask the Pharmacists, May 16, 2011, https://www.medscape.com/viewarticle/741999.

32. C. Hallert and J. Astrom, "Psychic Disturbances in Adult Coeliac Disease," *Scandinavian Journal of Gastroenterology* 17, no. 1 (January 1982): 21–24.

33. C. Ciacci, et al., "Depressive Symptoms in Adult Coeliac Disease," *Scandinavian Journal of Gastroenterology* 33, no. 3 (March 1998): 247–50; James M. Greenblatt, "Is Gluten Making You Depressed?" (see n. 8).

34. Fabiana Zingone, et al., "Psychological Morbidity of Celiac Disease: A Review of the Literature," *United European Gastroenterology Journal* 3, no. 2 (2015): 136–45.

35. J. F. Ludvigsson, et al., "Coeliac Disease and Risk of Mood Disorders: A General Population-Based Cohort Study," *Journal of Affective Disorders* 99, nos. 1–3 (April 2007): 117–26.

36. J. F. Ludvigsson, et al., "Increased Suicide Risk in Coeliac Disease: A Swedish Nationwide Cohort Study," *Digest of Liver Disorders* 43, no. 8 (August 2011): 616–22.

37. M. G. Carta, et al., "Recurrent Brief Depression in Celiac Disease," *Journal of Psychosomatic Research* 55, no. 6 (December 2003): 573–74.

38. R. Lasrado, et al., "Lineage-Dependent Spatial and Functional Organization of the Mammalian Enteric Nervous System," *Science* 356, no. 6339 (2017): 722–26.

39. M. Siwek, et al., "Zinc Supplementation Augments Efficacy of Imipramine in Treatment Resistant Patients: A Double Blind, Placebo-Controlled Study," *Journal of Affective Disorders* 118, nos. 1–3 (November 2009): 187–95.

40. Greenblatt, "Is Gluten Making You Depressed?" (see n. 8).

41. M. S. Cepeda, et al. "Depression Is Associated with High Levels of C-Reactive Protein and Low Levels of Fractional Exhaled Nitric Oxide: Results from the 2007–2012 National Health and Nutrition Examination Surveys," *Journal of Clinical Psychiatry* 77, no. 12 (2016): 1666–71; M. Berk, et al., "So Depression Is an Inflammatory Disease, but Where Does the Inflammation Come From?" *BMC Medicine* 11 (2013): 200.

42. Jennifer C. Felger and Francis E. Lotrich, "Inflammatory Cytokines in Depression: Neurobiological Mechanisms and Therapeutic Implications," *Neuroscience* 246 (2013): 199–229.

43. B. Gohier, et al., "Hepatitis C, Alpha Interferon, Anxiety and Depression Disorders: A Prospective Study of 71 Patients," *World Journal of Biological Psychiatry* 4, no. 3 (2003): 115–8.

44. H. Karlsson, et al., "Maternal Antibodies to Dietary Antigens and Risk for Nonaffective Psychosis in Offspring," *American Journal of Psychiatry* 169, no. 6 (June 2012): 625–32.

45. Grace Rattue, "Schizophrenia Risk in Kids Associated with Mothers' Gluten Antibodies," *Medical News Today*, May 16, 2012, http://www.medicalnewstoday.com/articles/245484.php.

46. Deborah R. Kim, Tracy L. Bale, and C. Neill Epperson, "Prenatal Programming of Mental Illness: Current Understanding of Relationship and Mechanisms," *Current Psychiatry Reports* 17, no. 2 (2015): 5.

47. D. J. Barker, "The Fetal and Infant Origins of Adult Disease," *BMJ* 301, no. 6761 (1990): 1111.

48. B. D. Kraft and E. C. Westman, "Schizophrenia, Gluten, and Low-Carbohydrate, Ketogenic Diets: A Case Report and Review of the Literature," *Nutrition & Metabolism* (London) 6 (February 26, 2009): 10.

49. Migraine Research Foundation, http://migraineresearchfoundation.org/.

50. Ibid.

51. A. K. Dimitrova, et al., "Prevalence of Migraine in Patients with Celiac Disease and Inflammatory Bowel Disease," *Headache* 53, no. 2 (February 2013): 344–55.

52. M. Hadjivassiliou and R. Grünewald, "The Neurology of Gluten Sensitivity: Science vs. Conviction," *Practical Neurology* 4 (2004): 124–26.

53. Center for Celiac Research and Treatment, http://www.celiaccenter.org/.

54. S. M. Wolf, et al., "Pediatric Migraine Management," *Pain Medicine News* (September/October 2003): 1–6.

55. E. Lionetti, et al. "Headache in Pediatric Patients with Celiac Disease and Its Prevalence as a Diagnostic Clue," *Journal of Pediatric Gastroenterology and Nutrition* 49, no. 2 (August 2009): 202–7; Benedetta Bellini, et al., "Headache and Comorbidity in Children and Adolescents," *Journal of Headache & Pain* 14, no. 1 (2013): 79.

56. D. Ferraro and G. Di Trapani, "Topiramate in the Prevention of Pediatric Migraine: Literature Review," *Journal of Headache Pain* 9, no. 3 (June 2008): 147–50.

57. E. Bakola, et al., "Anticonvulsant Drugs for Pediatric Migraine Prevention: An Evidence-Based Review," *European Journal of Pain* 13, no. 9 (October 2009): 893–901.

58. B. L. Peterlin, et al., "Obesity and Migraine: The Effect of Age, Gender, and Adipose Tissue Distribution," *Headache* 50, no. 1 (January 2010): 52–62.

59. M. E. Bigal, et al., "Obesity, Migraine, and Chronic Migraine: Possible Mechanisms of Interaction," *Neurology* 68, no. 27 (May 22, 2007): 1851–61.

60. M. E. Bigal and R. B. Lipton, "Obesity Is a Risk Factor for Transformed Migraine but Not Chronic Tension-Type Headache," *Neurology* 67, no. 2 (July 25, 2006): 252–57.

61. L. Robberstad, et al., "An Unfavorable Lifestyle and Recurrent Headaches among Adolescents: The HUNT Study," *Neurology* 75, no. 8 (August 24, 2010): 712–17.

Chapter 7

1. Perlmutter and Villoldo, *Power Up Your Brain* (see chap. 2, n. 10). Also see: A. Villoldo, "Size Does Matter!," April 25, 2011, https://www.healyourlife.com/size-does-matter.

2. G. F. Cahill and R. L. Veech Jr., "Ketoacids? Good Medicine?" *Transactions of the American Clinical and Climatological Association* 114 (2003): 149–61.

3. M. P. Mattson and R. Wan, "Beneficial Effects of Intermittent Fasting and Caloric Restriction on the Cardiovascular and Cerebrovascular Systems," *Journal of Nutritional Biochemistry* 16, no. 3 (March 2005): 129–37.

4. Valter D. Longo and Mark P. Mattson, "Fasting: Molecular Mechanisms and Clinical Applications," *Cell Metabolism* 19, no. 2 (2014): 181–92.

5. G. Zuccoli, et al., "Metabolic Management of Glioblastoma Multiforme Using Standard Therapy Together with a Restricted Ketogenic Diet: Case Report," *Nutrition & Metabolism* (London) 7 (April 22, 2010): 33.

6. M. Ota, et al., "Effect of a Ketogenic Meal on Cognitive Function in Elderly Adults: Potential for Cognitive Enhancement," *Psychopharmacology* (Berlin) 233, nos. 21–22 (2016): 3797–802.

7. S. J. Hallberg, et al., "Effectiveness and Safety of a Novel Care Model for the Management of Type 2 Diabetes at 1 Year: An Open-Label, Non-Randomized, Controlled Study," *Diabetes Therapy* 9, no. 2 (2018): 583–612.

8. T. Hallböök, et al., "The Effects of the Ketogenic Diet on Behavior and Cognition," *Epilepsy Research* 100, no. 3 (2012): 304–9.

9. N/A

10. T. P. Ng, et al., "Curry Consumption and Cognitive Function in the Elderly," *American Journal of Epidemiology* 164, no. 9 (November 1, 2006): 898–906.

11. K. Tillisch, et al., "Consumption of Fermented Milk Product with Probiotic Modulates Brain Activity," *Gastroenterology* (March 1, 2013). doi: 10.1053/ j.gastro .2013.02.043; J. A. Bravo, et al., "Ingestion of *Lactobacillus* Strain Regulates Emotional Behavior and Central GABA Receptor Expression in a Mouse via the Vagus Nerve," *Proceedings of the National Academy of Sciences* 108, no. 138 (September 20, 2011): 16050–55; A. C. Bested, et al., "Intestinal Microbiota, Probiotics and Mental Health: From Metchnikoff to Modern Advances: Part I—Autointoxication Revisited," *Gut Pathogens* 5, no. 1 (March 18, 2013): 5. See also Parts II and III of the same report.

12. J. F. Cryan and S. M. O'Mahony, "The Microbiome-Gut-Brain Axis: From Bowel to Behavior," *Neurogastroenterology and Motility* 23, no. 3 (March 2011): 187–92.

13. Michael Gershon, MD, *The Second Brain: The Scientific Basis of Gut Instinct and a Groundbreaking New Understanding of Nervous Disorders of the Stomach and Intestines* (New York: Harper, 1998).

14. For more about the brain-gut connection, check out the work of Dr. Emeran Mayer, MD, director of the University of California, Los Angeles's Center for Neurobiology of Stress. In particular, *The Mind Gut Connection: How the Hidden Conversation Within Our Bodies Impacts Our Mood, Our Choices, and Our Overall Health* (New York: Harper Wave, 2016).

15. Weinstein, et al., "Serum Brain-Derived Neurotrophic Factor and the Risk for Dementia: The Framingham Heart Study" (see chap. 5, no. 8).

16. L. Packer, et al., "Neuroprotection by the Metabolic Antioxidant Alpha-Lipoic Acid," *Free Radical Biology & Medicine* 22, nos. 1–2 (1997): 359–78.

17. Jun Sun, "Vitamin D and Mucosal Immune Function," *Current Opinion in Gastroenterology* 26, no. 6 (2010): 591–95.

18. For everything you want to know about vitamin D, including in-depth discussion of studies, refer to Dr. Michael Holick's seminal book *The Vitamin D Solution: A 3-Step Strategy to Cure Our Most Common Health Problems* (New York: Hudson Street Press, 2010).

19. D. J. Llewellyn, et al., "Vitamin D and Risk of Cognitive Decline in Elderly Persons," *Archives of Internal Medicine* 170, no. 13 (July 12, 2012): 1135–41; Elżbieta Kuźma, et al., "Vitamin D and Memory Decline: Two Population-based Prospective Studies," *Journal of Alzheimer's Disease* 50, no. 4 (2016): 1099–108.

20. Littlejohns, T. J., et al., "Vitamin D and the Risk of Dementia and Alzheimer Disease," *Neurology* 83, no. 10 (2014): 920–8.

21. C. Annweiler, et al., "Higher Vitamin D Dietary Intake Is Associated with Lower Risk of Alzheimer's Disease: A 7-Year Follow-Up," *Journals of Gerontology Series A: Biological Sciences and Medical Sciences* 67, no. 11 (November 2012): 1205–11.

22. Ruth Ann Marrie and Christopher A. Beck, "Preventing Multiple Sclerosis: To Take Vitamin D or Not to Take Vitamin D," *Neurology* 89, no. 15 (2017).

23. R. E. Anglin, et al., "Vitamin D Deficiency and Depression in Adults: Systematic Review and Meta-analysis," *British Journal of Psychiatry* 202 (February 2013): 100–107.

24. Willy Gomm, et al., "Association of Proton Pump Inhibitors with Risk of Dementia: A Pharmacoepidemiological Claims Data Analysis," *JAMA Neurology* 73, no. 4 (2016): 410–16.

25. G. R. Durso, et al., "Over-the-Counter Relief from Pains and Pleasures Alike: Acetaminophen Blunts Evaluation Sensitivity to Both Negative and Positive Stimuli," *Psychological Science* 26, no. 6 (June 2015): 750–58.

26. Liew et al., "Acetaminophen Use During Pregnancy, Behavioral Problems, and Hyperkinetic Disorders," *JAMA Pediatrics* 168, no. 4 (April 2014): 313–20.

27. D. Y. Graham et al., "Visible Small-Intestinal Mucosal Injury in Chronic NSAID Users," *Clinical Gastroenterology & Hepatology* 3, no. 1 (January 2005). 55–59.

28. G. Sigthorsson et al., "Intestinal Permeability and Inflammation in Patients on NSAIDs," *Gut* 43, no. 4 (October 1998): 506–11.

Chapter 8

1. J. Z. Willey, et al., "Leisure-Time Physical Activity Associates with Cognitive Decline: The Northern Manhattan Study," *Neurology* 86, no. 20 (2016): 1897–903.

2. C. A. Raji, et al., "Longitudinal Relationships between Caloric Expenditure and Gray Matter in the Cardiovascular Health Study," *Journal of Alzheimer's Disease* 52, no. 2 (2016): 719–29.

3. C. W. Cotman, et al., "Exercise Builds Brain Health: Key Roles of Growth Factor Cascades and Inflammation," *Trends in Neuroscience* 30, no. 9 (September 2007): 464–72. See also: University of Edinburgh, "Exercise the Body to Keep the Brain Healthy, Study Suggests," *Science Daily*, October 22, 2012, http://www.science daily.com/releases/2012/10/121022162647.htm; L. F. Defina, et al., "The Association Between Midlife Cardiorespiratory Fitness Levels and Later-life Dementia: A Cohort Study," *Annals of Internal Medicine* 158, no. 3 (February 5, 2013): 162–68.

4. Gretchen Reynolds, "How Exercise Could Lead to a Better Brain," *New York Times Magazine*, April 18, 2012, http://www.nytimes.com/2012/04/22/magazine/how -exercise-could-lead-to-a-better-brain.html.

5. A. S. Buchman, et al., "Total Daily Physical Activity and the Risk of AD and Cognitive Decline in Older Adults," *Neurology* 78, no. 17 (April 24, 2012): 1323–29.

6. D. M. Bramble and D. E. Lieberman, "Endurance Running and the Evolution of *Homo*," *Nature* 432, no. 7015 (November 18, 2004): 345–52.

7. D. A. Raichlen and A. D. Gordon, "Relationship between Exercise Capacity and Brain Size in Mammals," *PLOS One* 6, no. 6 (2011).

8. Gretchen Reynolds, "Exercise and the Ever-Smarter Human Brain," *New York Times*, December 26, 2012, https://well.blogs.nytimes.com/2012/12/26/exercise-and-the-ever -smarter-human-brain/; D. A. Raichlen and J. D. Polk, "Linking Brains and Brawn: Exercise and the Evolution of Human Neurobiology," *Proceedings of the Royal Society B: Biological Sciences* 280, no. 1750 (January 7, 2013): 2012–50.

9. Reynolds, "How Exercise Could Lead to a Better Brain" (see n. 4).

10. P. J. Clark, et al., "Genetic Influences on Exercise-Induced Adult Hippocampal Neurogenesis Across 12 Divergent Mouse Strains," *Genes, Brain and Behavior* 10, no. 3 (April 2011): 345–53. See also: R. A. Kohman, et al., "Voluntary Wheel Running Reverses Age-Induced Changes in Hippocampal Gene Expression," *PLOS One* 6, no. 8 (2011): e22654.

11. K. I. Erickson, et al., "Exercise Training Increases Size of Hippocampus and Improves Memory," *Proceedings of the National Academy of Sciences* 108, no. 7 (February 15, 2011): 3017–22.

12. N. Kee, et al., "Preferential Incorporation of Adult-Generated Granule Cells into Spatial Memory Networks in the Dentate Gyrus," *Nature Neuroscience* 10, no. 3 (March 2007): 355–62. See also: C. W. Wu, et al., "Treadmill Exercise Counteracts the Suppressive Effects of Peripheral Lipopolysaccharide on Hippocampal Neurogenesis and Learning and Memory," *Journal of Neurochemistry* 103, no. 6 (December 2007): 2471–81.

13. N. T. Lautenschlager, et al., "Effect of Physical Activity on Cognitive Function in Older Adults at Risk for Alzheimer Disease: A Randomized Trial," *JAMA* 300, no. 9 (September 3, 2008): 1027–37.

14. J. Weuve, et al., "Physical Activity, Including Walking, and Cognitive Function in Older Women," *JAMA* 292, no. 12 (September 22, 2004): 1454–61.

15. A. Yavari, et al., "The Effect of Aerobic Exercise on Glycosylated Hemoglobin Values in Type 2 Diabetes Patients," *Journal of Sports Medicine and Physical Fitness* 50, no. 4 (December 2010): 501–5.

16. Buchman, et al., "Total Daily Physical Activity and the Risk of AD and Cognitive Decline in Older Adults" (see chap. 8, n. 5). See also: Rush University Medical Center, "Daily Physical Activity May Reduce Alzheimer's Disease Risk at Any Age," *Science Daily*, April 18, 2012, http://www.sciencedaily.com/releases/2012/04/120418203530.htm (accessed April 23, 2018).

Chapter 9

1. For a general overview of the relationship between sleep and health, go to: National Institute of Neurological Disorders and Stroke, "Brain Basics: Understanding Sleep," https://www.ninds.nih.gov/Disorders/Patient-Caregiver-Education/Understanding -Sleep. Also refer to the works of Dr. Michael Breus, a noted authority on sleep medicine: http://www.thesleepdoctor.com/.

2. Benedict Carey, "Aging in Brain Found to Hurt Sleep Needed for Memory," *New York Times*, January 27, 2013, http://www.nytimes.com/2013/01/28/health/brain-aging-linked-to-sleep-related-memory-decline.html. See also: B. A. Mander, et al., "Prefrontal Atrophy, Disrupted NREM Slow Waves and Impaired Hippocampal-dependent Memory in Aging," *Nature Neuroscience* 16, no. 3 (March 2013): 357–64.

3. C. S. Möller-Levet, et al., "Effects of Insufficient Sleep on Circadian Rhythmicity and Expression Amplitude of the Human Blood Transcriptome," *Proceedings of the National Academy of Sciences* 110, no. 12 (March 19, 2013): E1132–41.

4. Andrew J. Westwood, et al., "Prolonged Sleep Duration as a Marker of Early Neuro-degeneration Predicting Incident Dementia," *Neurology* 88, no. 12 (2107): 1172–79.

5. For volumes of data about sleep and statistics about how much we get, refer to the National Sleep Foundation at https://sleepfoundation.org/.

6. Monica P. Mallampalli and Christine L. Carter, "Exploring Sex and Gender Differences in Sleep Health: A Society for Women's Health Research Report," *Journal of Women's Health* (Larchmont) 23, no. 7 (2014): 553–62.

7. T. Blackwell, et al., "Associations Between Sleep Architecture and Sleep-Disordered Breathing and Cognition in Older Community-Dwelling Men: The Osteoporotic Fractures in Men Sleep Study," *Journal of the American Geriatric Society* 59, no. 12 (December 2011): 2217–25. See also: K. Yaffe, et al., "Sleep-Disordered Breathing, Hypoxia, and Risk of Mild Cognitive Impairment and Dementia in Older Women," *JAMA* 306, no. 6 (August 10, 2011): 613–19; A. P. Spira, et al., "Sleep-Disordered Breathing and Cognition in Older Women," *Journal of the American Geriatric Society* 56, no. 1 (January 2008): 45–50.

8. Chunlong Mu, Yuxiang Yang, and Weiyun Zhu, "Gut Microbioa: The Brain Peace-keeper," *Frontiers in Microbiology* 7 (2016): 345; Leo Galland, "The Gut Microbiome and the Brain," *Journal of Medicinal Food* 17, no. 12 (2014): 1261–71.

9. Y. Zhang, et al., "Positional Cloning of the Mouse Obese Gene and Its Human Homologue," *Nature* 372, no. 6505 (December 1, 1994): 425–32; E. D. Green, et al., "The Human Obese (OB) Gene: RNA Expression Pattern and Mapping on the Physical, Cytogenetic, and Genetic Maps of Chromosome 7," *Genome Research* 5, no. 1 (August 1995): 5–12.

10. Nora T. Gedgaudas, *Primal Body, Primal Mind: Beyond the Paleo Diet for Total Health and a Longer Life* (Rochester, Vermont: Healing Arts Press, 2011).

11. K. Spiegel, et al., "Brief Communication: Sleep Curtailment in Healthy Young Men Is Associated with Decreased Leptin Levels, Elevated Ghrelin Levels, and Increased Hunger and Appetite," *Annals of Internal Medicine* 141, no. 11 (December 7, 2004): 846–50.

12. S. Taheri, et al., "Short Sleep Duration Is Associated with Reduced Leptin, Elevated Ghrelin, and Increased Body Mass Index," *PLOS Medicine* 1, no. 3 (December 2004): e62.

13. W. A. Banks, et al., "Triglycerides Induce Leptin Resistance at the Blood-Brain Barrier," *Diabetes* 53, no. 5 (May 2004): 1253–60.

14. Ron Rosedale and Carol Colman, *The Rosedale Diet* (New York: William Morrow, 2004).
15. Matthew Walker, *Why We Sleep: Unlocking the Power of Sleep and Dreams* (New York: Scribner, 2017).
16. National Sleep Foundation, https://sleepfoundation.org/.

Chapter 10

1. For access to studies and writings on glyphosate, go to DrPerlmutter.com and search under "glyphosate."
2. J. Gray and B. Griffin, "Eggs and Dietary Cholesterol—Dispelling the Myth," *Nutrition Bulletin* 34, no. 1 (March 2009): 66–70.
3. For more information and access to studies about eggs, go to The Incredible Egg, http://www.incredibleegg.org. See also: Janet Raloff, "Reevaluating Eggs' Cholesterol Risks," *Science News,* May 2, 2006, http://www.sciencenews.org/view/generic/id/7301/description/Reevaluating_Eggs_Cholesterol_Risks.
4. C. N. Blesso, et al., "Whole Egg Consumption Improves Lipoprotein Profiles and Insulin Sensitivity to a Greater Extent Than Yolk-free Egg Substitute in Individuals with Metabolic Syndrome," *Metabolism* 62, no. 3 (March 2013): 400–410.
5. J. K. Virtanen, et al., "Associations of Egg and Cholesterol Intakes with Carotid Intima-media Thickness and Risk of Incident Coronary Artery Disease According to Apolipoprotein E Phenotype in Men: The Kuopio Ischaemic Heart Disease Risk Factor Study," *American Journal of Clinical Nutrition* 103, no. 3 (2016): 895–901.

Chapter 11

1. Anya Topiwala, et al., "Moderate Alcohol Consumption as Risk Factor for Adverse Brain Outcomes and Cognitive Decline: Longitudinal Cohort Study," *BMJ* 357 (2017).
2. M. J. Gunter, et al., "Coffee Drinking and Mortality in 10 European Countries: A Multinational Cohort Study," *Annals of Internal Medicine* 167 no. 4 (2017): 236–47.

Epilogue

1. World Health Organization, "Measuring Overall Health System Performance for 191 Countries," http://www.who.int/healthinfo/paper30.pdf.
2. Aimee Cunningham, "U.S. Life Expectancy Drops for the Second Year in a Row," *Science News,* December 21, 2017; https://www.sciencenews.org/blog/science-ticker/us-life-expectancy-drops-second-year.

Index

About the Author

David Perlmutter, MD, is a board-certified neurologist and Fellow of the American College of Nutrition. He is a four-time *New York Times* bestselling author with his books translated into thirty languages. He is the recipient of the Linus Pauling Award for his pioneering research in neurodegenerative diseases. His writings appear extensively in medical publications and he lectures worldwide. Dr. Perlmutter serves on the Medical Advisory Board for *The Dr. Oz Show* and has appeared on many nationally syndicated radio and television programs, including *20/20*, *Today*, *Good Morning America*, *The Dr. Oz Show*, and *The Early Show* and on CNN and Fox News. He lives in Naples, Florida, with his wife and has two grown children.

If you enjoyed reading
Grain Brain, you may also enjoy
Dr David Perlmutter's other books:

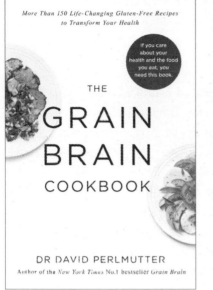

More Than 150 Life-Changing Gluten-Free Recipes
to Transform Your Health

If you care about your health and the food you eat, you need this book.

THE

GRAIN BRAIN

COOKBOOK

DR DAVID PERLMUTTER

Author of the *New York Times* No.1 bestseller *Grain Brain*

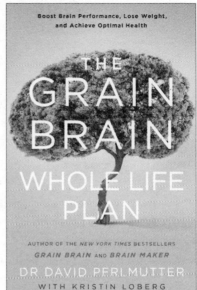

Boost Brain Performance, Lose Weight,
and Achieve Optimal Health

THE

GRAIN BRAIN

WHOLE LIFE
PLAN

AUTHOR OF THE *NEW YORK TIMES* BESTSELLERS
GRAIN BRAIN AND *BRAIN MAKER*

DR DAVID PERLMUTTER

WITH KRISTIN LOBERG

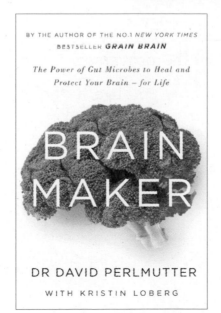

BY THE AUTHOR OF THE NO.1 *NEW YORK TIMES*
BESTSELLER *GRAIN BRAIN*

*The Power of Gut Microbes to Heal and
Protect Your Brain – for Life*

BRAIN MAKER

DR DAVID PERLMUTTER

WITH KRISTIN LOBERG

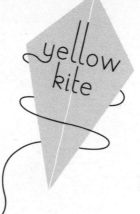

books to help you live a good life

Join the conversation and tell
us how you live a #goodlife

𝕏 @yellowkitebooks
f YellowKiteBooks
𝕡 Yellow Kite Books
📷 YellowKiteBooks